Pharmaceutical Waste Recycling: Opportunities and Challenges

Edited by

Suman Gautam
Department of Biochemistry,
Ganesh Shankar Vidyarthi Memorial Medical College,
Kanpur, Uttar Pradesh,
India

Jai Narayan Mishra
Department of Pharmacology,
Kailash Institute of Pharmacy and Management,
GIDA, Gorakhpur, Uttar Pradesh, India

Preeti Mishra
Department of Pharmacy,
Raja Balwant Singh Engineering Technical Campus,
Agra, Uttar Pradesh, India

Preeti Verma
Department of Pharmaceutical Chemistry,
Dr. M.C Saxena College of Pharmacy, Lucknow,
Uttar Pradesh, India

&

Sudhanshu Mishra
Faculty of Pharmaceutical Sciences,
Mahayogi Gorakhnath University, Gorakhpur,
Uttar Pradesh, India

Pharmaceutical Waste Recycling: Opportunities and Challenges

Editors: Suman Gautam, Jai Narayan Mishra, Preeti Mishra, Preeti Verma and

Sudhanshu Mishra

ISBN (Online): 979-8-89881-522-6

ISBN (Print): 979-8-89881-523-3

ISBN (Paperback): 979-8-89881-524-0

Published by Bentham Science Publishers Pte. Ltd. Singapore,

in collaboration with Eureka Conferences, USA.

First published in 2026.

need for a court order if at any point you breach any terms of this License Agreement. In no event will any delay or failure by Bentham Science Publishers in enforcing your compliance with this License Agreement constitute a waiver of any of its rights.

3. You acknowledge that you have read this License Agreement, and agree to be bound by its terms and conditions. To the extent that any other terms and conditions presented on any website of Bentham Science Publishers conflict with, or are inconsistent with, the terms and conditions set out in this License Agreement, you acknowledge that the terms and conditions set out in this License Agreement shall prevail.

Bentham Science Publishers Pte. Ltd.
No. 9 Raffles Place
Office No. 26-01
Singapore 048619
Singapore
Email: subscriptions@benthamscience.net

BENTHAM SCIENCE

CONTENTS

FOREWORD

The intersection of healthcare advancement and environmental sustainability poses a unique challenge: pharmaceutical waste. As the pharmaceutical industry expands to meet growing global needs, it also assumes a greater responsibility to mitigate environmental damage. The improper disposal of pharmaceutical products not only endangers ecosystems but also poses significant risks to human health, water sources, and biodiversity.

This book arrives at a pivotal time, providing critical perspectives on managing pharmaceutical waste through innovative and eco-conscious approaches. It thoughtfully explores topics ranging from classification and treatment processes to digital transformation, public awareness, and policy frameworks. What distinguishes this work is its multidisciplinary approach, which brings together the scientific, technological, and socio-political dimensions of waste management. Each chapter reflects the authors' academic rigor and commitment to real-world impact. Their work contributes meaningfully to ongoing efforts in making the pharmaceutical sector more responsible and sustainable.

I commend the editors and contributors for compiling this essential source of knowledge, and I am confident that readers will find in it both inspiration and practical guidance.

Raghav Mishra
Lloyd Institute of Management
and Technology,
Greater Noida, Uttar Pradesh,
India

PREFACE

Pharmaceutical waste management has become a pressing concern in today's rapidly evolving healthcare and pharmaceutical sectors. As the world becomes increasingly aware of the environmental and public health implications of improper waste disposal, the need for comprehensive, innovative, and sustainable strategies has never been more urgent. This book, "***Pharmaceutical Waste Recycling: Opportunities and Challenges***," was conceived to address these critical issues and provide a unified platform for knowledge, research, and real-world practices in this domain.

This collaborative volume brings together the expertise of distinguished contributors, each offering unique insights into various aspects of pharmaceutical waste—from classification and effects to advanced recycling technologies and policy frameworks. We hope that this book will serve not only as a valuable academic resource but also as a practical guide for industry professionals, environmentalists, policymakers, students, and researchers who are committed to fostering sustainable pharmaceutical waste management.

We would like to thank all the authors for their dedicated efforts, valuable contributions, and commitment to advancing this crucial field. We also extend our gratitude to the institutions and mentors who supported this endeavor.

Suman Gautam
Department of Biochemistry,
Ganesh Shankar Vidyarthi Memorial Medical College, Kanpur,
Uttar Pradesh, India

Jai Narayan Mishra
Department of Pharmacology
Kailash Institute of Pharmacy and Management,
GIDA, Gorakhpur, Uttar Pradesh, India

Preeti Mishra
Department of Pharmacy,
Raja Balwant Singh Engineering Technical Campus,
Agra, Uttar Pradesh, India

Preeti Verma
Department of Pharmaceutical Chemistry
Dr. M.C Saxena College of Pharmacy, Lucknow,
Uttar Pradesh, India

&

Sudhanshu Mishra
Faculty of Pharmaceutical Sciences,
Mahayogi Gorakhnath University, Gorakhpur,
Uttar Pradesh, India

List of Contributors

Aarti Tiwari	Institute of Pharmacy, Dr Rammanohar Lohia Avadh University, Ayodhya, Uttar Pradesh, India
Aastha Sharma	Department of Pharmacy, Institute of Pharmacy & Paramedical Sciences, Dr. Bhimrao Ambedkar University, Agra, Uttar Pradesh, India
Abdul Hafeez	Faculty of Pharmacy, Integral University, Dasauli, Lucknow, Uttar Pradesh, India
Ajay Kumar Shukla	Institute of Pharmacy, Dr Rammanohar Lohia Avadh University, Ayodhya, Uttar Pradesh, India
Akash Ved	Faculty of Pharmacy, Dr. A.P.J. Abdul Kalam Technical University, Lucknow, Uttar Pradesh, India
Akhalesh Kumar	Department of Pharmacy, Institute of Pharmacy & Paramedical Sciences, Dr. Bhimrao Ambedkar University, Agra, Uttar Pradesh, India
Anjali Chouhan	Department of Pharmacy, Institute of Pharmacy & Paramedical Sciences, Dr. Bhimrao Ambedkar University, Agra, Uttar Pradesh, India
Ankita Moharana	School of Pharmacy, ARKA JAIN University, Jamshedpur, Jharkhand, India
Arun Kumar	Faculty of Pharmacy, Integral University, Dasauli, Lucknow, Uttar Pradesh, India
Asheesh Kumar Singh	Department of Pharmacognosy, Buddia Institute of Pharmacy, GIDA, Gorakhpur, Uttar Pradesh, India
Ashruti Hor	Department of Pharmacy, Netaji Subhas University, Jamshedpur, Jharkhand, India
Deepak Kumar	Faculty of Pharmaceutical Sciences, Mahayogi Gorakhnath University, Gorakhpur, Uttar Pradesh, India
Dilip Kumar Mishra	Faculty of Pharmaceutical Sciences, Mahayogi Gorakhnath University, Gorakhpur, Uttar Pradesh, India
Jeet Kumar Ghosh	Department of Pharmacy, Usha Martin University, Ranchi, Jharkhand, India
Joohee Pradhan	Department of Pharmaceutical Sciences, Mohanlal Sukhadia University, Udaipur, Rajasthan, India
Juhi Tiwari	Faculty of Pharmaceutical Sciences, Mahayogi Gorakhnath University, Gorakhpur, Uttar Pradesh, India
Kuldeep Singh	Faculty of Pharmacy, Integral University, Dasauli, Lucknow, Uttar Pradesh, India
Mohammad Sufiyan Ashfaq	Amity Institute of Pharmacy, Amity University, Lucknow, Uttar Pradesh, India
Mukul Yadav	Department of Pharmacy, Institute of Pharmacy & Paramedical Sciences, Dr. Bhimrao Ambedkar University, Agra, Uttar Pradesh, India
Neha Mathur	Amity Institute of Pharmacy, Amity University, Lucknow, Uttar Pradesh, India

Neha Srivastava Department of Pharmacy, Buddha Institute of Pharmacy, GIDA, Gorakhpur, Uttar Pradesh, India

Nripendra Singh Department of Pharmacy, Veer Bahadur Singh Purvanchal University, Jaunpur, Uttar Pradesh, India

Piyush Anand Faculty of Pharmaceutical Sciences, Mahayogi Gorakhnath University, Gorakhpur, Uttar Pradesh, India

Pradeep Singh Department of Pharmaceutics, Sultanpur Institute of Pharmacy, Sultanpur, Uttar Pradesh, India

Poonam Kushwaha Faculty of Pharmacy, Integral University, Dasauli, Lucknow, Uttar Pradesh, India

Prashant Singh Department of Pharmaceutics, Buddha Institute of Pharmacy, GIDA, Gorakhpur, Uttar Pradesh, India

Prottay Dutta Department of Pharmacy, Usha Martin University, Ranchi, Jharkhand, India

Priya Rani Department of Nephrology, Kasturba Medical College, Manipal, Manipal Academy of Higher Education, Manipal, Karnataka, India

Pushpendra Soni Faculty of Pharmacy, Integral University, Dasauli, Lucknow, Uttar Pradesh, India

Rahul Kumar Maurya Department of Pharmacy, Madan Mohan Malaviya University of Technology, Gorakhpur, Uttar Pradesh, India

Rakesh Swain School of Pharmaceutical Sciences, Siksha O Anusandhan Deemed to be University, Bhubaneswar, Odisha, India

Rakhi Mishra Department of Pharmacy, Noida Institute of Engineering and Technology (Pharmacy Institute), Greater Noida, Uttar Pradesh, India

Rama Sankar Dubey Department of Anesthesiology Critical Care Medicine, University of New Mexico School of Medicine, Albuquerque, New Mexico, USA

Ravi Shekhar Department of Pharmacy, Institute of Pharmacy Paramedical Sciences, Dr. Bhimrao Ambedkar University, Agra, Uttar Pradesh, India

Rufaida Wasim Department of Pharmacology, Faculty of Pharmacy, Integral University, Lucknow, Uttar Pradesh, India

Saba Parveen Department of Pharmaceutical Science Technology, Madan Mohan Malaviya University of Technology, Gorakhpur, Uttar Pradesh, India

Sahi Hussain College of Health and Life Sciences, Hamad Bin Khalifa University, Doha, Qatar

Sakshi Verma Department of Pharmacy, Usha Martin University, Ranchi, Jharkhand, India

Shambaditya Goswami Department of Pharmaceutical Chemistry, Divine College of Pharmacy, Ziradei, Siwan, Bihar, India

Shashikant Singh Faculty of Pharmaceutical Sciences, Mahayogi Gorakhnath University, Gorakhpur, Uttar Pradesh, India

Shivali Singla Department of Anesthesiology Critical Care Medicine, University of New Mexico School of Medicine, Albuquerque, New Mexico, USA

Shobhit Raj Department of Endocrinology, Kasturba Medical College, Manipal, Manipal Academy of Higher Education, Manipal, Karnataka, India

Shom Prakash Kushwaha	Faculty of Pharmacy, Integral University, Dasauli, Lucknow, Uttar Pradesh, India
Shreya Maddesiya	Faculty of Pharmaceutical Sciences, Mahayogi Gorakhnath University, Gorakhpur, Uttar Pradesh, India
Shweta Yadav	Faculty of Pharmaceutical Sciences, Mahayogi Gorakhnath University, Gorakhpur, Uttar Pradesh, India
Snigdha Rani Behera	School of Pharmacy, ARKA JAIN University, Jamshedpur, Jharkhand, India
Sonali Dasgupta	Department of Pharmaceutics, Krishak College of Pharmacy, Rajgarh, Mirzapur, Uttar Pradesh, India
Sujit Kumar Martha	Department of Pharmaceutical Analysis, Jeypore College of Pharmacy, Jeypore, Odisha, India
Sumaiya Azmi	Department of Periodontics, Career Post Graduate Institute of Dental Sciences and Hospital, Lucknow, Uttar Pradesh, India
Swagatam Sahoo	School of Pharmacy, DRIEMS University, Tangi, Tangi, Cuttack, Odisha, India
Syed Misbahul Hasan	Faculty of Pharmacy, Integral University, Dasauli, Lucknow, Uttar Pradesh, India
Tarique Mahmood	Department of Pharmacology, Faculty of Pharmacy, Integral University, Lucknow, Uttar Pradesh, India

CHAPTER 1

Introduction of Pharmaceutical Waste: Sources and Classification

Shom Prakash Kushwaha[1], **Syed Misbahul Hasan**[1,*], **Pushpendra Soni**[1], **Kuldeep Singh**[1], **Arun Kumar**[1], **Abdul Hafeez**[1], **Poonam Kushwaha**[1], **Akash Ved**[2] and **Sahil Hussain**[3]

[1] *Faculty of Pharmacy, Integral University, Dasauli, Lucknow, Uttar Pradesh, India*

[2] *Faculty of Pharmacy, Dr. A.P.J. Abdul Kalam Technical University, Lucknow, Uttar Pradesh, India*

[3] *College of Health and Life Sciences, Hamad Bin Khalifa University, Doha, Qatar*

Abstract: Pharmaceutical waste is a major environmental and public health problem because it can pollute ecosystems and lead to problems such as antimicrobial resistance. This chapter defines pharmaceutical waste as unused medicine, personal care products, and accessories that need special collection and disposal. It discusses the main sources of pharmaceutical waste, ranging from healthcare facilities, drug manufacturing, homes, veterinary and agricultural sectors, to illegal drug markets. The chapter also explores several classification approaches for pharmaceutical waste by chemical composition, level of hazard, physical state, and regulatory classifications to guide suitable disposal and treatment. It also explores some of the challenges in determining and classifying pharmaceutical waste, including inconsistency in international regulations, non-uniform systems, analytical complexity in trace detection, and information gaps on pharmaceutical environmental fate. Based on notable academic research, the chapter emphasizes the importance of understanding pharmaceutical waste sources and classification to develop effective management practices and prevent their negative effects.

Keywords: Environmental contamination, Healthcare facilities, Pharmaceutical waste, Regulatory frameworks, Sustainable management, Waste classification.

INTRODUCTION

Pharmaceutical waste means unwanted, unused, or expired pharmaceutical products, drugs, and allied materials that are no longer effective for their purpose.

* **Corresponding author Syed Misbahul Hasan:** Faculty of Pharmacy, Integral University, Dasauli, Lucknow, Uttar Pradesh, India; E-mail: deanphar@iul.ac.in

Suman Gautam, Jai Narayan Mishra, Preeti Mishra, Preeti Verma & Sudhanshu Mishra (Eds.)

This group encompasses tablets, syrups, injectables, creams, and even the packaging or container of these products. The development of the pharmaceutical industry, wider availability of drugs, and modified patterns of healthcare have greatly added to the waste being generated in different sectors. Flushing drugs into sewage systems, open dumping in landfills, or burning them without environmental regulation can result in the contamination of soil, groundwater, and surface water [1]. Even tiny amounts of active pharmaceutical ingredients were found in drinking water supplies, resulting in ecological and health impacts. Pharmaceutical waste comes from a variety of sources. Hospitals, clinics, and other healthcare facilities, pharmaceutical companies and laboratories, veterinary clinics, retail pharmacies, and households are included among these [2].

BACKGROUND AND SIGNIFICANCE

Over the last several decades, the worldwide health care system has seen immense increases in the manufacture, prescription, and use of drugs. Though this advancement has brought about enhanced disease control and mortality, it has also introduced an unavoidable rise in drug waste. Frequently not considered in discussions of waste management, drug waste has recently been identified as a specific and dangerous waste stream that is causing severe risks to environmental and public health. Pharmaceutical waste consists of a broad array of chemicals from unused and out-of-date drugs to discarded packaging, soiled items, and production residues [3]. These chemicals may find their way into the environment as a result of uncontrolled disposal practices like flushing medication down the toilet, open dumping, or burning without effective filtration. Active pharmaceutical ingredients can persist in soil and water, have undesirable effects on aquatic ecosystems, and have the potential to enter the food chain. In addition, traditional wastewater treatment technologies are usually not optimized to eliminate completely the residues of pharmaceuticals, enabling their repeated circulation in natural resources [4].

Pharmaceutical waste is linked to antimicrobial resistance. Routine environmental exposure to diluted doses of antibiotics and other medicines can lead to the emergence of resistant microbial populations, which compromise the efficacy of life-saving medications and complicate the course of infectious diseases. Hormonal drugs, cytotoxics, and psychotropics can also have toxic impacts on non-target organisms and disrupt normal biological processes. The significance and background of pharmaceutical waste go beyond contamination of the environment. They also include economic, social, and regulatory aspects. Complete knowledge of the sources and forms of pharmaceutical waste is thus a prerequisite to the development of effective segregation, handling, treatment, and disposal strategies [5].

SOURCES OF PHARMACEUTICAL WASTE

Pharmaceutical waste comes from an assortment of industries engaged in drug manufacturing, distribution, administration, and disposal. These sources present unique types and amounts of waste, frequently necessitating sophisticated handling and disposal procedures. It is necessary to identify these sources to develop effective waste management plans.

Healthcare Facilities

Healthcare centers, including hospitals, clinics, and diagnostic laboratories, are major contributors of pharmaceutical waste. These institutions produce waste products, such as expired medicines, half-used ampoules, intravenous fluids contaminated with drugs, unused tablets, ampoules broken and crushed, and drug-contaminated protective gear [6]. Much of this waste is a consequence of regimen changes, patient discharge before completion of medication courses, or the keeping of emergency drug supplies that are unlikely to be consumed prior to expiration [7]. Cytotoxic and cytostatic agents for oncology, narcotics, antibiotics, and hormone treatments are some of the most toxic materials produced in these settings. Their improper disposal, like flushing down a drain or commingling with normal waste, results in the contamination of hospital effluents that end up being discharged into municipal sewage systems [8]. The majority of wastewater treatment facilities are unable to screen out pharmaceutical residues, and as a result, active drug compounds end up being discharged into natural water bodies. Standardized protocols and training programs must be put in place to ensure safe, environmentally friendly waste disposal in such high-risk facilities [9].

Pharmaceutical Manufacturing

Pharmaceutical production facilities are another major contributor to pharmaceutical waste. These facilities generate waste at nearly every phase of drug production, such as synthesis, formulation, quality control testing, and packaging [10]. The waste produced could be active pharmaceutical ingredients (APIs), solvents, intermediates, degraded products, cleaning agents, and off-specification or rejected batches of drugs. The volumes of materials involved can be huge, particularly in production on a mass scale, where even a small fraction of rejected materials or spillage translates into huge quantities [11]. Inadequately treated industrial effluents have been found to discharge pharmaceutical compounds directly into surrounding rivers and lakes, resulting in intense concentrations of antibiotics, analgesics, and hormones within the environment. Such pollutants remain in the environment for extended periods, transform aquatic organisms, and stimulate the growth of resistant bacterial strains in water bodies

[12]. Although regulatory systems exist in most countries, enforcement and compliance are extremely variable, particularly in developing areas where monitoring infrastructure is scarce [13].

Households

Household pharmaceutical waste is usually underestimated, but it makes up a significant proportion of the total amount of pharmaceutical waste that is produced around the world. In households, waste is usually generated when people are unable to follow through with prescribed medication regimens, buy drugs in excess, improperly store drugs, or hold expired and unused drugs for an extended duration [3].

These household disposal practices are largely uncontrolled, with most individuals being unaware of the dangers of inappropriate disposal. Typical household practices include discarding tablets and syrups in trash, flushing drugs down a toilet or sink, and discarding medicines along with domestic waste. These disposal activities release pharmaceutical residues into sewage systems, landfills, and the wider environment without any treatment or neutralization [14]. Over-the-counter medications like analgesics, antibiotics, hormone pills, and cough syrups are commonly part of such waste streams. The environmental effect is also problematic, as these chemicals can remain biologically active and can contaminate water bodies, interfere with aquatic food, and be a major cause of the growth of drug resistance [15].

Drug Retail Stores and Drug Distributors

Retail drug distribution centers and retail pharmacies are the biggest contributors of pharmaceutical waste, primarily in the form of spent, returned, or damaged items. These centers handle enormous quantities of pharmaceutical stock in the form of prescription drugs, over-the-counter drugs, and special forms of preparations such as cold-chain dependent vaccines or insulin [16]. Products that have expired from shelf life, are returned by customers, or get damaged while in transit or storage, are usually thrown away [17]. Without a proper system of collection and disposal of these pharmaceutical wastes in most locations, improper disposal takes place by mixing expired drugs with regular trash or by flushing liquid preparations through sewerage systems [18]. Such disposal not only contaminates the environment but also poses a public health risk, especially when such wastes are accessible to scavengers or children. Another concern is regulatory constraints that prevent pharmacies from re-dispensing returned meds even when found complete in packaging due to storage conditions and tampering issues [19]. Consequently, enormous quantities of potentially useful drugs go down the drain. Furthermore, improper awareness among pharmacy staff regarding segregation and documentation of waste also renders safe disposal challenging [20]. In locations lacking take-back programs or specific regulatory guidelines, retail pharmacy pharmaceutical waste predominantly goes uncontrolled and unmonitored. This spilling of waste into landfills or municipal sewerage systems contaminates the soil and water resources. Therefore, it is important to include pharmacy-level waste management practices in national pharmaceutical policies for reducing the environmental footprint of retail pharmaceutical waste [21].

Veterinary Clinics and Farm Use

Veterinary clinics, animal farms, poultry farms, and aquaculture farms are major contributors of pharmaceutical waste through the application of veterinary medicines. These are antiparasitics, antibiotics, vaccines, hormones, sedatives, and topical formulations that are applied to prevent disease, cure disease, and increase productivity in animals [22]. Pharmaceutical waste from the industry arises from expired drugs, unused supplies, spillage during administration, and residues in animal feces and urine. One of the biggest problems of veterinary pharmaceutical waste is its dispersal in the environment, especially in intensive agricultural production systems where wastewater and manure from treated animals are released into water bodies and land [23]. Antibiotic residues destroyed in animal excreta are frequently present in untreated or poorly managed animal waste, which may be used directly as fertilizer in farms, leading to the contamination of agricultural land and nearby water bodies. This leads to the emergence of antimicrobial resistance in environmental microbial populations, which can ultimately be transmitted to human populations *via* food, water, or direct contact [24]. In aquaculture, medicated feeds and medicated water additives deposit residues in fishponds or are released into natural water bodies. Veterinary clinics and rural facilities also lack good waste disposal facilities (Table **1**), especially in low-resource settings, and therefore dispose of pharmaceutical waste directly into open fields, pit latrines, or surface drains. In comparison with human health industries, veterinary pharmaceutical waste is less regulated, and adherence to guidelines of disposal is low [25].

Table 1. Comparative analysis and disposal methods.

Category	Examples	Regulatory Authority	Disposal Methods
Controlled Substances	Morphine, Diazepam	DEA (US), National Agencies	Incineration at permitted facilities, non-retrievable destruction [40].

(Table 1) cont.....

Category	Examples	Regulatory Authority	Disposal Methods
Non-Controlled: Hazardous Waste	Cyclophosphamide, Mercury-containing vaccines	EPA (RCRA)	High-temperature incineration, chemical neutralization, secure landfilling [41].
Non-Controlled: Non-Hazardous Waste	Ibuprofen, Acetaminophen	EPA, Local Regulations	Municipal waste, take-back programs, designated disposal sites [42].
Special: Cytotoxic/ Antineoplastic	Methotrexate, Doxorubicin	WHO, National Guidelines	Encapsulation, inertization, high-temperature incineration (not to sewer/landfill) [43].
Special: Anti-Infective Drugs	Amoxicillin, Fluconazole	WHO	Encapsulation, incineration, diluted sewer disposal (liquids) [44].
Special: Controlled Drugs	Codeine, Alprazolam	WHO, National Agencies	Encapsulation, incineration, secure storage [45].

Educational and Research Institutions

Educational and research centers, especially those dealing with pharmaceutical, biomedical, and life science research, also contribute to pharmaceutical waste, though in limited quantity as opposed to hospitals or production units [26]. Universities, pharmacy schools, and science laboratories also produce waste while making experimental drugs, synthesizing chemicals, conducting pharmacological tests, and conducting practical sessions. Waste in these environments may comprise active pharmaceutical ingredients, organic solvents, reagents, and small-scale preparations, many of which are chemically complex and potentially toxic [27]. While the quantity of pharmaceutical waste in academic and research institutions may be small, its chemical heterogeneity and complexity present certain challenges to segregation, identification, and disposal. In addition, incorrect labeling or storage, spillage during handling, and commingling of pharmaceutical waste with laboratory general waste may cause environmental pollution or risk of occupational exposure [28]. Insufficient training of students and research personnel in waste management protocol leads to poor adherence to institutional guidelines. Moreover, budgetary constraints in educational institutions can limit the number of special pharmaceutical waste collection and disposal systems available. Unused or expired instructional materials, in some instances, are dumped in regular trash receptacles or flushed down laboratory drains, circumventing treatment processes [29].

CLASSIFICATION OF PHARMACEUTICAL WASTE

The proper classification of pharmaceutical waste is of paramount importance in determining its proper safe handling, segregation, storage, transport, and ultimate disposal. Because of the wide range of pharmaceutical products with reference to chemical structure, therapeutic use, and physical state, a standardized classification scheme is indispensable in order to reduce risk to human beings and the environment to a minimum [30]. Misclassification commonly leads to inadmissible disposal methods, which can result in natural resource contamination, the dissemination of antimicrobial resistance, and even inadvertent human or animal exposure. Worldwide, regulatory agencies and healthcare facilities utilize a combination of chemical, pharmacological, physical, and regulatory factors for pharmaceutical waste classification, each with unique merits for operational and safety considerations.

Classification Based on Hazardous Nature

One of the most common ways of categorizing pharmaceutical waste is based on its potential hazard. Under this scheme, waste is normally separated into hazardous and non-hazardous wastes. Hazardous pharmaceutical waste consists of medications and chemicals that have a high potential of causing serious harm to human health and the environment, even at low levels. These chemicals are toxic, carcinogenic, teratogenic, mutagenic, flammable, corrosive, or reactive. Examples are cytotoxic agents that are administered in cancer therapy (such as cyclophosphamide), some antibiotic classes (such as vancomycin), hormonal medications, and anesthetics. These wastes have to be treated with great caution, usually being incinerated at temperatures over 1,200°C or using chemical neutralization processes to make them safe [31].

Non-hazardous pharmaceutical wastes, on the other hand, are expired multivitamins, electrolyte solutions, saline infusions, and non-toxic over-the-counter medications. Although deemed to be of low risk, their uncontrolled disposal can still lead to the pollution of the environment and long-term ecological damage. For instance, disposing of huge quantities of unused painkillers in landfills may lead to groundwater pollution [32].

Hazardous Waste: Hazardous non-controlled substances meet RCRA criteria for toxicity, ignitability, corrosivity, or reactivity, or are listed as P- or U-listed wastes. P-listed wastes, such as arsenic trioxide (P012), are acutely hazardous, while U-listed wastes, like cyclophosphamide (U058), are non-acute but still hazardous. Characteristic hazardous wastes include drugs with high alcohol content (ignitable, D001) or those failing the Toxicity Characteristic Leaching Procedure (TCLP) for substances like mercury (D009. For example, multi-dose flu vaccines containing thimerosal may be classified as D009 due to mercury content. These wastes require management under RCRA Subpart P, which mandates secure storage, transportation, and disposal, often *via* high-temperature incineration or chemical neutralization [33].

Non-Hazardous Waste: Non-hazardous non-controlled substances, such as most OTC medications (*e.g.*, ibuprofen, acetaminophen), do not meet RCRA hazardous waste criteria. These can often be disposed of through municipal waste systems or take-back programs, though improper disposal, such as flushing, can still contribute to environmental contamination. Best practices recommend using designated disposal sites to minimize ecological impact, aligning with circular economy principles. State and local regulations may impose additional requirements, such as segregation from general waste [34].

Classified according to Pharmacological or Therapeutic Category

Pharmaceutical waste can be effectively sorted into pharmacological categories, where therapeutic function is usually aligned with environmental or safety hazards. Cytotoxic medications like methotrexate or doxorubicin for cancer treatment are high-risk drugs because of their genotoxic properties and have to be handled using PPE and disposed of by high-temperature incineration. Antimicrobials, like tetracycline and fluoroquinolones, are under scrutiny because of their role in antimicrobial resistance; minimal environmental exposure can interfere with microbial ecology. Controlled drugs, like morphine, fentanyl, and lorazepam, are illegally controlled because of their potential for abuse and must be rigorously monitored, usually incinerated in DEA-approved facilities in the United States or analogous regulations in other countries [35]. Hormone-type drugs such as estradiol and levonorgestrel are endocrine disruptors that have been known to modify reproductive cycles in aquatic organisms; sealed containment and chemical neutralization are generally necessary. Non-essential medicines such as paracetamol or antacids are of minimal individual hazard but collectively may pollute water or add to non-biodegradable pharmaceutical loads. This classification is operationally convenient in hospitals, pharmacies, and research facilities where segregation of drugs needs to be compatible with therapeutic risk profiles [36].

Classification According to Shape

Pharmaceutical waste is also categorized based on its physical state because this will influence the selection of containers, transportation, treatment technologies, and ultimate disposal. The principal physical forms are solid, liquid, semi-solid, and gaseous or pressurized. Liquid waste comprises oral syrups, injectable medication, IV solutions, antiseptics, and chemical reagents. Liquids are more likely to contaminate the environment when spilled or leaked and should thus be contained in leak-proof containers and processed with chemical neutralization or high-temperature incineration.

Semi-solid waste, like creams, ointments, gels, and suppositories, sticks to the surface if not disposed of properly. Pressurized medication containers, such as aerosol sprays, inhalers, and anesthetic gas cylinders, represent another group that has specific needs. These materials pose explosion or fire risks and should be punctured, decompressed, and discarded in regulated situations. These materials, incorrectly disposed of, will result in work-related injuries or environmental incidents [37].

According to the Source of Generation

Pharmaceutical waste is highly variable by source, each with unique types and hazards. Healthcare facilities and hospitals produce the largest amount, such as expired inventory, unused doses, cytotoxic waste from cancer centers, and antibiotic residues. It takes an average of 0.5 to 2 kg of pharmaceutical waste per bed per day for the hospitals in developed nations. Manufacturing facilities generate batch rejects, API residues, solvents, and cleaning agents. In industrial areas, production unit effluents have recorded antibiotic concentrations thousands of times higher than environmental safety levels. Retailers and distributors waste expired, recalled, or spoiled medicines, particularly following regulatory labeling adjustments or market removal.

Households are decentralized but significant sources of environmental drug load. Surveys indicate that 60–70% of households dispose of unused medicines in waste or toilets because return schemes are not available. Veterinary clinics and farms dispose of dewormers, growth-promoting hormones, and antibiotics, with manure runoff being a significant environmental route. Academic and research institutions generate small volumes but chemically complex waste, sometimes containing experimental or unlisted drugs [38].

CHALLENGES IN IDENTIFYING AND CLASSIFYING

Chemical and Formulation Complexity

Pharmaceutical waste originates from thousands of drug molecules with unique physicochemical, pharmacokinetic, and toxicological characteristics. Such variety makes classification at the time of disposal challenging. Most products are formulated as fixed-dose combinations—two or more APIs with different hazard levels. An example is a tablet that combines paracetamol (low-risk) and tramadol (controlled drug) with a dual classification challenge. In addition, numerous formulations are encapsulated, enteric-coated, or formulated in biodegradable polymers, which conceal their chemical nature on inspection. The advent of biosimilars, monoclonal antibodies, gene therapies, and RNA drugs has brought into play molecular entities that are not well reflected within conventional classification schemes. Even with standard APIs, differences in salt forms (*e.g.*, amlodipine besylate *vs.* amlodipine maleate) can influence reactivity and disposal needs [39].

In other instances, products of degradation or metabolites that have formed during storage are more environmentally or health-hazardous than the parent compound. For instancc, some tetracyclines turn nephrotoxic once they expire. Lacking real-time chemical analytical tools such as FTIR, Raman spectroscopy, or LC-MS, these conversions go unnoticed in most clinical or pharmacy environments. In addition, most excipients, preservatives, coloring agents, or solvents can be dangerous or flammable in themselves, but, through a lack of complete formulation openness, fall undetected. High-rate settings, such as hospitals and factories, create the demand for rapid processing of waste, where the danger of misclassifying such a complicated material is greater. The absence of dynamic, formulation-informed waste classification tools is still a paramount impediment in waste segregation [46].

Partial or Absent Label Information

One of the most direct obstacles to the proper classification of pharmaceutical waste is the common lack of labeling or readable identification on discarded items. Medications in hospitals, clinics, and homes tend to be removed from their original containers at the time of use. Strips are cut, vials opened, and ampoules broken—often leaving no evidence of the product's identity. This is most prevalent with loose tablets, unit doses, or intravenous medications packaged in generic IV syringes and bags. After being removed from barcodes, batch numbers, or product names, proper classification becomes virtually impossible to achieve without laboratory assistance.

Other compounded products, particularly in hospital pharmacies, have non-standard labels and may contain combinations of two or more active ingredients. These are dangerous, especially when they contain cytotoxic compounds, but without a descriptive label, their contents cannot be confirmed. Likewise, old drugs that have been stored for extended periods tend to have illegible or faded labels, while spills can lead to unidentified powders or liquids for handling as unknown waste. Lacking label data also makes traceability and documentation difficult, both of which are needed for regulated drugs. For instance, with opioids or psychotropics, not being able to verify identity can cause legal issues during an audit or inspection [47].

Mixed Waste Streams

One of the biggest operational problems in the classification of pharmaceutical waste is that more than one category of waste is co-mingled within a single disposal stream. In high-volume clinical settings, particularly high-turnover wards such as emergency departments and oncology wards, pharmaceutical waste is frequently thrown away into common containers with biomedical, sharps, or hospital general waste. Such blending can encompass hazardous and non-hazardous drugs, cytotoxic agents with general drugs, or even narcotics with standard disposables, thereby making post-disposal segregation almost impossible and unsafe. Waste that is not segregated appropriately poses several risks. For example, if cytotoxic waste is sent to a landfill with non-infectious general waste, it might get incinerated at low temperatures, producing genotoxic fumes [48].

Conversely, treating all mixed waste as hazardous, common in facilities lacking training, leads to overclassification and dramatically increases treatment costs. For reference, hazardous waste disposal can cost 5 to 10 times more per kilogram than non-hazardous waste. Moreover, when controlled substances are co-mingled with other waste types, regulatory tracking and accountability are compromised, potentially resulting in legal violations. Pharmacies and laboratory centers are also vulnerable to co-mingling errors, especially during clean-outs or bulk stock returns. Leftover vials, expired specimens, and damaged containers can be thrown together, particularly if their original containers are compromised. Shortages of color-coded bins, inadequate signposting, and a lack of designated collection areas worsen the problem [49].

Inadequate Staff Training

Lack of proper training among healthcare workers (Table **2**) has also remained one of the most consistent problems in identifying and classifying pharmaceutical waste appropriately. Even though national health institutions and agencies have released guidelines, frontline workers often have not received formal education about waste classification. This problem is particularly acute in low-resource environments, where medical waste is more viewed as a logistically burdensome aspect of clinical practice than an essential component of clinical safety.

Table 2. Comparative analysis of classification challenges and practical implications.

Challenge	Examples	Implications
Variability in Global Regulations	US RCRA *vs.* EU directives, Canadian provincial variations	Inconsistent classification, compliance issues for multinational operations [52].
Lack of Standardized Classification	US P/U lists *vs.* UK codes, WHO dosage-based categories.	Misclassification, challenges in data comparison, and international trade [53].
Analytical Detection Challenges	Low concentrations (ng/L–µg/L), complex wastewater matrices.	High costs, need for advanced equipment, and potential under-detection [54].
Knowledge Gaps in Environmental Fate	Mixture toxicity, antimicrobial resistance, and long-term ecological effects.	Limited risk assessment, ineffective waste management strategies [55].

Most institutions do not have waste sorting modules as part of routine orientation or continuing education curricula. Even in training-differentiated facilities, it is mostly vague biomedical waste segregation, with a little focus on pharmaceutical subgroups such as cytotoxic, controlled substances, or flammable agents. Consequently, personnel might dispose of high-risk waste in the general waste bins or misbelieve that expired medications can be sent out with house trash or biological waste [50].

Restricted Access to Analytical and Identification Equipment

Accurate pharmaceutical waste categorization normally involves chemical confirmation, particularly when labels are absent, drugs are mixed, or physical form is changed. In the majority of healthcare and institutional environments, though, access to analytical equipment is nonexistent or highly restricted. In the vast majority of instances, except for a few, namely cytotoxic or biologically derived agents, rough visual inspection is insufficient to define the chemical nature of the waste. The same clear solution in a syringe can be an innocuous saline flush or an extremely active chemotherapeutic agent without equipment or verified labels; the identification is a guess. In the event of uncertain identification, waste is often treated as hazardous by default, which significantly increases disposal expense and overwhelms hazardous waste facilities.

Also, where technologies are available, the operators may not be knowledgeable in drug analysis. The equipment is not cost-effective for regular use in the determination of waste and is rarely a part of regular waste management procedures. Drug residue mobile kits or field-screening technology are not in place and are not a regular practice. This technology gap results in overclassification, late disposal, and safety hazards. Closing the gap requires investment in low-cost, portable identification instruments, real-time drug databases, and training staff to enable on-site verification and classification [51].

NEED FOR PHARMACEUTICAL WASTE MANAGEMENT

Pharmaceutical waste, even though commonly produced in small quantities relative to other health wastes, presents disproportionately significant risks on account of its chemical reactivity, toxicity, and environmental persistence. As production and consumption of drugs increase worldwide, including hospital-derived, prescription, and over-the-counter drugs, their incorrect disposal poses an emerging issue that needs to be addressed through organized interventions.

Prevention of environmental pollution is one of the major needs in the management of drug waste. Pharmaceutical residues such as analgesics, antibiotics, antiepileptics, and hormonal drugs have been found in surface water, groundwater, and even drinking water supplies through various studies across the world. These residues tend to find their way into the environment through sewage, leachate from landfills, and inappropriate disposal into sinks or toilets. Traditional wastewater treatment facilities do not have the capability to completely remove drug products, enabling bioactive molecules to remain present in aquatic environments. This may result in changed reproductive cycles in aquatic organisms, changes in the behavior of fish, and bioaccumulation in food chains [56].

Discarding antibiotics into the environment, even in low levels, imposes selective pressure on the microbial population. This favors the survival and dissemination of resistant populations that can share resistance determinants with human pathogens. The World Health Organization and the United Nations identify environmental AMR as one of the greatest threats to future healthcare and food security. Pharmaceutical waste disposal is a strategic element of containing AMR. Occupational safety and public health also require effective waste procedures. Unused medication remaining in homes is a frequent source of childhood and elderly accidental poisoning. In pharmacies and hospitals, poor segregation exposes hospital cleaning staff and waste handlers to addictive or cytotoxic materials, allowing for a higher risk of exposure-related disease or drug abuse. Trace exposure to anticancer chemotherapy drugs has been associated with reproductive and genetic hazards among medical personnel [57].

Economically, inefficient waste disposal costs more. Misclassified hazardous waste or co-mingled waste needs expensive disposal, such as incineration or chemical neutralization. A mixture of pharmaceutical waste with general biomedical waste can cause the whole collection to be treated as hazardous, which has a heavier burden on waste treatment facilities and costs more in disposal for health care institutions. From an ethical and regulatory perspective, pharmaceutical waste disposal supports compliance with international and national legislation. Violation of waste management standards can lead to legal sanctions, the loss of licenses, and reputational loss for health providers and industries. The management of pharmaceuticals is critical for environmental conservation, control of AMR, public health, cost-effectiveness, and legality [58].

REVIEW OF KEY STUDIES ON PHARMACEUTICAL WASTE SOURCES

Hospital waste audits are essential for understanding the volume and composition of pharmaceutical waste generated in medical settings. A systematic review by Slutzman *et al.* (2023) [59] analyzed 156 studies from 37 countries, finding that 24% (37 studies) specifically assessed pharmaceutical waste. These studies aimed to improve local waste sorting policies (74%, 116 studies), reduce waste generation (45%, 70 studies), and inform regulatory policy development (42%, 65 studies). The review highlighted the significant contribution of hospitals to pharmaceutical waste, emphasizing the need for standardized auditing and reporting practices to enhance waste management efficiency.

Another pivotal study by Voudrias *et al.* [60] examined pharmaceutical and chemical waste from Xanthi General Hospital in Greece. Over five weeks, 233 kg of pharmaceutical waste and 110 kg of chemical waste were collected, with pharmaceutical waste comprising 3.9% of total hazardous medical waste. The waste was categorized into vial waste (51.1%), syringe waste (11.4%), and intravenous therapy waste (37.5%), with vial waste further classified into antibiotics, digestive system drugs, analgesics, hormones, circulatory system drugs, and others. The study reported a production rate of 14421452 kg/year, underscoring the importance of hospital-specific data for designing cost-effective waste management systems.

Wastewater analyses have revealed WWTPs as major pathways for pharmaceutical residues entering aquatic environments. Fatta-Kassinos, Meric, and Nikolaou [61] conducted a comprehensive review, documenting the presence of antibiotics (*e.g.*, ciprofloxacin, sulfamethoxazole) and analgesics (*e.g.*, ibuprofen, diclofenac) in WWTP effluents at concentrations ranging from ng/L to μg/L. Specific findings included sulfonamide concentrations of 0.01568.8 ng/L in Catalonia, Spain, and ibuprofen influent concentrations up to 115 g/L in Seville, Spain, with removal rates of 8088%. High concentrations of ciprofloxacin (751101, 000 ng/L) in hospital effluents further highlighted healthcare facilities as significant contributors to environmental contamination.

Hejna, Kapuścińska, and Aksmann [62] reviewed the eco-toxicological impacts of pharmaceuticals, focusing on ibuprofen and diclofenac. Ibuprofen was found to affect algal growth (Desmodeus subspicatus, EC50 315.0 mg/L) and cause genotoxic effects in zebrafish (*Danio rerio*) at 0.000092 mg/L. These findings indicate that pharmaceuticals can disrupt physiological processes, such as antioxidant enzyme activity and reproductive health, posing risks to aquatic ecosystems and necessitating further research into long-term ecological impacts.

Sapkota and Pariatamby [63] reviewed current techniques, such as incineration for solid and semi-solid wastes (*e.g.*, tablets, capsules), encapsulation, and landfilling, with disposal costs estimated at $ 790/ton in the USA and £450/ton in the UK. The study proposed sustainable alternatives, including medicine take back programs, eco-pharmacovigilance, extended producer responsibility, co-payment models, and life cycle analysis focusing on reduction and reuse.

Alshemari *et al.* [64] explored a circular pharmaceutical supply chain to reduce medicine waste, advocating for waste minimization, reuse/re-dispensing, and optimized stock management. A case study in Ethiopia reported a 3.68% wastage rate at public health facilities, costing $ 14, 339.93, highlighting the potential for circular economy principles to enhance sustainability.

Despite significant progress, several research gaps persist, limiting the ability to fully address pharmaceutical waste challenges. Kummerer [65] identified sparse knowledge on long-term ecological effects, mixture toxicity, and the environmental fate of biopharmaceuticals. The study noted that while pharmaceuticals are detected in the environment, their chronic impacts, particularly from low-level exposure, remain poorly understood. Mixture toxicity, where pharmaceuticals interact with other pollutants, may lead to synergistic or antagonistic effects not captured by standard tests. Additionally, the biodegradability of biopharmaceuticals and the nomenclature of metabolites *versus* transformation products require clarification.

Research on antibiotic resistance development due to pharmaceutical residues is also critical, given its public health implications. Future investigations should focus on developing cost-effective, green analytical techniques, conducting long-term ecological studies, and assessing the environmental behavior of emerging biopharmaceuticals to support comprehensive risk assessments and sustainable management strategies [65].

CONCLUSION

Pharmaceutical waste is becoming an important concern in healthcare and environmental protection. With the increasing use of medicines in hospitals, homes, and industries, there is more remaining or expired medicine. This waste, if improperly managed, will have harmful effects on people, animals, and the environment. The chapter considers the sources of pharmaceutical waste, such as hospitals, factories, homes, veterinary clinics, and laboratories, and why each source requires its own means of managing the waste. Proper identification and characterization of this waste is extremely critical. Most drugs are chemically complex, sometimes labels are incomplete or unclear, and various types of waste are commingled. Many facilities do not have the equipment to analyze or identify the waste in-house. To rectify this, we require a regulatory firm, national guidelines, electronic tools that are able to detect drugs, routine training for healthcare professionals, color-coded bins for simplicity of sorting, and improved technology to analyze unfamiliar waste. Regular inspections and improved coordination among healthcare, environmental, and waste management staff can also make a difference. Bottom line: handling pharmaceutical waste is not simply about compliance; it is about safeguarding public health and the environment. A transparent, efficient, and well-structured system is required to get it right.

REFERENCES

[1] Kayode-Afolayan SD, Ahuekwe EF, Nwinyi OC. Impacts of pharmaceutical effluents on aquatic ecosystems. Sci Afr 2022; 17: e01288.
[http://dx.doi.org/10.1016/j.sciaf.2022.e01288]

[2] Kadam A, Patil SS, Patil SV, Tumikar A. Pharmaceutical waste management an overview. Indian J Pharm Pract 2016; 9(1): 2-8.

[3] Rogowska J, Zimmermann A. Household pharmaceutical waste disposal as a global problem—a review. Int J Environ Res Public Health 2022; 19(23): 15798.
[http://dx.doi.org/10.3390/ijerph192315798] [PMID: 36497873]

[4] Castensson S. Pharmaceutical waste. In: Kümmerer K, Ed. Pharmaceuticals in the environment: sources, fate, effects and risks. 3. Berlin, Heidelberg: Springer 2008; pp. 489-99.
[http://dx.doi.org/10.1007/978-3-540-74664-5_31]

[5] Sreekanth K, Vishal G, Raghunandan H, *et al.* A review on managing of pharmaceutical waste in industry. Int J Pharm Tech Res 2014; 6: 899-907.

[6] Caban M, Stepnowski P. How to decrease pharmaceuticals in the environment? A review. Environ Chem Lett 2021; 19(4): 3115-38.
[http://dx.doi.org/10.1007/s10311-021-01194-y]

[7] Hiew SY, Low BY. A systematic review of the knowledge, attitude and practice of healthcare professionals and healthcare professional students towards household pharmaceutical waste disposal. Explor Res Clin Soc Pharm 2025; 17: 100556.
[http://dx.doi.org/10.1016/j.rcsop.2024.100556] [PMID: 39877296]

[8] Vatovec C, Kolodinsky J, Callas P, Hart C, Gallagher K. Pharmaceutical pollution sources and solutions: Survey of human and veterinary medication purchasing, use, and disposal. J Environ Manage 2021; 285: 112106.
[http://dx.doi.org/10.1016/j.jenvman.2021.112106] [PMID: 33588165]

[9] Janik-Karpinska E, Brancaleoni R, Niemcewicz M, *et al.* Healthcare waste—a serious problem for global health. Healthcare 2023; 11(2): 242.

[10] khalidi-idrissi A, Madinzi A, Anouzla A, *et al.* Recent advances in the biological treatment of

wastewater rich in emerging pollutants produced by pharmaceutical industrial discharges. Int J Environ Sci Technol 2023; 20(10): 11719-40.
[http://dx.doi.org/10.1007/s13762-023-04867-z] [PMID: 37360558]

[11] Okeke ES, Ezeorba TPC, Okoye CO, *et al.* Environmental and health impact of unrecovered API from pharmaceutical manufacturing wastes: A review of contemporary treatment, recycling and management strategies. Sustain Chem Pharm 2022; 30: 100865.
[http://dx.doi.org/10.1016/j.scp.2022.100865]

[12] Ai X, Zhang X, Tian Y, *et al.* Research status, key technologies and development trends of pharmaceutical waste salt treatment technology: A review. Waste Manag Res: The J Sus Circular Eco 2025; 43(10): 1525-1547.
[http://dx.doi.org/10.1177/0734242X251326271]

[13] Smale EM, Egberts TCG, Heerdink ER, van den Bemt BJF, Bekker CL. Waste-minimising measures to achieve sustainable supply and use of medication. Sustain Chem Pharm 2021; 20: 100400.
[http://dx.doi.org/10.1016/j.scp.2021.100400]

[14] Bankole DT, Oluyori AP, Inyinbor AA. The removal of pharmaceutical pollutants from aqueous solution by Agro-waste. Arab J Chem 2023; 16(5): 104699.
[http://dx.doi.org/10.1016/j.arabjc.2023.104699]

[15] Magagula BK, Rampedi IT, Yessoufou K. Household pharmaceutical waste management practices in the Johannesburg Area, South Africa. Int J Environ Res Public Health 2022; 19(12): 7484.
[http://dx.doi.org/10.3390/ijerph19127484] [PMID: 35742731]

[16] Balakumar J. Waste disposition management: an enabler to achieve the United Nations' SDG #3 within the pharmaceutical industry [master's thesis]. Richardson (TX): University of Texas at Dallas; 2023.

[17] Miettinen M, Khan SA. Pharmaceutical pollution: A weakly regulated global environmental risk. Rev Eur Comp Int Environ Law 2022; 31(1): 75-88.
[http://dx.doi.org/10.1111/reel.12422]

[18] Tat R, Heydari J. Avoiding medicine wastes: Introducing a sustainable approach in the pharmaceutical supply chain. J Clean Prod 2021; 320: 128698.
[http://dx.doi.org/10.1016/j.jclepro.2021.128698]

[19] Desai M, Njoku A, Nimo-Sefah L. Comparing environmental policies to reduce pharmaceutical pollution and address disparities. Int J Environ Res Public Health 2022; 19(14): 8292.
[http://dx.doi.org/10.3390/ijerph19148292] [PMID: 35886145]

[20] Huq T, Khan A, Brown D, Dhayagude N, He Z, Ni Y. Sources, production and commercial applications of fungal chitosan: A review. Journal of Bioresources and Bioproducts 2022; 7(2): 85-98.
[http://dx.doi.org/10.1016/j.jobab.2022.01.002]

[21] Sazvar Z, Zokaee M, Tavakkoli-Moghaddam R, Salari SA, Nayeri S. Designing a sustainable closed-loop pharmaceutical supply chain in a competitive market considering demand uncertainty, manufacturer's brand and waste management. Ann Oper Res 2022; 315(2): 2057-88.
[http://dx.doi.org/10.1007/s10479-021-03961-0] [PMID: 33583989]

[22] Valsson O, Tayler E, Kitutu F E, *et al.* Antibiotic surveillance: an action-oriented integrated approach. Wellcome Open Research 2026; 11: 55.

[23] Carrasco Menzir A, Adeladlw T A. A review on veterinary medical waste disposal and management. J Pharm Drug Dev 2022; 9(1): 102.

[24] Koytcheva MK, Sauerwein LK, Webb TL, Baumgarn SA, Skeels SA, Duncan CG. A systematic review of environmental sustainability in veterinary practice. Top Companion Anim Med 2021; 44: 100550.
[http://dx.doi.org/10.1016/j.tcam.2021.100550] [PMID: 34051396]

[25] Khalifa HO, Shikoray L, Mohamed MYI, Habib I, Matsumoto T. Veterinary drug residues in the food

chain as an emerging public health threat: Sources, analytical methods, health impacts, and preventive measures. Foods 2024; 13(11): 1629.
[http://dx.doi.org/10.3390/foods13111629] [PMID: 38890858]

[26] Agarwal S, Saha H, Kaushik S, Patil VM, Verma S. Critical review of biomedical waste management for future pandemics: Pharmaceutical perspective. J Chem Health Saf 2024; 31(6): 444-67.
[http://dx.doi.org/10.1021/acs.chas.4c00067]

[27] Andeobu L, Wibowo S, Grandhi S. Medical waste from COVID-19 pandemic—a systematic review of management and environmental impacts in Australia. Int J Environ Res Public Health 2022; 19(3): 1381.
[http://dx.doi.org/10.3390/ijerph19031381] [PMID: 35162400]

[28] Essam O, Elmahdy MA, Elmenshawy Y, Elshami AA, Ahmad SS, Aboubakr A. Experimental investigation on the recycling of medical waste for sustainable fiber-reinforced concrete production. Case Stud Constr Mater 2025; 22: e04675.

[29] Deepika Kanyal , Ranjit Ambad , Ambad R. Biomedical waste management in India-a review. Indian J Forensic Med Toxicol 2021; 15(2): 108-13.
[http://dx.doi.org/10.37506/ijfmt.v15i2.14285]

[30] Zhang J, Yu X, Wang J, Sui Q, Zhao W. Impacts of garbage classification and disposal on the occurrence of pharmaceutical and personal care products in municipal solid waste leachates: A case study in Shanghai. Sci Total Environ 2023; 874: 162467.
[http://dx.doi.org/10.1016/j.scitotenv.2023.162467] [PMID: 36842588]

[31] Menda C, Ramakrishna C. A review: Analytical methods in pharmaceutical waste and its chemical hazards in environmental management.

[32] Sungur Ş. Pharmaceutical and personal care products in the environment: occurrence and impact on the functioning of the ecosystem. In: Sarma H, Dominguez DC, Lee WY, eds. Emerging contaminants in the environment. Elsevier 2022; pp. 137-57.
[http://dx.doi.org/10.1016/B978-0-323-85160-2.00009-3]

[33] Patel M, Kumar R, Kishor K, Mlsna T, Pittman CU Jr, Mohan D. Pharmaceuticals of emerging concern in aquatic systems: Chemistry, occurrence, effects, and removal methods. Chem Rev 2019; 119(6): 3510-673.
[http://dx.doi.org/10.1021/acs.chemrev.8b00299] [PMID: 30830758]

[34] Destroyer Rx. DEA Compliant Pharmaceutical Disposal Regulations. Rx Destroyer; 2023 [Internet]. Avaiilable from: https://www.rxdestroyer.com/dea-compliant-pharmaceutical-disposal-regulations/

[35] Zhou H, Yu X, Alhaskawi A, *et al.* A deep learning approach for medical waste classification. Sci Rep 2022; 12(1): 2159.
[http://dx.doi.org/10.1038/s41598-022-06146-2] [PMID: 35140263]

[36] Hanning SM, Hua C, Baroutian S, *et al.* Quantification and composition of pharmaceutical waste in New Zealand. J Mater Cycles Waste Manag 2022; 24(4): 1603-11.
[http://dx.doi.org/10.1007/s10163-022-01410-z] [PMID: 35570848]

[37] Ulusoy U. A Review of Particle Shape Effects on Material Properties for Various Engineering Applications: From Macro to Nanoscale. Minerals (Basel) 2023; 13(1): 91.
[http://dx.doi.org/10.3390/min13010091]

[38] Kobayashi N, Tsuchiya Y, Kosugi Y, Suzuki T. Occurrence and fate of pharmaceuticals and personal care products in river water, lake water, sewage effluent, tap water, and groundwater in Japan. Environmental Toxicology and Chemistry. 2026 Jan;45(1):45-56.

[39] Kumar D, Malviya R, Singh DP. Innovative Techniques for Pharmaceutical Waste Management: Enhancing Drug Recovery and Environmental Sustainability. Curr Green Chem 2025; 12(2): 138-45.
[http://dx.doi.org/10.2174/0122133461322762240926072018]

[40] Choudhury M, Majumdar S, Sillanpää M. Understanding waste management: a comprehensive

overview of environmental, economic, and social implications. In: Choudhury M, Majumdar S, Sillanpää M, Eds. The circular path: waste as a resource. Cham: Springer 2026; pp. 1-28.

[41] Breve F, LeQuang J K, Batastini L. Controlled Substance Waste: Concerns, Controversies, Solutions. Cureus 2022; 14(2): e22564.
[http://dx.doi.org/10.7759/cureus.22564]

[42] Chaudhary R. Pharmaceutical waste management in pharmaceutical industries of Kathmandu, Nepal [bachelor's thesis]. Vantaa (FI): Laurea University of Applied Sciences; 2021. Available from: https://urn.fi/URN:NBN:fi:amk-2021062116467

[43] Capoor MR, Bhowmik KT. Cytotoxic Drug Dispersal, Cytotoxic Safety, and Cytotoxic Waste Management: Practices and Proposed India-specific Guidelines. Indian J Med Paediatr Oncol 2017; 38(2): 190-7.
[PMID: 28900329]

[44] MacBrayne CE, Williams MC, Obermeier H, *et al.* Anti-infective waste in a pediatric institution: pinpointing problems in the process. Hosp Pharm 2020; 55(4): 220-3.
[http://dx.doi.org/10.1177/0018578719844164] [PMID: 32742009]

[45] Ahmed I, Majeed A. The safe and responsible disposal of unused controlled drugs. Br J Nurs 2007; 16(21): 1318-22.
[http://dx.doi.org/10.12968/bjon.2007.16.21.27717] [PMID: 18073668]

[46] Nguyen MK, Lin C, Nguyen HL, *et al.* Occurrence, fate, and potential risk of pharmaceutical pollutants in agriculture: Challenges and environmentally friendly solutions. Sci Total Environ 2023; 899: 165323.
[http://dx.doi.org/10.1016/j.scitotenv.2023.165323] [PMID: 37422238]

[47] Mohammed SA, Kahissay MH, Hailu AD. Pharmaceuticals wastage and pharmaceuticals waste management in public health facilities of Dessie town, North East Ethiopia. PLoS ONE 2021; 16(10): e0259160.
[http://dx.doi.org/10.1371/journal.pone.0259160]

[48] Fradinho J, Allegue LD, Ventura M, Melero JA, Reis MAM, Puyol D. Up-scale challenges on biopolymer production from waste streams by Purple Phototrophic Bacteria mixed cultures: A critical review. Bioresour Technol 2021; 327: 124820.
[http://dx.doi.org/10.1016/j.biortech.2021.124820] [PMID: 33578354]

[49] Hemidat S, Achouri O, El Fels L, *et al.* Solid Waste Management in the Context of a Circular Economy in the MENA Region. Sustainability (Basel) 2022; 14(1): 480.
[http://dx.doi.org/10.3390/su14010480]

[50] Olaniyi FC, Ogola JS, Tshitangano TG. Challenges of effective management of medical waste in low-resource settings: perception of healthcare workers in Vhembe district healthcare facilities, South Africa. Trans R Soc S Afr 2021; 76(1): 81-8.
[http://dx.doi.org/10.1080/0035919X.2021.1900949]

[51] Jæger B, Menebo MM, Upadhyay A. Identification of environmental supply chain bottlenecks: a case study of the Ethiopian healthcare supply chain. Manag Environ Qual 2021; 32(6): 1233-54.
[http://dx.doi.org/10.1108/MEQ-12-2019-0277]

[52] Pezzola A, Sweet CM. Global pharmaceutical regulation: the challenge of integration for developing states. Global Health 2016; 12(1): 85.
[http://dx.doi.org/10.1186/s12992-016-0208-2] [PMID: 27998293]

[53] Brechtelsbauer E, Shah S. Update on pharmaceutical waste disposal regulations: Strategies for success. Am J Health Syst Pharm 2020; 77(7): 574-82.
[http://dx.doi.org/10.1093/ajhp/zxz360] [PMID: 32050015]

[54] Dogan A, Płotka-Wasylka J, Kempińska-Kupczyk D, Namieśnik J, Kot-Wasik A. Detection, identification and determination of chiral pharmaceutical residues in wastewater: Problems and

challenges. Trends Analyt Chem 2020; 122: 115710.
[http://dx.doi.org/10.1016/j.trac.2019.115710]

[55] Hiew SY, Low BY. The knowledge, attitude, and practice of the public regarding household pharmaceutical waste disposal: a systematic review (2013–2023). Int J Pharm Pract 2024; 32(2): 120-32.
[http://dx.doi.org/10.1093/ijpp/riae001] [PMID: 38300734]

[56] de Campos EAR, ten Caten CS, de Paula IC. End-of-use and end-of-life medicines—insights from pharmaceutical care process into waste medicines management. Environ Sci Pollut Res Int 2021; 28(41): 58170-88.
[http://dx.doi.org/10.1007/s11356-021-14661-4] [PMID: 34105077]

[57] Kumar A, Thakur AK, Gaurav GK, *et al.* A critical review on sustainable hazardous waste management strategies: a step towards a circular economy. Environ Sci Pollut Res Int 2023; 30(48): 105030-55.
[http://dx.doi.org/10.1007/s11356-023-29511-8] [PMID: 37725301]

[58] Chisholm JM, Zamani R, Negm AM, *et al.* Sustainable waste management of medical waste in African developing countries: A narrative review. Waste Manag Res 2021; 39(9): 1149-63.
[http://dx.doi.org/10.1177/0734242X211029175] [PMID: 34218734]

[59] Slutzman JE, Bockius H, Gordon IO, *et al.* Waste audits in healthcare: A systematic review and description of best practices. Waste Manag Res 2023; 41(1): 3-17.
[http://dx.doi.org/10.1177/0734242X221101531] [PMID: 35652693]

[60] Voudrias E, Goudakou L, Kermenidou M, Softa A. Composition and production rate of pharmaceutical and chemical waste from Xanthi General Hospital in Greece. Waste Manag 2012; 32(7): 1442-52.
[http://dx.doi.org/10.1016/j.wasman.2012.01.027] [PMID: 22365264]

[61] Fatta-Kassinos D, Meric S, Nikolaou A. Pharmaceutical residues in environmental waters and wastewater: current state of knowledge and future research. Anal Bioanal Chem 2011; 399(1): 251-75.
[http://dx.doi.org/10.1007/s00216-010-4300-9] [PMID: 21063687]

[62] Hejna M, Kapuścińska D, Aksmann A. Pharmaceuticals in the aquatic environment: A review on eco-toxicology and the remediation potential of algae. Int J Environ Res Public Health 2022; 19(13): 7717.
[http://dx.doi.org/10.3390/ijerph19137717] [PMID: 35805373]

[63] Sapkota B, Pariatamby A. Pharmaceutical waste management system – Are the current techniques sustainable, eco-friendly and circular? A review. Waste Manag 2023; 168: 83-97.
[http://dx.doi.org/10.1016/j.wasman.2023.05.052] [PMID: 37285639]

[64] Alshemari A, Breen L, Quinn G, Sivarajah U. Can we create a circular pharmaceutical supply chain (CPSC) to reduce medicines waste?. Pharmacy (Basel) 2020; 8(4): 221.
[http://dx.doi.org/10.3390/pharmacy8040221] [PMID: 33218038]

[65] Kümmerer K. The presence of pharmaceuticals in the environment due to human use – present knowledge and future challenges. J Environ Manage 2009; 90(8): 2354-66.
[http://dx.doi.org/10.1016/j.jenvman.2009.01.023] [PMID: 19261375]

CHAPTER 2

Effects of Improper Pharmaceutical Waste Disposal

Shreya Maddesiya[1], **Piyush Anand**[1], **Shweta Yadav**[1], **Juhi Tiwari**[1], **Deepak Kumar**[1] and **Shashikant Singh**[1,*]

[1] *Faculty of Pharmaceutical Sciences, Mahayogi Gorakhnath University, Gorakhpur, Uttar Pradesh, India*

Abstract: The substantial effects that inappropriate disposal of pharmaceutical waste has on ecosystems and public health have drawn more attention to the environmental effects of this practice. Pharmaceutical waste includes unwanted, outdated, or unused drugs that can be harmful if not disposed of properly. These materials are frequently improperly disposed of, which allows them to enter soil, water bodies, and the air. This contamination endangers aquatic life, terrestrial organisms, and human health. Data suggest that pharmaceutical residues, particularly those from antibiotics, and endocrine disruptors may negatively affect aquatic ecosystems, leading to antibiotic resistance and biodiversity loss. These substances, for example, can increase biological oxygen demand in water bodies, lowering oxygen levels that are vital for aquatic life. Environmentally Persistent Pharmaceutical Products (ERPs), which are medications that linger in the environment, can also interfere with wildlife's physiological functions, altering behavior and causing reproductive problems. Many nations lack comprehensive frameworks to address the complexities of pharmaceutical contamination, and the regulatory environment for pharmaceutical waste disposal is often insufficient. Unknowingly contributing to environmental degradation, many people treat pharmaceutical waste as regular household waste. The public's ignorance and lack of education about proper disposal practices exacerbate this issue. The problem is further compounded by research indicating that healthcare providers and community pharmacies frequently lack sufficient understanding of appropriate disposal techniques. Implementing robust waste management measures, such as public education campaigns, regulatory reforms, and the creation of appropriate disposal facilities, is crucial to reducing the environmental impacts of pharmaceutical waste. To encourage sustainable practices and lessen the environmental impact of pharmaceutical waste, legislators, healthcare professionals, and the general public must work together. Ultimately, a multifaceted approach to addressing the issues caused by pharmaceutical waste is needed, emphasizing public safety and environmental well-being.

* **Corresponding author Shashikant Singh:** Faculty of Pharmaceutical Sciences, Mahayogi Gorakhnath University, Gorakhpur, Uttar Pradesh, India; E-mail: Shashikantsingh59@gmail.com

Suman Gautam, Jai Narayan Mishra, Preeti Mishra, Preeti Verma & Sudhanshu Mishra (Eds.)

Keywords: Antibiotic resistance (amr), Aquatic ecosystem toxicity, Biological oxygen demand (BOD), Endocrine-disrupting chemicals, Environmental contamination, Environmentally persistent pharmaceutical products (EPPS), Pharmaceutical waste disposal, Soil contamination, Water pollution from pharmaceuticals, Wildlife behavioral changes.

INTRODUCTION

Pharmaceutical waste refers to unused, expired, spilled, or contaminated pharmaceutical products, vaccines, drugs, and sera that are no longer needed and must be disposed of. These are acquired from various sources such as clinics, hospitals, pharmacies, veterinary clinics, and homes. They consist of different forms of materials—injectables, ointments, syrups, capsules, tablets, and even packs with drug residues. Increased use of drugs around the globe has been driven by population growth, aging, and rising health needs. Inadequate disposal and handling of drug waste pose a serious threat to environmental sustainability and human health. The pollutants in the wastes can be absorbed into the soil and water bodies, endangering terrestrial and aquatic life. Most active pharmaceutical ingredients (APIs) are meant to act on biological levels at low levels of concentration and can remain in the environment for long periods owing to their chemical stability. An example is antibiotics released into water bodies, which can disorganize microbial communities and further drive the development of antimicrobial resistance (AMR), an increasing concern worldwide. Hormonal drugs, such as estrogens, may be endocrine-disrupting chemicals, disrupting the reproductive cycles of aquatic organisms. Further, EPPP drugs can accumulate in the ecosystem and interfere with wildlife's physiological functioning, including altered mating behavior and reproductive defects. In light of these observations, the ecological effects of pharmaceutical waste are an immediate concern that necessitates an immediate response from scientists, doctors, regulators, and society in general [1].

CURRENT METHODS OF DISPOSAL

The practices adopted for the disposal of pharmaceutical waste today are extremely diverse, depending on the country's regulatory environment, infrastructure, and public awareness. The usual methods of disposal are landfilling, incineration, sewer disposal, and chemical treatment. All of these have their strengths and weaknesses regarding efficiency, cost, and environmental concerns [1].

LANDFILLING

Landfill disposal of drug waste is the most frequent. It is generally inexpensive and easy to accomplish, but it involves the danger of leachate creation. Water passes over rubbish and acts upon drug products to migrate into groundwater systems, where drugs become entrained within those aquifer systems to persist over extensive timeframes [1].

INCINERATION

High-temperature incineration is considered one of the most effective technologies for destroying drug compounds. Effective incinerators can minimize the environmental impact of toxic waste. But when operated under suboptimal conditions, it can emit harmful air pollutants such as dioxins and furans. Operation of incineration plants is extremely expensive, hence an unsustainable option in the majority of developing countries [1]

SEWER DISPOSAL

Unused or expired drugs are, in certain cases, discarded by flushing them down sinks or toilets, especially in residential areas and small clinics. Such practice is highly discouraged because wastewater treatment plants cannot destroy complex drug residues. This causes the pollution of rivers, lakes, and sources of water [1].

CHEMICAL DEACTIVATION AND ENCAPSULATION

Some institutions dispose of drug waste, especially cytotoxic and harmful drugs, by using chemical neutralization technology or encapsulation. These techniques work but depend heavily on qualified professionals and adequate facilities. Even though such processes are available, the lack of uniform regulations and enforcement in most places has resulted in unequal practices. Lack of public awareness, poor segregation at the source, and inadequate disposal facilities aggravate the situation, resulting in ongoing environmental pollution. Therefore, concerted action through improved public education, green disposal methods, and rigorous regulation is needed to prevent the adverse environmental consequences of pharmaceutical waste [1].

CONTAMINATION PATHWAYS IN THE ENVIRONMENT

The Contamination of Water

The problem of water pollution from the wrong disposal of pharmaceutical waste is becoming a serious environmental issue deserving serious academic scrutiny. Pharmaceutical waste, including unused or expired drugs, tends to be disposed of improperly by community households and health centers. Because of inadequate dumping procedures, toxic chemicals become part of the water sources and hence present hazards to life in the waters and human well-being [2, 3].

Pharmaceuticals can travel *via* various systems of water through various routes. Specifically, wastewater treatment plants (WWTPs) are being identified as critical sites wherein such pollutants enter undetected or untreated in effluents and subsequently reach surface waters [4, 5]. One disturbing feature of this pollution is that most pharmaceuticals have low aqueous solubility, enabling them to remain in environmental waters, and possibly causing damage to aquatic life and ecosystems [6, 7]. Significantly, environmental agencies have pointed out that antibiotics and hormones present in most of these compounds can cause such effects as antibiotic resistance in microbial communities, with implications not only for wildlife but also for human populations when entering drinking water supplies [8, 9]

The pathways of contamination are intricate and multifaceted. Misuse of disposal habits by consumers, such as disposing of drugs in the garbage or flushing them down the toilet, allows for direct access to water supply. High percentages of these discarded drugs evade efficient elimination measures throughout wastewater treatment and end up polluting surrounding streams, rivers, and groundwater [10, 11]. Research demonstrates that trace amounts of these micropollutants can interfere with aquatic ecosystems, giving rise to altered reproductive processes and wildlife habits [12, 13]. The broader implications of improper pharmaceutical waste handling practices highlight the significance of effective public health policies. Initiatives taken to promote awareness of pharmaceutical disposal and the related health effects of water pollution are desperately needed [14]. In addition, the development of strict regulatory systems would greatly reduce these environmental hazards by imposing improved pharmaceutical waste-handling standards across the board among all stakeholders, ranging from healthcare facilities to homes [15, 16].

The Contamination of Soil

Soil pollution by pharmaceutical waste is a serious and emerging environmental issue. The routes by which pharmaceuticals find their way into soil ecosystems are varied and often involve both direct and indirect pathways. Littering of unused and expired drugs, either through water runoff, landfilling, or incineration, leads to the entry of pharmaceutical pollutants into the soil [17 - 19]. Additionally, agricultural applications of treated waste or effluent from pharmaceutical manufacturing plants further increase contamination levels [20, 21].

Pharmaceuticals in the environment may occur due to direct application as well as human and animal metabolism. Upon ingestion of medications, a large amount is eliminated in their intact forms *via* urine and feces, resulting in environmental exposure when such waste products are poorly controlled [22].

The use of antibiotics and hormones in agriculture also adds to the soil burden of such pollutants since runoff and manure handling procedures can unintentionally spread active pharmaceutical ingredients (APIs) into adjacent soil matrices [23, 24].

The effects of soil contamination with pharmaceuticals are manifold, affecting the environment and human health. Soil microorganisms play a key role in the breakdown of pharmaceutical products; nevertheless, the recalcitrance of a few drugs, particularly the highly polar ones, may lead to significant soil buildup due to a lack of adsorption [25, 26]. For example, research shows that some drugs can persist and remain bioavailable in soils, thus disrupting local microbial communities and hindering their vital processes like nutrient cycling [27]. Such eco-disruption of soil can result in decreased soil fertility, inhibited plant growth, and possible bioaccumulation in food webs, potentially harming human health through contaminated crops [28, 29].

Other than that, the presence of pharmaceutical contaminants in soil has the potential to induce antimicrobial resistance through the selection of microbial communities. This presents important questions concerning the safety of agro-products and points to the need for sustainable pharmaceutical waste management strategies to mitigate this issue. Better public education and regulation must be instituted to stop improper disposal methods that cause soil contamination, so that the environmental pathways of pharmacy waste are regulated appropriately [29].

Atmospheric Dispersion

The atmospheric dispersion and environmental impact of pharmaceutical waste are shown in Table **1** below.

Table 1. Atmospheric dispersion and environmental impact of pharmaceutical waste.

S.No	Aspect	Description	References
1.	**Improper Disposal of Pharmaceutical Waste**	Improper disposal of pharmaceutical waste. Improper disposal results in environmental pollution by atmospheric dispersion, affecting public health and ecosystems.	[30, 31]
2.	**Incineration as a Disposal Method**	Incineration releases pollutants like NO_2, SO_2, CO, and particulate matter (PM), deteriorating air quality and causing health hazards.	[32]
3.	**Pollutants Released**	Toxic chemicals released include: Nitrogen dioxide (NO_2) Sulfur dioxide (SO_2) Carbon monoxide (CO)	[32]

(Table 1) cont.....

S.No	Aspect	Description	References
4.	**Effect on Ecosystems**	Pharmaceutical pollutants are a risk to biodiversity and food safety by way of introduction into the food chain through contaminated biomass.	[32]
5.	**Acute toxicity to aquatic life**	Household waste of antidepressants and antibiotics is harmful to aquatic life.	[32]
6.	**Bioaccumulation Effects**	Contaminants bioaccumulate, resulting in biodiversity loss and public health issues (*e.g.*, the Death of Asian vultures from diclofenac).	[32]
7.	**Regulatory Challenges**	Developing countries usually have weak frameworks for managing pharmaceutical waste, exacerbating environmental degradation.	[33]
8.	**Landfill Pollution**	Pharmaceuticals disposed of in landfills generate leachate, polluting agricultural land and soil.	[33]
9.	**Public Health Issue**	Drugs' environmental persistence enhances the risk of disease transmission and antimicrobial resistance.	[33]
10.	**Need for Sustainable Practices**	Effective policies, public knowledge, and sustainable waste management practices must be in place to reduce risks.	[34]

EVALUATION OF THE ENVIRONMENTAL IMPACT

Demand for Biological Oxygen in Water Bodies

Poor pharmaceutical waste disposal is one of the greatest environmental issues, especially regarding the biological oxygen demand in water bodies. Pharmaceutical waste from domestic or medical environments can cause acute water pollution, impacting ecosystems and human health. This test discusses the mechanism by which improper disposal causes environmental degradation, through biological oxygen demand (BOD). Pharmaceutical waste, when disposed of improperly, usually ends up in water bodies, leading to contamination that impacts water and aquatic life quality. Misdisposal through unsuitable disposal of unused medicines into domestic waste or flushing them down toilets contributes to the discharge of pharmaceutical residues into the environment. They are usually found in rivers, streams, and groundwater at levels capable of having a drastic impact on aquatic ecosystems. A review has revealed that effluent from hospitals and homes accounts for a significant share of drugs entering water bodies, leading to increased BOD as microbial communities respond to extraneous chemicals [35]. In particular, the introduction of organic chemicals like anti-inflammatory drugs and antibiotics disrupts the indigenous balance of aquatic organisms, thereby increasing biological oxygen demand because microorganisms reproduce to biodegrade the chemicals [36]. This process extracts dissolved oxygen content, creating a challenge for aquatic organisms that thrive on abundant oxygen. Besides, the presence of "drug pollutants" in the environment has a lot to do with disrupting aquatic food webs and the "potential to exert long-term ecological effects" on the environment [37, 38]. Reports have proven that more than 631 different pharmaceuticals have been detected in environmental samples in many countries, indicating a worldwide crisis in pharmaceutical waste as shown in Table **2,** which describes various environmental impacts of pharmaceutical waste [39, 40]. In certain regions, particularly where regulatory frameworks are lacking, pharmaceuticals can reach the environment at alarming rates, with household disposal being a leading contributor. This rampant disposal reflects a failure to implement adequate waste management practices and to educate the public about the risks associated with improper [41]. In addition, the consequences of these practices have implications beyond environmental effects; they result in health risks, such as the creation of antibiotic resistance because of the constant occurrence of these chemicals in ecosystems. The requirement for biological oxygen in contaminated water bodies can be used as an indicator of the level of pharmaceutical contamination, highlighting the necessity for enhanced regulatory controls and community participation in pharmaceutical waste management. To properly counteract these environmental effects, overall strategies need to be implemented that include improved disposal protocols, the avoidance of unnecessary pharmaceutical use, and proper segregation of waste at the source. Policymakers, clinicians, and communities have to come together to set sustainable practices to keep pharmaceuticals from entering the environment and to defend our water systems [42, 43].

Table 2. Various environmental impacts of pharmaceutical waste.

S. No	Impact	Description	Source of Contamination	Affected Environment	Reference
1	Water Pollution	Due to the pharmaceuticals entering rivers, lakes, and groundwater.	Improper sink disposal	Freshwater bodies	[99]
2	Soil Contamination	All the medicines dumped in landfills leach into the soil.	Illegal Landfills, dumping	Agricultural lands, forests	[100]
3	Bioaccumulation	Accumulation of drugs in organisms over time.	Contaminated water & soil	Aquatic & terrestrial animals	[101]
4	Hormonal Disruption in Wildlife	Various synthetic hormones affect the reproductive systems.	All Birth control residues	Fish, amphibians	[102]

(Table 2) cont.....

S. No	Impact	Description	Source of Contamination	Affected Environment	Reference
5	Antibiotic Resistance	Antibiotics in the environment promote resistant bacteria.	Various Hospitals, agriculture	Water and soil microbiomes	[103]
6	Algal Blooms	Stimulation of Nutrients and chemicals causes harmful algae growth.	Due to Wastewater treatment failures	Lakes, rivers, and coasts	[104]
7	Aquatic Toxicity	Causing direct poisoning of fish and aquatic organisms.	Various Expired drugs were dumped in the water	Oceans, rivers	[22]
8	Decreased Biodiversity	Sensitive species decline due to contamination.	Long-term exposure to pollutants and waste	Ecosystems	[105]
9	Disruption of Food Chains	Toxins travel up the food chain, affecting predators.	Persistent chemicals in prey	Entire ecosystems	[106]
10	Genetic Mutations in Aquatic Life	Exposure to certain chemicals causes mutations.	Endocrine disruptors	Fish, amphibians	[107]
11	Soil Microbe Disruption	Antibiotics kill beneficial soil bacteria.	Veterinary waste, agriculture	Farmlands	[108]
12	Surface Water Contamination	Rainwater runoff carries pharmaceuticals into rivers.	Improper waste handling	Streams, lakes	[109]
13	Groundwater Contamination	Leaching through soil affects drinking water sources.	Landfills, septic systems	Aquifers	[109]
14	Air Pollution	Burning of pharmaceuticals releases toxic gases.	Open burning/incineration	Atmosphere	[109]
15	Wildlife Poisoning	Animals consume discarded drugs or contaminated water.	Various Improper disposal in nature	Forests, wetlands	[110]
16	Developmental Issues in Animals	Deformities or stunted growth in animals that are exposed.	Various Hormonal drugs, sedatives	Rivers, lakes	[110]
17	Coral Reef Degradation	Chemicals have an impact on coral growth and reproduction.	Marine runoff	Ocean reefs	[110]
18	Disruption of Plant Growth	Drug residues prevent roots from growing or seeds from germinating.	All Contaminated irrigation water	Agricultural fields	[111]

(Table 2) cont.....

S. No	Impact	Description	Source of Contamination	Affected Environment	Reference
19	Changes in pH and Water Quality	Certain substances change the chemistry of water.	Various Industrial and household waste	Freshwater sources	[111]
20	Eutrophication	Drug waste increases nutrient loads and encourages algal blooms that deplete oxygen.	improper disposal sites	Lakes, ponds	[112]

Pharmaceuticals with an Environmental Persistence (ERPs)

Environmental persistence of drugs, or Environmentally Persistent Pharmacological Products (EPPPs) as they are referred to, has become an important issue across the disciplines of environmental science and public health. Drugs have a variety of environmental behaviors, with some remaining in the environment much longer than they were intended to [44, 45]. They are naturally chemically stable and biodegradable, and are continuously introduced into aquatic environments through various routes, including wastewater effluents from treatment plants and pharmaceutical production facilities. These factors can all contribute to their long-term environmental persistence. Drugs are categorized according to the PBT criterion, which considers toxicity, bioaccumulation potential, and persistence [46, 47]. The drug carbamazepine, for instance, has been shown to have a considerable mean dissipation time, indicating that although many medications may break down rapidly, their ongoing release into the environment maintains their ecological influence and presence. This classification is important because it helps identify potential environmental hazards [48]. One such important route for EPPP release into the environment is through wastewater treatment plants (WWTPs), where most pharmaceuticals are not effectively removed [49]. The inefficiency of existing treatment processes results in active pharmaceutical ingredients (APIs) remaining in effluents, which are then continuously discharged into surface waters [50]. Studies have shown that pharmaceutical concentrations can become alarming due to inefficiencies in wastewater treatment degradation processes, underscoring the need to enhance treatment technologies to reduce these impacts. In addition, incorrect disposal practices, such as the over-excretion of non-absorbed pharmaceuticals by patients, worsen the situation [51, 52]. One of the key features of the environmental impact of pharmaceuticals is their ecological risk. Various studies have established that these chemicals harm aquatic organisms, leading to chronic exposure effects that can disrupt endocrine processes and contribute to the development of antibiotic-resistant bacteria [53]. This underscores the importance of evaluating the risks of pharmaceuticals not only based on their chemical characteristics but also taking into account their biological impacts on ecosystems [54]. The global increase in pharmaceutical consumption, alongside insufficient regulatory measures and awareness, underscores the urgency of the issue [55]. With rising pharmaceutical production linked to increased environmental presence, there is an alarming gap in ecotoxicological data necessary for risk assessment, prompting calls for more comprehensive studies to understand their long-term effects on both ecosystems and human health. This knowledge is crucial for developing effective monitoring and mitigation strategies to protect environmental health in the face of growing pharmaceutical contaminants [56].

Changes in Wildlife Behavior

The effects of pharmaceutical pollution on wildlife behavior are a critical ecological issue that is receiving increasing attention in environmental science. As active biological substances, pharmaceuticals can interfere with normal behaviors among wildlife, especially in aquatic systems where such compounds often enter as wastewater effluent and agricultural runoff. The phenomenon highlights the critical need to track and curb the effects of these environmental pollutants [57]. Numerous studies have revealed how drugs affect animal behaviors, especially in aquatic animals like fish. Some drugs, such as psychoactive drugs, have been discovered to change essential behaviors like feeding, mating, and predator defense [58, 59]. As an example, the antidepressant drug fluoxetine has been known to affect anxiety-related behavior among mosquitofish, exhibiting less threat response. These kinds of changes in behavior can considerably affect the reproductive success and survival of such creatures and, therefore, the population dynamics [60]. Pharmaceuticals are sometimes classified by their persistence in the environment. Some chemicals, especially those that are non-degradable, have very adverse ecological effects due to their longevity. They are known as Environmentally Persistent Pharmaceutical Pollutants (EPPPs) that can also accumulate within biological systems and thus cause different behaviors and even physiological changes within wildlife [61]. The action of these chemicals on evolutionarily conserved physiological receptors across species indicates that non-target organisms are susceptible to comparable effects as exhibited in humans [62]. Moreover, changes in chemical communication in ecosystems caused by pharmaceutical contaminants can result in larger-scale ecological changes. Research shows that behavioral changes in individual organisms destabilize social structure and community life, such as changes in social rank in fish treated with certain drugs [63]. Accumulation of these contaminants threatens not only the individual level but may also have cascading impacts on the ecosystem, resulting in the loss of biodiversity and habitat instability. Additionally, drugs can heighten wildlife's vulnerability to antibiotic resistance, further complicating the ecological impacts of these contaminants. Such a trend has dire implications for food web and ecosystem resilience, necessitating awareness of and a response to the multidimensional impacts of drug pollution on wildlife behavior [64 - 66].

Effects on Reproduction in Organisms

The effects of pharmaceuticals on the reproductive health of wildlife are increasingly emerging as a cause of concern as these chemicals continue to persist in different ecosystems. Pharmaceuticals, especially those that fall under the category of endocrine-disrupting chemicals (EDCs), can disrupt the endocrine systems of organisms, resulting in reproductive and developmental abnormalities. Once these chemicals reach the environment through effluents of wastewater, agricultural run-off, or improper disposal of unused drugs, they accumulate in aquatic organisms and pose enormous threats [67, 68]. It is proven through scientific research that the intake of some pharmaceuticals results in reproductive failures in wildlife populations. One of the most alarming examples is the drug ethynylestradiol (EE2), which has been found to induce reproductive failure in zebrafish following exposure to environmentally realistic concentrations over several generations (Nash *et al.*, 2004). This implies that the combined effects of pharmaceuticals in the environment not only influence individual reproductive success but may also contribute to broader population decline and reduce biodiversity. The mechanisms through which pharmaceuticals cause these reproductive impacts are diverse. EDCs disrupt normal hormonal signaling, and this results in changes in sexual development, infertility, and atypical gamete quality [69]. The disruptions may take different forms, such as reduced fertility, changes in mating behavior, and disruptions in parental care, further impacting population dynamics and ecological balance [70]. For example, hormonal contaminants in sewage have been linked to widespread sexual disruption in fish populations in natural water bodies [71]. Amphibians, a second group of organisms highly vulnerable to the effects of environmental contaminants, have shown reproductive problems related to exposure to EDCs [72]. Chemical exposure as an estrogen mimic has been reported in the scientific literature to correspond with altered gonadal development and altered expression of vitellogenin in female amphibians, once more illustrating the hazard posed by human-made pollutants in interfering with other taxa's reproductive health [73, 74]. In broader ecological settings, these chemicals have cascading impacts across food webs, affecting predator-prey relationships and community structure due to impaired reproductive success in keystone species [75 - 77].

AWARENESS OF PROFESSIONALS AND THE PUBLIC

Gaps in Community Pharmacy Knowledge

The disposal of pharmaceutical waste poses a serious threat to public health and the environment. Community pharmacists are essential in reducing the dangers of inappropriate disposal because they are easily available to healthcare professionals. However, several investigations have found significant gaps in their understanding and procedures:

Limited Awareness of Environmental Impact

Many community pharmacists lack a thorough understanding of the negative environmental impacts of improper pharmaceutical disposal. Common habits, such as throwing prescription drugs in the trash can contaminate land and water sources with pharmaceutical residues. Community pharmacists' knowledge and procedures for disposing of unnecessary medications were found to be inadequate in a Karachi-based study. Most participants, however, had a positive attitude toward learning safe disposal techniques and were aware of the adverse environmental effects that improper disposal causes [78].

Inadequate Training on Disposal Protocols

Pharmacists frequently complain that they were not given enough instruction on how to manage pharmaceutical waste during their schooling and career advancement properly. As a result of this lack of training, disposal procedures are irregular or antiquated. During their academic careers, less than half of students and healthcare professionals received formal instruction on safe pharmaceutical disposal methods, according to a comprehensive review. This gap makes it more difficult for them to advise patients on appropriate disposal techniques [79].

Poor Understanding of Regulatory Guidelines

Pharmacists are generally unaware of the laws at the local and federal levels that control the disposal of pharmaceutical waste. For example, 75% of pharmacists were not aware of the proper way to dispose of expired medications, according to a study evaluating how registered pharmacists in urban areas dispose of pharmaceutical waste. This ignorance may fail to comply with legal requirements and miss opportunities to participate in appropriate incineration procedures or take-back initiatives [80].

Lack of Knowledge of Health Risks

Pharmacists might not be completely aware of the health hazards, like the emergence of antimicrobial resistance (AMR), that come with pharmaceutical pollution in the environment. According to research, only 45.2% of pharmacists believed that antibiotics disposed of inappropriately could result in AMR. Inadequate attention to appropriate disposal procedures may arise from underestimating these hazards [81].

Minimal Public Education Efforts

The public is often not actively informed by pharmacists about safe disposal practices or accessible community resources, even though pharmacists are well positioned to educate patients. According to research evaluating community pharmacists' knowledge, attitudes, and practices regarding the disposal of domestic pharmaceutical waste, few had signage in their pharmacies promoting proper medication disposal. This lack of proactive involvement encourages patients to continue their inappropriate disposal practices [82].

Limited Access to or Awareness of Disposal Resources

It can be challenging for pharmacists in some areas to provide patients with appropriate disposal services because they lack access to drug take-back bins or are unaware of local disposal programs. For instance, a study conducted in Kuwait found that insufficient training, inappropriate waste management, and a lack of knowledge about the health risks associated with medical waste are the main causes of improper waste management. Pharmacists are unable to properly advise the public or carry out appropriate disposal procedures without these resources [83].

Training for Healthcare Professionals

Pharmaceutical waste must be managed effectively to protect human health and reduce environmental damage. A key role in this process is played by healthcare personnel, who require thorough training to improve their knowledge and disposal procedures for pharmaceutical waste. In addition to enhancing adherence to legal requirements, this kind of training enables experts to inform the public about appropriate disposal practices [84].

Importance of Training Healthcare Professionals

To fill in knowledge gaps and advance best practices in pharmaceutical waste management, healthcare workers must participate in training programs. Systematic research found that healthcare workers' perspectives and understanding of drug disposal are insufficient due to a lack of formal education and shortcomings in the academic curriculum. Due to this deficiency, patients are frequently not informed of appropriate disposal techniques, which encourages the community to continue using inappropriate disposal methods [84].

The implementation of focused educational initiatives has demonstrated notable advancements in the management of medical waste and according to one study evaluating the effects of training on healthcare personnel, sorting procedures and general adherence to waste management guidelines significantly improved. Nonetheless, the study also identified recurring issues in areas such as the timeliness of garbage collection and container labeling, highlighting the necessity of ongoing system enhancements and training [84].

Techniques for Raising Public and Professional Awareness

The following tactics can be used to successfully increase awareness of the effects of disposing of pharmaceutical waste:

1. **Include Comprehensive Waste Management Training in Curricula:** Including comprehensive modules on pharmaceutical waste management in healthcare education guarantees that future practitioners are knowledgeable about appropriate disposal procedures right away [85].
2. **Hold Regular Courses for Continuing Education:** Providing workshops and seminars helps healthcare workers stay current on the laws, disposal methods, and environmental effects of pharmaceutical waste. Programs like these have been demonstrated to greatly increase employee awareness and adherence to waste management procedures [85].
3. **Create Unambiguous Institutional Rules and Regulations:** Healthcare facilities can guarantee uniform and legal waste disposal procedures by establishing and sharing standardized procedures. To help healthcare institutions properly manage pharmaceutical waste, the U.S. Environmental Protection Agency offers a thorough 10-step guide.
4. **Take Part in Public Awareness Campaigns:** Medical practitioners can spearhead neighborhood campaigns to inform people about the dangers posed by improper disposal of pharmaceutical waste to the environment and human health. These initiatives can be strengthened through partnerships with groups like the International Pharmaceutical Students' Federation, which runs campaigns to raise awareness of medicine.
5. **Make Use of Digital Platforms for Greater Reach:** By utilizing social media, webinars, and online courses, knowledge may be efficiently distributed to professionals and the general public, catering to a range of learning styles and enhancing accessibility [85].

6. **Put Feedback Mechanisms in Place:** Creating avenues for the public and healthcare professionals to offer input on waste management procedures can help pinpoint problem areas and promote a culture of ongoing learning and adaptation.

Promoting appropriate pharmaceutical waste disposal procedures requires extensive training and awareness campaigns for medical personnel. Giving professionals the right information and abilities would enable them to manage waste in healthcare settings efficiently and act as public educators and role models. This two-pronged strategy guarantees a team effort to reduce the adverse effects of pharmaceutical waste on the environment and human health.

Procedures for Public Disposal

WHO-recommended Methods for Getting Rid of Pharmaceutical Waste

When disposing of unneeded medicines, follow these seven key procedures.

Decision: When to get rid of collected pharmaceutical waste should be decided by the pharmacy or medical facility [86].

Approval: The relevant authorities are consulted to obtain permission to dispose of pharmaceutical waste. In Kenya, disposal is done under the supervision of the PPB and the National Environment Management Authority (NEMA). The trash generator must pay the PPB 2,500 Ksh and correctly complete the disposal form. Upon disposal, a Drug Safe Disposal Certificate is issued by the PPB. In Hong Kong, a chemical waste generator must apply to the Environmental Protection Department (EPD) and then receive a waste generator number. Within a month following collection, the waste generator receives the charges. When the generator is picked up, the waste collector gives it a trip ticket.

Planning: To make resources like money, human capital, skills, time, equipment, and disposal techniques available, planning is essential. It is necessary to estimate the amount of pharmaceutical waste at this point, which is calculated in weights per quantity using 0.2 metric tons per m3.

Creating working teams: Pharmacists, pharmacist technicians, and employees of pharmaceutical warehouses should make up the disposal teams. Workplace conditions, pharmaceutical waste type, and volume all influence the number of employees and their ratio.

Work teams devoted to safety and health: Teams in charge of disposal should be provided with protective gear, including masks, gloves, helmets, boots, and overalls.

Sorting: Drugs come in a variety of pharmacological and dosage forms.

Some categories can be securely reintroduced into the supply chain, while others require alternative disposal methods, which is why sorting is required.

Pharmaceutical waste needs to be properly labeled, stored, and separated before being disposed of [86].

Disposal: Several waste disposal choices should be evaluated based on considerations such as cost, safety, ease of use, and practicality. Keep track of the following: the date and place of destruction, the method of disposal, the name of the pharmaceutical, the dosage form and quantity, the goods' worth, the reasons for disposal, the name and signature of the pharmacist disposing of the things, and a witness before destruction.

Security: Strict precautions and regulations must be followed when handling drugs, psychotropics, and antineoplastics to prevent distractions during sorting, scavenging, and theft.

Techniques for Getting Rid of Pharmaceutical Waste

Pharmaceutical waste can be disposed of in eight different ways: incineration, immobilization, landfill, sewage, chemical decomposition, burning in open containers, fast-flowing watercourses, and return to the donor [87].

Give Back to the Donor

Unwanted or outdated donations and large medications that are difficult to dispose of, including antineoplastics, should be returned to the manufacturer or donor. Pharmaceutical waste can be disposed of through cross-border exchanges. This strategy entails transporting hazardous material across national borders. The Basel Convention on the Transboundary Transfer of Hazardous Wastes governs it. The processes involved in this approach, however, require a long time to justify the transfer [87].

A landfill- When pharmaceutical waste is dumped directly into a landfill, it is referred to as landfilling. The most popular way of disposal is a landfill. Landfills fall into one of three types.

Uncontrolled, Open, Non-engineered Dump

It is a common practice in poor nations. Waste that has not been processed should not be disposed of using this method. As a final resort, it might be used after immobilization. Watercourses should be kept separate from open landfills to avoid contamination [87].

A landfill that has been engineered: This is the second-best way to get rid of pharmaceutical waste that has been immobilized. Features of the method reduce the release into the aquifer.

Sanitary landfill with heavy-duty construction: These locations are above the water table, well-managed, and kept away from watercourses. Because it protects the aquifer, this is the safest way to get rid of waste. To maintain the conditions for waste, garbage is compacted and covered with soil [88].

Being Immobilized

There are two ways to immobilize waste: inertization and encapsulation.

Encapsulation is the process of immobilizing garbage inside a drum as a block of concrete. The process that follows is employed:

1. Drums should be clean. Drums that have previously held explosive materials should not be used.
2. Bend the drum lids back after cutting them open.
3. Fill drums 75% of the way to the top with liquids, powders, antineoplastics, prohibited drugs, or solid or semi-solid trash.
4. Pour cement, lime, and water into the drum in a 15:15:5 ratio. To get uniformity, add a sizable amount of water.
5. Weld the lid after bending it back.
6. Fill the landfill with fresh municipal rubbish after placing the drums at the bottom.

Inertization is a low-cost technique that can be carried out with simple tools. A grinder, cement, lime, water supply, and concrete mixture are among the materials needed. It can be used to dispose of powders, antineoplastics, regulated drugs, and solid or semi-solid waste. The process that follows is employed:

1. Put on protective gear, like masks and gloves.
2. Keep pharmaceutical packaging materials, including blister packs, cardboard, plastics, and papers, separate.

3. To create a uniform waste, combine pharmaceutical waste, water, cement, and lime in the following ratio: 65%: 15%: 15%: 5%.
4. Use a concrete mixer truck to transport the trash to a landfill.
5. Disperse into municipal waste or decant into urban waste.

The Sewer

Small amounts of diluted garbage are released into sewers when disposed of in drains. The technique works well for getting rid of liquids, intravenous fluids, and trace levels of antiseptics or disinfectants. Antiseptics, disinfectants, and antineoplastics should not be disposed of in this manner [88].

Burning in Open Containers

Small amounts of pharmaceutical waste should be disposed of using this method. To prevent air pollution, medications disposed of in this way shouldn't be burned at low temperatures. It works well with drugs that are stored in cabinets and papers. Polyvinyl chloride (PVC)-containing items should not be burned.

Decomposition by Chemicals

It is only practical in cases where incineration is not an option and chemical competence is available. It requires constant access to chemicals and is laborious and time-consuming. It is suitable for getting rid of antineoplastic weighing less than 50 kg. Ought to be done under the manufacturer's advice [89].

Burning Up

The two techniques for incineration are medium and innovative high-temperature combustion.

Medium-temperature incineration- If high-temperature incinerators are not accessible or there are less secure alternatives, medium-temperature incineration can be utilized to get rid of solids, semi-solids, powders, and regulated chemicals. Two chambers in the incinerator reach $8500^{\circ C}$. The combustion retention duration of the second chamber is two seconds. It is recommended that pharmaceutical and municipal garbage be combined in a 1:1000 ratio. Because very small levels of halogen end up in combustion gases, medium-temperature incinerators should not be utilized to dispose of halogenated compounds (>1% halogenated chemicals).

Novel high-temperature incineration- Using new high-temperature incineration, solids, semi-solids, liquids, powders, regulated chemicals, and antineoplastics can all be disposed of. For example, cement kilns are incinerators that run at temperatures higher than 12,000 degrees Celsius, have extended combustion retention times, short gas residence times, appropriate pollution controls, and are costly and employ advanced technology. Every component of organic waste is broken down in this incinerator, which also absorbs any hazardous combustion byproducts. They can quickly and efficiently get rid of large amounts of pharmaceutical waste. It is recommended that pharmaceuticals be added to the furnace in smaller doses (5%) than fuel feed (95%). Remove package materials and ground the medications before burning them to prevent fuel feed blockage [89].

Risks Associated with Inappropriate Disposal

The economy, the environment, and human and animal life are all at risk from improper handling, storage, and disposal practices. Pharmaceutical waste leaks from landfills into aquifers or ends up in rivers and lakes. Pharmaceutical companies, homes, and medical facilities should nt flush their waste into sewer systems or pour it down the drain. While solid waste was disposed of in garbage or bins, the majority of liquid dosage forms were disposed of through the sink and toilet, according to a study done to assess disposal habits in South and Southeast Asia. The study's recommended disposal practices could harm the environment. Some of the repercussions of inappropriate disposal include the following:

- Contamination of residential and wildlife water sources. After consuming water tainted with Viagra, lambs showed signs of uncontrollable sex drive.
- Because teens believe prescription medicines are safer than other narcotics, improper opioid disposal can result in drug abuse.
- Children who come into contact with improperly disposed of medications may accidentally become poisoned. Pills might end up in the wrong hands of people or dogs since they are colorful and resemble candy. Children may inadvertently ingest medication if they are not careful, which could result in overdosing [89, 90].
- Aquatic life is affected by improper disposal. Because of ethyl estradiol contamination, male fish have become intersex by exhibiting sexual traits. Androgens cause female fish to become more masculine. Fish have experienced less hatching and organ damage as a result of analgesics. When fluoxetine was dumped into waterways, it changed fish behavior, disrupted their hormones, and caused frogs to produce tadpoles without legs. Decreased growth of algae and aquatic plants (Daphnia, Artemia) as a result of antifungals and antibiotics. Tramadol, carbamazepine, and felodipine were detected in blue mussels at amounts greater than 100 µg/kg, according to data gathered by the Helsinki Commission (HELCOM) in cooperation with Baltic Sea states. Many of these medications were found in seabirds, such as common eiders, indicating that they may be passed down through food chains [91].

- Antineoplastics, antibiotics, and non-biodegradable disinfectants destroy bacteria needed for sewage treatment, impacting nitrification, denitrification, and organic degradation processes.
- Antimicrobial resistance and the emergence of superbugs as a result of abuse, overuse, animal growth promotion, and the discharge of large amounts of antibiotics into freshwater environments. According to a survey by medical staff at pediatric wards at São Paulo University Hospital, antimicrobials (22.7%) were the most often disposed of medications, with the sink drain being the second most popular disposal technique. In their physical form, the majority of the medications were disposed of. Furthermore, 48% of the medications disposed of were hazardous to the health of people and the environment.
- When medications are burned in open containers or at low temperatures, harmful carbon emissions are released into the air, contributing to pollution.
- Encouragement of illicit activity, such as scavenging, reselling, and diversion of outdated medications to the general population.
- The soil is damaged. Because the soil is unable to sustain plant growth, the resulting plants contain harmful compounds. Plants are harmed by the phytotoxic effects of pharmaceutical compounds in the soil. The root growth of carrots and lettuce was found to be impacted by 1000 μg/L of the antibiotic amoxicillin. Horseradish viability was 65% of the nonsteroidal anti-inflammatory drug diclofenac.
- The design of landfills results in leaching and sluggish waste decomposition, which contaminates the soil and hinders output.
- The disposal of infectious blood in landfills and the washing up of syringes on beaches are two examples.
- When vultures were fed carcasses, the high dosage of diclofenac (Cataflam, Voltaren) in cattle resulted in renal failure.
- Rising medical expenses, as well as the needless waste of money.
- Loss of the waste generator's license, penalties, and reputation.

Difficulties in Managing Home Waste

The general lack of knowledge about the proper ways to dispose of unused or expired pharmaceuticals is one of the main problems with home pharmaceutical waste management. Many people don't know that throwing medications in the trash or flushing them down the toilet can contaminate the environment and pose health hazards. According to Tong *et al.* (2011), the majority of people in New Zealand admitted to using sewer systems or general garbage bins, indicating that a sizable section of the population was ignorant about proper medicine disposal techniques. This practice is replicated throughout the world and is associated with a lack of pharmaceutical waste-related public health campaigns or educational programs [92].

Restricted Access to Infrastructure for Safe Disposal

Drug disposal kiosks and appropriate take-back schemes are frequently inaccessible to home users. Many nations either have little coverage or no organized household disposal system. Because of this infrastructure deficiency, people resort to risky disposal methods. Inappropriate disposal procedures are exacerbated by the lack of community-level systems, according to the World Health Organization (WHO), which highlights the significance of adequate disposal facilities.

Even in wealthy nations, access to collection sites can be irregular or poorly publicized.

Poor Storage and the Chance of Unintentional Exposure or Abuse

Due to "just in case" mentalities or simple forgetfulness, medications are frequently kept in homes for a long time after they are no longer needed. Long-term storage raises the possibility of misuse by other family members as well as unintentional consumption by kids or pets. It is discovered that elderly persons in the community seldom properly dispose of their expired prescriptions and frequently hoard them. This contributes to the long-term accumulation of pharmaceutical waste at home, in addition to posing health risks [93].

Pollution of the Environment

Pharmaceutical substances leak into soil and water systems due to improper disposal practices, such as flushing or throwing them down the drain. These pharmaceutical residues are frequently found in rivers, lakes, and even drinking water sources since wastewater treatment facilities are ill-equipped to remove them. According to a review, human disposal practices are mostly to blame for the ubiquitous presence of medicines in aquatic environments worldwide. These leftovers have the potential to bioaccumulate in organisms and disturb aquatic ecosystems [94].

Gaps in Regulation and Policy

Clear government regulations or guidelines about how customers should dispose of pharmaceuticals are frequently lacking. Laws that manage pharmaceutical waste at the household level are either nonexistent or insufficient in many areas, which causes people to behave inconsistently. The disarray of regulations and the absence of universally accepted guidelines for disposing of drugs. Households resort to handy yet environmentally poor disposal methods when there are unclear guidelines.

Social and Cultural Attitudes

In some cultures, retaining medications for future use is seen as practical or necessary due to limited access to healthcare or the high costs of medicines. This cultural norm can contribute to large accumulations of unused medicines, which are then disposed of unsafely.

Various local studies in developing countries support this behavioral trend, though global-scale data is still emerging. Social perceptions and mistrust of disposal systems can also discourage participation in official take-back programs.

EFFECTS OF IMPROPER PHARMACEUTICAL WASTE DISPOSAL

Structure of Regulations

Present Deficits

Inadequate infrastructure for safe collection and disposal, poor disposal practices, and a lack of awareness are the main causes of the current gap in pharmaceutical waste disposal. Contamination of the environment and possible harm to human health result from this. Rules governing the disposal of pharmaceutical waste can differ by nation, state, and even locality. By ensuring that pharmaceutical waste is disposed of properly and safely, these rules aim to safeguard the environment and public health. These rules specify how drugs should be disposed of and how healthcare facilities must handle and dispose of their pharmaceutical waste responsibly and safely.

Furthermore, disposing of pharmaceutical waste is subject to laws in many states and localities. For instance, certain jurisdictions could mandate that pharmacies or medical facilities dispose of pharmaceutical waste using specific techniques or participate in take-back programs. To guarantee safe and responsible waste management, people and healthcare facilities must understand and abide by local laws about the disposal of pharmaceutical waste. Regulation noncompliance can harm the environment and public health in addition to fines and other penalties. People lack direction on proper disposal methods when there are no government disposal systems in place. To give citizens efficient disposal methods, community education must be improved. Additionally, the recovery of valuable materials from discarded pharmaceuticals and public awareness campaigns are hampered by the absence of disposal procedures [95].

Implementation Difficulties

The implementation of appropriate pharmaceutical waste disposal is complicated by regulatory loopholes, poor infrastructure, limited public awareness, and a lack of funding for waste management. These challenges make it more difficult to dispose of pharmaceutical waste in a safe and environmentally responsible manner, which could result in health hazards and environmental damage. Comprehensive laws and regulations that particularly handle the disposal of pharmaceutical waste are lacking in many areas. Even in cases when restrictions are in place, non-compliance may result from lax enforcement. There is often a lack of coordination and cooperation among parties, including waste management services, government organizations, medical facilities, and pharmaceutical corporations [84, 96].

Cross-border Concerns

The importance of international cooperation and the implementation of the Basel Convention on the Transboundary Movement of Hazardous Wastes are the main cross-border issues in the disposal of pharmaceutical waste. Ensuring the safe and responsible transportation and disposal of expired or unwanted medications, which are classified as hazardous waste, across international boundaries is at the heart of these issues. This entails securing the required authorizations, providing thorough documentation, and obtaining prior informed consent from both the importing and exporting nations [97, 98].

There are protocols in place for obtaining permissions and supplying documentation for the international transportation of hazardous waste. Numerous nations have ratified this international agreement, which governs the transboundary transportation of hazardous waste, including pharmaceutical waste. If pharmaceutical waste is not managed following international standards, there is a chance that it will be disposed of incorrectly. In certa*in situ*ations, investigating alternative disposal techniques, such as encapsulation or other technologies, may be required [98].

Techniques for Mitigation

Initiatives for Public Education

There are serious concerns for human health and the environment when pharmaceutical waste is improperly disposed of. Initiatives for public education are essential to reducing this problem since they raise awareness and promote safe disposal practices. The following tactics demonstrate successful methods for informing the public on how to properly dispose of pharmaceutical waste:

Campaigns in the Mass Media

When it comes to reaching a large audience with information, the mass media is essential. Public awareness of the environmental risks associated with flushing pharmaceuticals or disposing of them in home trash is increased through campaigns on television, radio, newspapers, and social media.

Campaigns in the Mass Media

When it comes to reaching a large audience with information, the mass media is essential. Public awareness of the environmental risks associated with flushing pharmaceuticals or disposing of them in home trash is increased through campaigns on television, radio, newspapers, and social media [113].

Education Based on Pharmacy

As reputable medical experts, pharmacists are in a unique position to inform the public at the point of dispensing. It is timely and effective to counsel patients on appropriate disposal during medicine distribution.

School Programs and Community Workshops

Raising awareness at the local level is accomplished by involving the community through informational seminars, school visits, and educational workshops. These initiatives promote communication and information exchange between various age groups [113].

Printed Learning Resources

Visual reminders are provided by leaflets, posters, and brochures displayed at pharmacies, clinics, and community centers. These materials ought to be created with culturally relevant messaging and in a variety of languages.

Utilizing Online Resources

Social media, smartphone apps, and websites can be used to find local take-back locations and distribute disposal instructions. Interactive tools, infographics, and brief movies make the information more approachable and interesting [114].

Drug Take-Back Events and Programs

The public is encouraged to safely return unwanted or expired prescriptions by regularly planned take-back days, which are frequently organized in collaboration with local authorities or pharmacists.

Changes to Regulations

There are now serious concerns about the effects of improper pharmaceutical waste disposal on the environment and human health, driven by growing evidence of pharmaceutical residues in drinking water sources, groundwater, and surface waterways [115].

It has been discovered that medications such as hormones, antidepressants, analgesics, and antibiotics can linger in aquatic habitats, harming aquatic life and fostering the emergence of antibiotic resistance. A strong regulatory framework that covers every stage of the pharmaceutical life cycle, from manufacturing and prescription to disposal, is necessary to address this problem. As part of mitigation efforts, several changes to the laws governing the disposal of pharmaceutical waste have been implemented globally throughout the last 20 years. The goal of these reforms is to manage pharmaceutical waste in a way that is consistent, legally binding, and ecologically friendly [115].

Reforms in Law and Institutions

Establishing a Regulatory Category for Pharmaceutical Waste

Pharmaceutical waste has historically been governed by general hazardous or medical waste regulations in many nations. However, particular legal definitions and management procedures are required due to the intricacy and distinct environmental behavior of medications.

- Under the Resource Conservation and Recovery Act (RCRA), the US Environmental Protection Agency (EPA) lists some medications as "listed hazardous wastes." The following are included in the Pharmaceuticals Rule that the EPA issued in 2019: A nationwide prohibition on pharmaceutical hazardous waste going down the sewage. Reverse distributors and healthcare facilities are subject to specific criteria. Nicotine over-the-counter products are not included in the list of hazardous waste [115].
- According to Directive 2008/98/EC (Waste Framework Directive), pharmaceutical waste is classified as potentially hazardous waste by the European Union. Together with Directive 2001/83/EC on medicinal products, the framework requires member states to set up secure disposal methods for pharmaceuticals that are no longer needed or have expired [116].

Comparing Centralized and Decentralized Regulatory Methods

Decentralized models (like the U.S., where states freely adopt and enforce EPA rules) and centralized ones (like France, where the central government manages take-back programs) have different regulatory frameworks.

Centralized systems might provide greater consistency and responsibility, even while decentralized alternatives can provide flexibility.

EXTENDED PRODUCER RESPONSIBILITY (EPR) AND TAKE-BACK PROGRAMS

The Extended Producer Responsibility Principle

Pharmaceutical producers are held responsible for the post-consumer phase of their products under the EPR policy approach. This involves providing funds and overseeing mechanisms for collecting and disposing of leftover medication. The Cyclamed program in France was established in 1993 and is a nationwide system in which pharmacists gather outdated medications, which are subsequently burned at energy recovery facilities. In Canada, province-wide EPR programs are run by the Health Products Stewardship Association (HPSA). In British Columbia, for example, pharmaceutical companies are obligated to finance and oversee take-back initiatives [117].

Permanent Collection Locations and National Drug Take-Back Days

The Drug Enforcement Administration (DEA) in the United States hosts National Prescription Drug Take-Back Days every two years. These gatherings have gathered more than 16.6 million pounds (7,520 tons) of unwanted medications as of 2023. Permanent pharmaceutical collecting systems are incorporated into community pharmacies in nations like Sweden and Germany to guarantee ongoing availability and public convenience [117].

ENVIRONMENTALLY CONSCIOUS INCINERATION AND DISPOSAL GUIDELINES

Incineration at High Temperatures

The most dependable and environmentally friendly way to get rid of pharmaceutical waste, especially dangerous materials, is by incineration. However, total thermal annihilation of APIs can only be guaranteed by specialist high-temperature incinerators (over 1,100°C). According to the Biomedical Waste

Management Rules, 2016 (modified in 2018), nations such as India require that abandoned and expired medications be disposed of at Common Biomedical Waste Treatment Facilities (CBWTFs) [118].

Ban on Flushing and Landfilling

The FDA "Flush List" (updated 2023) limits flushing to specific controlled substances (such as opioids), but only in cases where take-back programs are not available, and prompt disposal is essential to prevent abuse. The U.S. EPA's 2019 Rule forbids healthcare facilities and retail pharmacies from storing hazardous pharmaceuticals [119].

COMBINING PUBLIC HEALTH AND ENVIRONMENTAL POLICIES

Antimicrobial Resistance (AMR) and Pharmaceuticals

When discharged into the environment in sub-therapeutic doses, pharmaceuticals, particularly antibiotics, play a major role in the AMR epidemic. The WHO and UNEP have suggested national strategies that incorporate pharmaceutical waste management into AMR action plans [120, 121].

Assessment of Environmental Risk and Monitoring (ERA)

All new medications must undergo Environmental Risk Assessments (ERA), which are required by the European Medicines Agency (EMA). Older items, however, are still excluded. To evaluate legacy APIs, some nations are shifting to retrospective ERA reviews [122].

INTERNATIONAL COOPERATION AND HARMONIZATION

International Organizations and Multilateral Projects

- UNEP created the Strategic Approach to International Chemicals Management (SAICM), which assists low- and middle-income nations in creating policies for pharmaceutical waste.
- With an emphasis on responsible life-cycle management and pollution reduction, the OECD has created guidelines for standardizing pharmaceutical regulations across nations [123, 124].

Reform Initiatives Support the Following Sustainable Development Goals (SDGs)

- SDG 3: Ensure healthy lifestyles and promote well-being (goal 3.9: minimize illnesses from hazardous substances) [125].
- SDG 6: Make sure everyone has access to sanitary facilities and clean water [125].
- SDG 12: Make sure patterns of production and consumption are sustainable [125].

Disposal Infrastructure Development

One important strategy for reducing the threats to the environment and public health that improper disposal of pharmaceutical products poses is the construction of infrastructure for the disposal of pharmaceutical waste. This infrastructure must facilitate the safe collection, conveyance, processing, and ultimate disposal of pharmaceutical waste while adhering to environmental and legal requirements [126].

Waste Segregation and Classification

Segregation at the source, such as in manufacturing facilities, pharmacies, and hospitals, is the first step toward proper infrastructure. Pharmaceutical waste is divided into two categories: non-hazardous (*e.g.*, expired over-the-counter medications) and hazardous (*e.g.*, cytotoxic pharmaceuticals, antibiotics, and opioids). To guarantee appropriate separation and reduce the possibility of chemical reactions or environmental contamination, the World Health Organization (WHO, 2017) advises the use of color-coded waste containers, such as blue for non-hazardous pharmaceutical waste and yellow for cytotoxic waste. Fig. (**1**) describes the Segregation of Hospital biomedical waste through the Biomedical waste management system [126].

Transportation and Collection

After being separated, pharmaceutical waste needs to be gathered and transported in vehicles and approved containers that adhere to hazardous material laws.

Unauthorized entry, spills, and leaks must be avoided by these vehicles. Licensed waste handlers must ensure compliance with the Resource Conservation and Recovery Act (RCRA) and maintain paperwork for the chain of custody, according to the US Environmental Protection Agency (EPA, 2019) [127].

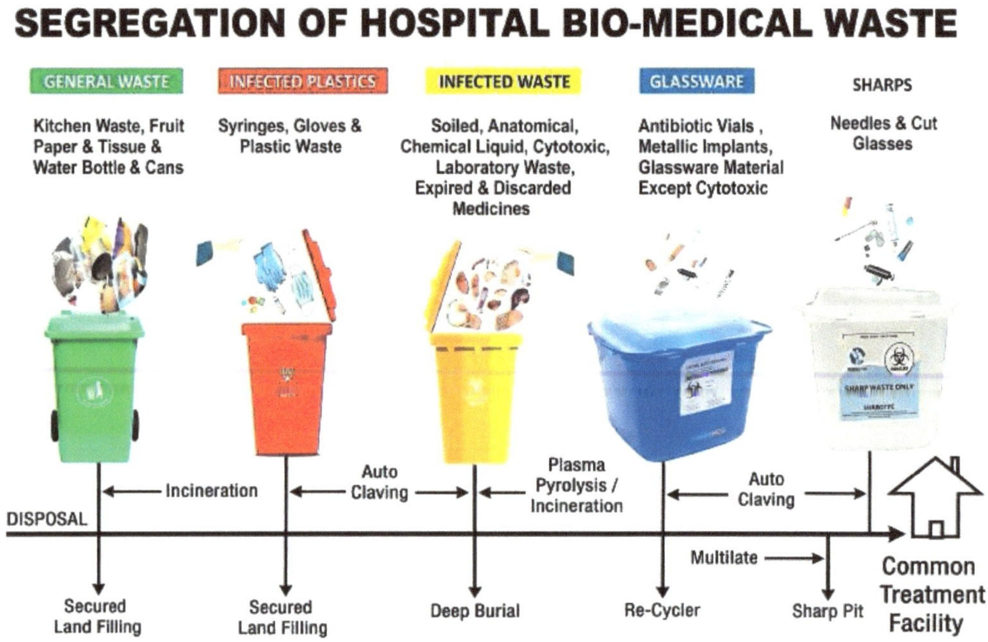

Fig. (1). Segregation of hospital bio-medical waste.

Programs for Drug Returns and Reverse Logistics

To prevent stockpiling and the flushing or discarding of medications into household waste streams, drug take-back programs (DTBPs) are crucial parts of pharmaceutical waste infrastructure. They give the public and healthcare institutions a way to return unused or expired medications to authorized collection points, such as France's Cyclamed system, which allows consumers to return unused medications to pharmacies where they are collected and sent to incineration facilities.

Technologies of Treatment

A safe and efficient treatment system is the foundation of the disposal infrastructure. High-temperature incineration (HTI), typically above 1100°C is the most widely used technique because it ensures the complete destruction of active pharmaceutical ingredients (APIs), particularly cytotoxic and hormonally active substances. In Sweden, for example, pharmaceutical waste is neutralized, and energy is recovered through the use of centralized high-efficiency incineration units. Encapsulation, in which medications are embedded in cement or inert materials, is utilized in low-resource environments to keep waste contained and stop environmental leaching. For facilities without access to advanced incineration, the WHO recommends this as a temporary solution [128, 129].

Safe Landfilling

After treatment, any remaining pharmaceutical waste needs to be dumped in sanitary landfills that have been constructed to contain groundwater monitoring systems, leachate collection systems, and impermeable liners. Antimicrobial resistance and endocrine disruption are caused by the improper disposal of unprocessed pharmaceutical waste, which contaminates the soil and water [130].

Utilizing Digital Infrastructure

Pharmaceutical waste management is made more transparent and efficient by digital infrastructure. Traceability is improved by systems like barcode tracking, inventory alerts for expired medications, and electronic waste movement documentation. To maintain real-time monitoring and regulatory compliance, the Central Pollution Control Board (CPCB) in India uses a digital tracking system for pharmaceutical and biomedical waste [131].

Facilities in Low- and Middle-Income Nations (LMICs)

Regional treatment centers, solar-powered autoclaves, and mobile incinerators are being encouraged in LMICs where permanent facilities can be scarce. With backing from the UN and WHO, these technologies provide rural and underserved areas with scalable and affordable solutions [132].

Options for Mitigating the Environmental Impact of Pharmaceutical Waste

There are a few studies examining the negative environmental consequences of medications. 88% of human medications lack environmental toxicity data, and pharmaceutical corporations prioritize patient health, dose, and efficacy during clinical trials. A strategy to address pharmaceutical waste in the environment has been created by nations such as Sweden, Germany, France, and the Netherlands. To obtain long-term advantages and cost-effectiveness in the subsequent steps, mitigation methods should be tailored particularly to a pharmaceutical's lifetime [133].

Cross-cutting: In collaboration with pharmaceutical and research institutions, the government should prioritize high-risk APIs and create monitoring programs for water quality, risk assessment, and modeling. Standards for pharmaceuticals' water and environmental quality should be defined by guidelines [134].

Design: Pharmaceutical businesses should provide effective or tailored medications and biological therapies in addition to creating a green pharmacy. Authorization: The government should monitor rules and assess environmental risks before authorizing a prescription medication. Strict requirements should be met before medications with a high ecological risk are introduced to the market. The sector ought to provide choices for mitigation, post-approval monitoring, eco-labeling, and risk intervention.

Production: The Government and the pharmaceutical sector should develop an environmental criterion describing effluent discharge limits, disclosure of wastewater discharge, and ethical production practices [134].

Consumption: To reduce unnecessary prescribing, the health sector could recommend customized medications, environmentally friendly drugs, and targeted delivery systems. The health and business sectors should raise consumer awareness and choice through the use of eco-labeling for personal consumption. The use of hormones to promote cattle growth and antibiotics for prophylactic purposes are examples of high-risk activities that the government ought to outlaw. To prevent emissions, healthcare facilities must have safe management procedures, acceptable livestock handling techniques, and enhanced hygiene and diagnosis [134].

Collection and disposal: Solid waste utilities are interested in using anaerobic biogas fermentation and passive manure storage to improve manure management. Plans should be put in place by the industry for dealing with expired or no longer-needed drugs. People must be cautioned not to use sinks and toilets to dispose of unneeded or expired drugs.

Wastewater treatment: To improve the detection of pharmaceutical substances, WWTPs should modernize their wastewater utilities. Chlorhexidine digluconate and methylene blue have been destroyed by more than 40% and 30%, respectively, when photocatalytic-ultrafiltration membranes immobilized by sol-gel are used in wastewater treatment facilities. 90% of the pantoprazole in wastewater was effectively eliminated by a combination of biochemical, Fenton's, and ozone treatment, according to a toxicological investigation. The integrated process uses less energy, is safe, and is inexpensive [135]. Pharmaceutical compounds in wastewater can be reduced by using the laccase enzyme that is isolated from the Trametes fungus. Through a hydroxylation process, the enzyme breaks down medications like ibuprofen and diclofenac in wastewater [136].

Due to their cheap operating costs, high organic loading, and reduced sludge production, modern anaerobic technologies, such as hybrid anaerobic-chemical and anaerobic-aerobic systems, help treat wastewater. Amoxicillin and sulfamerazine have been removed by the designs with >90% and 97% success, respectively [137]. Under ideal circumstances, the content of ibuprofen in wastewater was reduced from 400 parts per million to 6.8 parts per million by modern wastewater technology, such as the electron-Fenton process [138].

RECOMMENDATIONS

Collaborative Methods

Effective drug waste management calls for a collaborative, multi-stakeholder approach involving government agencies, health facilities, drug producers, regulatory agencies, environmental groups, universities, and the public. A multi-stakeholder task force is critical to creating standard policies and structures that allow environmentally sustainable waste management practices. Governments, in association with pharmaceutical companies, can institute product stewardship schemes that encourage take-back programs, reverse logistics, and sustainable packaging. Enhanced coordination between healthcare institutions and waste management agencies is crucial for effective collection and treatment. Incorporating pharmaceutical waste management training into healthcare and environmental science curricula will help improve long-term awareness and compliance. Public-private partnerships will also help develop necessary infrastructure, such as centralized disposal facilities and advanced treatment facilities. Society-level operations through campaigns for raising awareness, training courses, and workshops will also help cultivate better waste disposal practices [139].

Sustainable Methods

On the sustainability side, efforts must be made for environmentally friendly methodologies such as green pharmacy, which encourages the formulation of drugs that are more biodegradable and less harmful. Electronic stock systems can be accessed by hospitals and pharmacies to reduce wastage of stock, and customers can be encouraged to return drugs to special points instead of dumping them in household trash or sewage. Plasma pyrolysis and advanced oxidation processes are environmentally friendly disposal technologies with substitute options that substitute the conventional alternatives of landfilling and burning, though they might have huge capital investment needs [139].

Ecological Health Priorities

Ecological health should be a long-term focus. Drug residue, as trace as it is, has the potential to disrupt non-target organisms' biological functions. Conservation of aquatic systems through the enforcement of more stringent effluent treatment practices and expanding wastewater facilities is critical. Implementing routine environmental monitoring regimes will allow for the quantification of pollution levels and guide enlightened policymaking. Minimization of AMR environmental dissemination is also imperative, such as safe disposal of antibiotics and mass education. Promoting research toward the creation of eco-friendly drug compounds will also align drug innovation with ecological soundness, ensuring an ecologically sustainable and healthier future [140].

CONCLUSION

Pharmaceutical waste is a major and increasing hazard to environmental sustainability and public health. As elaborated in this chapter, pharmaceuticals can be present in ecosystems for extended periods through soil, water, and air dispersion, causing extensive contamination. These pollutants adversely affect aquatic and terrestrial flora and fauna, change reproduction and behavioral patterns in animals, and are also behind general issues like antibiotic resistance and hormonal interference in living things. Environmentally Persistent Pharmaceutical Pollutants (EPPPs) in particular are ecologically long-term issues due to their chemical stability and non-biodegradability. The lack of standardized disposal habits, unfavourable regulatory regimes, inadequate public awareness, and limited infrastructure, most particularly in developing nations, have heightened the environmental burden. Unfavorable practices such as open incineration, dumping of sewage, and unregulated landfills continue to be used extensively. Furthermore, poor health workers' knowledge and inadequate public education continue to undermine safe disposal operations. To counter these effects, an integrated strategy is necessary. This encompasses more efficient legal regulations, more pharmaceutical take-back initiatives, high-efficiency treatment technologies, and large-scale training of medical professionals. Public education campaigns and organizational restructuring must be accorded top priority to facilitate responsible waste-handling practices. Furthermore, the application of green pharmacy principles, investment in next-generation wastewater treatments, and the use of eco-friendly drug designs are essential to reduce the environmental footprint of pharmaceuticals. Policy coordination involving policymakers, healthcare professionals, the pharmaceutical industry, and the general public is needed. Pharmaceutical waste reduction is not merely an environmental imperative but also a public health requirement for future and current generations.

REFERENCES

[1] Eniola JO, Kumar R, Barakat MA, Rashid J. A review on conventional and advanced hybrid technologies for pharmaceutical wastewater treatment. J Clean Prod 2022; 356: 131826. [http://dx.doi.org/10.1016/j.jclepro.2022.131826]

[2] Kaimuri M, Mwangi E, Karani C. Methods of pharmaceutical waste management disposal practiced in sanitation value chain by community pharmacies and households in Nkubu town: Health interventions for sustainable development amidst global crises. African Journal of Science. Technology and Social Sciences 2022; 1(2): 46-51.

[3] Ingale MH, Tayade MC, Patil YP, Salunkhe RH. Pharmaceutical waste disposal current practices and regulations: rewiev. Int J Pharm Qual Assur 2023; 14(3): 821-4. [http://dx.doi.org/10.25258/ijpqa.14.3.59]

[4] aus der Beek T, Weber FA, Bergmann A, *et al.* Pharmaceuticals in the environment—Global occurrences and perspectives. Environ Toxicol Chem 2015; 35(4): 823-35. [http://dx.doi.org/10.1002/*etc.*3339] [PMID: 26666847]

[5] Chander V, Sharma B, Negi V, *et al.* Pharmaceutical compounds in drinking water. J Xenobiot 2016; 6(1): 5774. [http://dx.doi.org/10.4081/xeno.2016.5774] [PMID: 30701048]

[6] Kanama KM, Daso AP, Mpenyana-Monyatsi L, Coetzee MAA. Assessment of pharmaceuticals, personal care products, and hormones in wastewater treatment plants receiving inflows from health facilities in North West Province, South Africa. J Toxicol 2018; 2018(1): 1-15. [http://dx.doi.org/10.1155/2018/3751930] [PMID: 30510574]

[7] Adewuyi A, Ogunkunle OA, Oderinde RA. Zirconium ferrite incorporated zeolitic imidazolate framework-8: a suitable photocatalyst for degradation of dopamine and sulfamethoxazole in aqueous solution. RSC Advances 2023; 13(14): 9563-75. [http://dx.doi.org/10.1039/D3RA01055D] [PMID: 36968036]

[8] Akash MSH, Rehman K, Sabir S, Gul J, Hussain I. Review potential risk assessment of pharmaceutical waste: Critical review and analysis. Pak J Sci Ind Res Ser A Phys Sci 2020; 63(3): 209-19. [http://dx.doi.org/10.52763/PJSIR.PHYS.SCI.63.3.2020.209.219]

[9] Gupta A, Kumar S, Bajpai Y, *et al.* Pharmaceutically active micropollutants: origin, hazards and removal. Front Microbiol 2024; 15: 1339469. [http://dx.doi.org/10.3389/fmicb.2024.1339469] [PMID: 38419628]

[10] Adesina A, Sanni F. Pharmaceutical wastes management and the presence of pharmaceuticals in the environment of health facilities in Lagos state, Nigeria. Texila International Journal of Public Health 2018; 6(3): 104-18. [http://dx.doi.org/10.21522/TIJPH.2013.06.03.Art011]

[11] Richmond EK, Rosi EJ, Walters DM, *et al.* A diverse suite of pharmaceuticals contaminates stream and riparian food webs. Nat Commun 2018; 9(1): 4491. [http://dx.doi.org/10.1038/s41467-018-06822-w] [PMID: 30401828]

[12] Desai M, Njoku A, Nimo-Sefah L. Comparing environmental policies to reduce pharmaceutical pollution and address disparities. Int J Environ Res Public Health 2022; 19(14): 8292. [http://dx.doi.org/10.3390/ijerph19148292] [PMID: 35886145]

[13] Nastiti A, *et al.* Self-Reported Pharmaceutical Storage, Use, and Improper Disposal to The Environment Among Urban Parents in Indonesia. 2022. [http://dx.doi.org/10.1088/1755-1315/1111/1/012045]

[14] Esseku YY, Mante PK, Dodoo ANO, Woode E. Drug disposal and ecopharmacovigilance practices in the Krowor Municipality, Ghana. J Toxicol 2022; 2022(1): 1-12. [http://dx.doi.org/10.1155/2022/7674701] [PMID: 36619292]

[15] Alshemari A, Breen L, Quinn G, Sivarajah U. Can we create a circular pharmaceutical supply chain (CPSC) to reduce medicines waste? Pharmacy (Basel) 2020; 8(4): 221. [http://dx.doi.org/10.3390/pharmacy8040221] [PMID: 33218038]

[16] Gupta S, Sesai S. Environmental impact and regulatory compliance: a comprehensive approach in managing institutional pharmaceutical waste. 2024.

[17] Alnahas F, Yeboah P, Fliedel L, Abdin AY, Alhareth K. Expired medication: Societal, regulatory and ethical aspects of a wasted opportunity. Int J Environ Res Public Health 2020; 17(3): 787. [http://dx.doi.org/10.3390/ijerph17030787] [PMID: 32012703]

[18] Freitas LAA, Radis-Baptista G. Pharmaceutical pollution and disposal of expired, unused, and unwanted medicines in the Brazilian context. J Xenobiot 2021; 11(2): 61-76. [http://dx.doi.org/10.3390/jox11020005] [PMID: 34069823]

[19] Seehusen DA, Edwards J. Patient practices and beliefs concerning disposal of medications. J Am Board Fam Med 2006; 19(6): 542-7. [http://dx.doi.org/10.3122/jabfm.19.6.542] [PMID: 17090787]

[20] Su Q, Zhang X, Zhang Y, *et al.* Risk assessment of heavy metal pollution in agricultural soil surrounding a typical pharmaceutical manufacturing complex. Front Environ Sci 2023; 10: 1105910. [http://dx.doi.org/10.3389/fenvs.2022.1105910]

[21] Selwe KP, Thorn JPR, Desrousseaux AOS, Dessent CEH, Sallach JB. Emerging contaminant exposure to aquatic systems in the Southern African Development Community. Environ Toxicol Chem 2022; 41(2): 382-95. [http://dx.doi.org/10.1002/*etc.*5284] [PMID: 35020964]

[22] Khan AHA, Barros R. Pharmaceuticals in water: risks to aquatic life and remediation strategies. Hydrobiology 2023; 2(2): 395-409. [http://dx.doi.org/10.3390/hydrobiology2020026]

[23] Garazade N, Nightingale J, Kay P, Varank G, Carter J L. Pharmaceuticals and their transformation products in agroecosystems: Threats to plant–soil sustainability. Crit Rev Environ Sci Technol 2026; 56(6): 269-99. [http://dx.doi.org/10.1080/10643389.2025.2585891]

[24] Fernandes JP, Almeida CMR, Salgado MA, Carvalho MF, Mucha AP. Pharmaceutical compounds in aquatic environments—occurrence, fate and bioremediation prospective. Toxics 2021; 9(10): 257. [http://dx.doi.org/10.3390/toxics9100257] [PMID: 34678953]

[25] Ternes TA, Meisenheimer M, McDowell D, *et al.* Removal of pharmaceuticals during drinking water treatment. Environ Sci Technol 2002; 36(17): 3855-63. [http://dx.doi.org/10.1021/es015757k] [PMID: 12322761]

[26] Beaumelle L, Thouvenot L, Hines J, Jochum M, Eisenhauer N, Phillips HRP. Soil fauna diversity and chemical stressors: a review of knowledge gaps and roadmap for future research. Ecography 2021; 44(6): 845-59. [http://dx.doi.org/10.1111/ecog.05627]

[27] Efremenko E, Stepanov N, Senko O, Maslova O, Lyagin I, Aslanli A. Progressive biocatalysts for the treatment of aqueous systems containing pharmaceutical pollutants. Life (Basel) 2023; 13(3): 841. [http://dx.doi.org/10.3390/life13030841] [PMID: 36983996]

[28] Eapen JV, Thomas S, Antony S, George P, Antony J. A review of the effects of pharmaceutical pollutants on humans and aquatic ecosystem. Exploration of Drug Science 2024; 2(5): 484-507. [http://dx.doi.org/10.37349/eds.2024.00058]

[29] Candello FP, Guimarães JR, Nour EAA. Earthworm avoidance behavior to antimicrobial sulfadiazine on tropical artificial soil. Ecotoxicol Environ Contam 2018; 13(2): 69-75. [http://dx.doi.org/10.5132/eec.2018.02.09]

[30] Pollyana DC, Lúcia MM. Evaluation of pharmaceuticals in household waste in Senador Canedo, State of Gois, Brazil. Afr J Pharm Pharmacol 2020; 14(1): 20-8. [http://dx.doi.org/10.5897/AJPP2019.5108]

[31] Arnold K E, Boxall A B A, Brown A R, *et al.* Assessing the exposure risk and impacts of pharmaceuticals in the environment on individuals and ecosystems. Biology Letters. 2013; 9: p. (4)20130492. [http://dx.doi.org/10.1098/rsbl.2013.0492]

[32] Joyosemito I S, Meilani S S, Azmi . Clearing the air: assessing air quality impact from a proposed medical waste incinerator using Gaussian dispersion modeling. Research Square [Preprint] 2023; 21. [http://dx.doi.org/10.21203/rs.3.rs-3392460/v1]

[33] Jahan E, Nessa A, Hossain MF, Parveen Z. Characteristics of municipal landfill leachate and its impact on surrounding agricultural land. Bangladesh J Sci Res 2016; 29(1): 31-9.

[http://dx.doi.org/10.3329/bjsr.v29i1.29755]

[34] Smith M. Reusing medicines to mitigate their environmental impact. Prescriber 2024; 35(3): 5-8. [http://dx.doi.org/10.1002/psb.2124]

[35] Bain K T. Public Health Implications of Household Pharmaceutical Waste in the United States. Health Services Insights 2010; 3: 9-15. [http://dx.doi.org/10.4137/HSI.S4673]

[36] Yuan X, Qiang Z, Ben W, Zhu B, Qu J. Distribution, mass load and environmental impact of multiple-class pharmaceuticals in conventional and upgraded municipal wastewater treatment plants in East China. Environ Sci Process Impacts 2015; 17(3): 596-605. [http://dx.doi.org/10.1039/C4EM00596A] [PMID: 25614232]

[37] Karimi KJ, Ahmad A, Duse A, Mwanthi M, Ayah R. Prevalence of antibiotic use and disposal at household level in informal settlements of Kisumu, Kenya. Int J Environ Res Public Health 2022; 20(1): 287. [http://dx.doi.org/10.3390/ijerph20010287] [PMID: 36612608]

[38] Renata V, Parker J, Loganathar S, *et al.* Tossing your Tylenol: supporting sustainable behavior in medication disposal through label design. In: Proceedings of the Human Factors and Ergonomics Society Annual Meeting; 2023; pp. 67(1): 2466-71. [http://dx.doi.org/10.1177/21695067231192218]

[39] Vijayalakshmi M K, Priyan S. Endangerment of Pharmaceutical Waste Disposal in the Environment. Medico-Legal Update 2020; 20(4): 420-4.

[40] Dias-Ferreira C, Valente S, Vaz J. Practices of pharmaceutical waste generation and discarding in households across Portugal. Waste Manag Res 2016; 34(10): 1006-13. [http://dx.doi.org/10.1177/0734242X16639388] [PMID: 27026517]

[41] Paut Kusturica M, Jevtic M, Ristovski JT. Minimizing the environmental impact of unused pharmaceuticals: Review focused on prevention. Front Environ Sci 2022; 10: 1077974. [http://dx.doi.org/10.3389/fenvs.2022.1077974]

[42] Ugoeze K, Alalor C, Ibezim C, *et al.* Environmental and human health impact of antibiotics waste mismanagement: a review. Advances in Environmental and Engineering Research 2024; 5(1): 1-21. [http://dx.doi.org/10.21926/aeer.2401005]

[43] Abubakar AM, *et al.* Unlocking biogas production potential: Evaluating the environmental impact and biodegradability of pharmaceutical and medical wastes. Sigma Journal of Engineering and Natural Sciences – Sigma Mühendislik ve Fen Bilimleri Dergisi 2024; 42(4): 1194-224. [http://dx.doi.org/10.14744/sigma.2024.00096]

[44] Löffler D, Römbke J, Meller M, Ternes TA. Environmental fate of pharmaceuticals in water/sediment systems. Environ Sci Technol 2005; 39(14): 5209-18. [http://dx.doi.org/10.1021/es0484146] [PMID: 16082949]

[45] Gros M, Petrović M, Barceló D. Wastewater treatment plants as a pathway for aquatic contamination by pharmaceuticals in the Ebro river basin (Northeast Spain). Environ Toxicol Chem 2007; 26(8): 1553-62. [http://dx.doi.org/10.1897/06-495R.1] [PMID: 17702326]

[46] Kairigo P, Ngumba E, Sundberg L-R, Gachanja A, Tuhkanen T. Contamination of surface water and river sediments by antibiotic and antiretroviral drug cocktails in low and middle-income countries: occurrence, risk and mitigation strategies. Water 2020; 12(5): 1376. [http://dx.doi.org/10.3390/w12051376]

[47] Luís S, Moura R, Lima ML, Poggio L, Aragonés JI, Camilo C. Judging pharmaceutical environmental risk by its cover? The effects of prescription medication and disease severity on environmental risk perception. Risk Anal 2022; 42(10): 2231-42. [http://dx.doi.org/10.1111/risa.13856] [PMID: 34791702]

[48] Kar S, Roy K, Leszczynski J. Impact of Pharmaceuticals on the Environment: Risk Assessment Using QSAR Modeling Approach. In: Nicolotti O, Ed. Computational Toxicology. New York, NY: Humana Press 2018; pp. 439-67.
[http://dx.doi.org/10.1007/978-1-4939-7899-1_19]

[49] Bagnis S, Fitzsimons MF, Snape J, Tappin A, Comber S. Processes of distribution of pharmaceuticals in surface freshwaters: implications for risk assessment. Environ Chem Lett 2018; 16(4): 1193-216.
[http://dx.doi.org/10.1007/s10311-018-0742-7]

[50] Fick J, Söderström H, Lindberg RH, Phan C, Tysklind M, Larsson DGJ. Contamination of surface, ground, and drinking water from pharmaceutical production. Environ Toxicol Chem 2009; 28(12): 2522-7.
[http://dx.doi.org/10.1897/09-073.1] [PMID: 19449981]

[51] Neibergs M, Strade E, Nikolajeva V, Susinskis I, Rozitis D, Kalnina D. Application of bioaugmentation to improve pharmaceutical wastewater treatment efficiency. Key Eng Mater 2019; 800: 122-31.
[http://dx.doi.org/10.4028/www.scientific.net/KEM.800.122]

[52] Deshmukh G, Umap S, Bhapkar T, *et al.* Pharmaceutical waste a global challenge to ecosystem. Chron Aquat Sci 2024; 1(10): 53-64.

[53] Ripanda AS, Rwiza MJ, Nyanza EC, Machunda RL, Vuai SH. Contribution of Illicit Drug Use to Pharmaceutical Load in the Environment: A Focus on Sub-Saharan Africa. J Environ Public Health 2022; 2022(1): 9056476.
[http://dx.doi.org/10.1155/2022/9056476] [PMID: 35719855]

[54] Bustos Bustos E, Sandoval-González A, Martínez-Sánchez C. Detection and treatment of persistent pollutants in water: general review of pharmaceutical products. ChemElectroChem 2022; 9(12): e202200188.
[http://dx.doi.org/10.1002/celc.202200188]

[55] Fabbri E. Pharmaceuticals in the environment: expected and unexpected effects on aquatic fauna. Ann N Y Acad Sci 2015; 1340(1): 20-8.
[http://dx.doi.org/10.1111/nyas.12605] [PMID: 25557669]

[56] Welch SA, Moe SJ, Sharikabad MN, Tollefsen KE, Olsen K, Grung M. Predicting environmental risks of pharmaceuticals from wholesale data: An example from Norway. Environ Toxicol Chem 2023; 42(10): 2253-70.
[http://dx.doi.org/10.1002/*etc.*5702] [PMID: 37341554]

[57] Domínguez-García P, Fernández-Ruano L, Báguena J, Cuadros J, Gómez-Canela C. Assessing the pharmaceutical residues as hotspots of the main rivers of Catalonia, Spain. Environ Sci Pollut Res Int 2024; 31(31): 44080-95.
[http://dx.doi.org/10.1007/s11356-024-33967-7] [PMID: 38926308]

[58] Polverino G, Aich U, Brand JA, *et al.* Sex-specific effects of psychoactive pollution on behavioral individuality and plasticity in fish. Behav Ecol 2023; 34(6): 969-78.
[http://dx.doi.org/10.1093/beheco/arad065] [PMID: 37969553]

[59] Brodin T, Fick J, Jonsson M, Klaminder J. Dilute concentrations of a psychiatric drug alter behavior of fish from natural populations. Science 2013; 339(6121): 814-5.
[http://dx.doi.org/10.1126/science.1226850] [PMID: 23413353]

[60] Martin JM, Bertram MG, Saaristo M, *et al.* Antidepressants in surface waters: fluoxetine influences mosquitofish anxiety-related behavior at environmentally relevant levels. Environ Sci Technol 2019; 53(10): 6035-43.
[http://dx.doi.org/10.1021/acs.est.9b00944] [PMID: 31034220]

[61] Punginelli D, Maccotta A, Savoca D. Biological and Environmental Impact of Pharmaceuticals on Marine Fishes: A Review. J Mar Sci Eng 2024; 12(7): 1133.

[http://dx.doi.org/10.3390/jmse12071133]

[62] Saaristo M, Brodin T, Balshine S, *et al.* Direct and indirect effects of chemical contaminants on the behaviour, ecology and evolution of wildlife. Proc Biol Sci 2018; 285(1885): 20181297.
[http://dx.doi.org/10.1098/rspb.2018.1297] [PMID: 30135169]

[63] Gurgenidze D, Romanovski V. The pharmaceutical pollution of water resources using the example of the Kura River (Tbilisi, Georgia). Water 2023; 15(14): 2574.
[http://dx.doi.org/10.3390/w15142574]

[64] Burns EE, Carter LJ, Snape J, Thomas-Oates J, Boxall ABA. Application of prioritization approaches to optimize environmental monitoring and testing of pharmaceuticals. J Toxicol Environ Health B Crit Rev 2018; 21(3): 115-41.
[http://dx.doi.org/10.1080/10937404.2018.1465873] [PMID: 29714645]

[65] Wang J, Hu X. Ecopharmacovigilance: Current state, challenges, and opportunities in China. Indian J Pharmacol 2014; 46(1): 13-7.
[http://dx.doi.org/10.4103/0253-7613.125158] [PMID: 24550578]

[66] Cabrera-Campos I, Ávila-Flores R, Rivera-Ruiz DA, Herrera M LG. Pernicious liaisons: antibiotic-depressed immune response of a livestock micropredator, the common vampire bat (Desmodus rotundus). Mamm Biol 2025; 105(3): 283-90.
[http://dx.doi.org/10.1007/s42991-025-00476-0]

[67] Nash JP, Kime DE, Van der Ven LTM, *et al.* Long-term exposure to environmental concentrations of the pharmaceutical ethynylestradiol causes reproductive failure in fish. Environ Health Perspect 2004; 112(17): 1725-33.
[http://dx.doi.org/10.1289/ehp.7209] [PMID: 15579420]

[68] Brown AR, Hosken DJ, Balloux F, *et al.* Genetic variation, inbreeding and chemical exposure—combined effects in wildlife and critical considerations for ecotoxicology. Philos Trans R Soc Lond B Biol Sci 2009; 364(1534): 3377-90.
[http://dx.doi.org/10.1098/rstb.2009.0126] [PMID: 19833649]

[69] Aulsebrook LC, Bertram MG, Martin JM, *et al.* Reproduction in a polluted world: implications for wildlife. Reproduction 2020; 160(2): R13-23.
[http://dx.doi.org/10.1530/REP-20-0154] [PMID: 32442963]

[70] Hamlin HJ, Guillette LJ Jr. Embryos as targets of endocrine disrupting contaminants in wildlife. Birth Defects Res C Embryo Today 2011; 93(1): 19-33.
[http://dx.doi.org/10.1002/bdrc.20202] [PMID: 21425439]

[71] Jobling S, Nolan M, Tyler CR, Brighty G, Sumpter JP. Widespread sexual disruption in wild fish. Environ Sci Technol 1998; 32(17): 2498-506.
[http://dx.doi.org/10.1021/es9710870]

[72] Orton F, Tyler CR. Do hormone-modulating chemicals impact on reproduction and development of wild amphibians? Biol Rev Camb Philos Soc 2015; 90(4): 1100-17.
[http://dx.doi.org/10.1111/brv.12147] [PMID: 25335651]

[73] Fort DJ, Stover EL, Bantle JA, Dumont JN, Finch RA. Evaluation of a reproductive toxicity assay using *Xenopus laevis:* boric acid, cadmium and ethylene glycol monomethyl ether. J Appl Toxicol 2001; 21(1): 41-52.
[http://dx.doi.org/10.1002/jat.731] [PMID: 11180279]

[74] Huang Y, Twidwell DL, Elrod JC. Occurrence and effects of endocrine disrupting chemicals in the environment. Pract Period Hazard Toxic Radioact Waste Manage 2003; 7(4): 241-52.
[http://dx.doi.org/10.1061/(ASCE)1090-025X(2003)7:4(241)]

[75] Bustnes JO, Bourgeon S, Leat EHK, *et al.* Multiple stressors in a top predator seabird: potential ecological consequences of environmental contaminants, population health and breeding conditions. PLoS One 2015; 10(7): e0131769.

[http://dx.doi.org/10.1371/journal.pone.0131769] [PMID: 26172383]

[76] Rhind SM. Anthropogenic pollutants: a threat to ecosystem sustainability? Philos Trans R Soc Lond B Biol Sci 2009; 364(1534): 3391-401.
[http://dx.doi.org/10.1098/rstb.2009.0122] [PMID: 19833650]

[77] Milligan SR, Holt WV, Lloyd R. Impacts of climate change and environmental factors on reproduction and development in wildlife. The Royal Society 2009; pp. 3313-9.

[78] Khan A, Jaffar N, Razzak S, Zeesahn F, Shabbir A, Ishaque SM. Knowledge, attitude and practices of pharmaceutical waste disposal in community pharmacies of Karachi. Annals of Jinnah Sindh Medical University 2020; 6(2): 54-9.
[http://dx.doi.org/10.46663/ajsmu.v6i2.54-59]

[79] Jarvis CI, Seed SM, Silva M, Sullivan KM. Educational campaign for proper medication disposal. J Am Pharm Assoc (Wash DC) 2009; 49(1): 65-8.
[http://dx.doi.org/10.1331/JAPhA.2009.08032] [PMID: 19196599]

[80] Hagawane D B, Parihar N B, Parihar S N. Assessment of methods used by registered pharmacists for disposing of the pharmaceutical waste and expired medicines at community pharmacies in urban area. Int J Res Pharm Pharm Sci 2022; 7(2): 16-20.

[81] Jankie S, Stuart A V, Barsatee N, *et al.* Pharmacists knowledge, perception and practice regarding medication disposal. Exploratory Research in Clinical and Social Pharmacy 2022; 8: 100202.
[http://dx.doi.org/10.1016/j.rcsop.2022.100202]

[82] Low BY, Ting KN, Lee MK. Knowledge, attitude and practice of community pharmacists towards household pharmaceutical waste disposal. Int J Pharm Pract 2023; 31(2): 261-5.
[http://dx.doi.org/10.1093/ijpp/riac101] [PMID: 36534990]

[83] Abahussain E, Waheedi M, Koshy S. Practice, awareness and opinion of pharmacists toward disposal of unwanted medications in Kuwait. Saudi Pharm J 2012; 20(3): 195-201.
[http://dx.doi.org/10.1016/j.jsps.2012.04.001] [PMID: 23960793]

[84] Hiew S Y, Low B Y. A systematic review of the knowledge, attitude and practice of healthcare professionals and healthcare professional students towards household pharmaceutical waste disposal. Exploratory Research in Clinical and Social Pharmacy 2025; 17: 100556.

[85] Sapkota B, Pariatamby A. Pharmaceutical waste management system – Are the current techniques sustainable, eco-friendly and circular? A review. Waste Manag 2023; 168: 83-97.
[http://dx.doi.org/10.1016/j.wasman.2023.05.052] [PMID: 37285639]

[86] Nyagah D M, Njagi A, Nyaga M N. Pharmaceutical waste: overview, management and impact of improper disposal. Journal of PeerSci 2020; 3(2): e1000028.

[87] Rajbongshi S, Shah YD, Sajib AU. Pharmaceutical waste management: a review. European Journal of Biomedical and Pharmaceutical Sciences 2016; 3(12): 192-206.

[88] Kadam A, Patil S, Patil S, Tumkur A. Pharmaceutical waste management an overview. Indian Journal of Pharmacy Practice 2016; 9(1): 2-8.
[http://dx.doi.org/10.5530/ijopp.9.1.2]

[89] Nipa N Y, Ahmed S, Shahariar M D, *et al.* Improper Management of Pharmaceutical Waste in South and South-East Asian Regions. J Environ Stud 2017; 3(1): 7.

[90] Di Russo M, Heidar Alizadeh A, Nurchis M C, *et al.* Hospital waste management before and during COVID-19 pandemic: an analysis of the environmental impact of CO emissions in four Italian facilities. Int J Healthc Manag 2025; 18(4): 663-73.

[91] Coskun M, Coskun M, Cayir A, Ozdemir O. Frequencies of micronuclei (MNi), nucleoplasmic bridges (NPBs), and nuclear buds (NBUDs) in farmers exposed to pesticides in Çanakkale, Turkey. Environ Int 2011; 37(1): 93-6.
[http://dx.doi.org/10.1016/j.envint.2010.08.002] [PMID: 20739066]

[92] Kümmerer K. The presence of pharmaceuticals in the environment due to human use – present knowledge and future challenges. J Environ Manage 2009; 90(8): 2354-66.
[http://dx.doi.org/10.1016/j.jenvman.2009.01.023] [PMID: 19261375]

[93] Eckstein M, Eleazer R, Rea M, Fondufe-Mittendorf Y. Epigenomic reprogramming in inorganic arsenic-mediated gene expression patterns during carcinogenesis. Rev Environ Health 2017; 32(1-2): 93-103.
[http://dx.doi.org/10.1515/reveh-2016-0025] [PMID: 27701139]

[94] Christensen KY, Maisonet M, Rubin C, *et al.* Exposure to polyfluoroalkyl chemicals during pregnancy is not associated with offspring age at menarche in a contemporary British cohort. Environ Int 2011; 37(1): 129-35.
[http://dx.doi.org/10.1016/j.envint.2010.08.007] [PMID: 20843552]

[95] Ionescu A M, Cazan C. Pharmaceutical Waste Management: A Comprehensive Analysis of Romanian Practices and Perspectives. Sustainability 2024; 16(15): 6571.
[http://dx.doi.org/10.3390/su16156571]

[96] Karungamye P, Rugaika A, Mtei K, Machunda R. The pharmaceutical disposal practices and environmental contamination: A review in East African countries. HydroResearch 2022; 5: 99-107.
[http://dx.doi.org/10.1016/j.hydres.2022.11.001]

[97] Rogowska J, Zimmermann A. Household pharmaceutical waste disposal as a global problem—a review. Int J Environ Res Public Health 2022; 19(23): 15798.
[http://dx.doi.org/10.3390/ijerph192315798] [PMID: 36497873]

[98] Abbott FM, Reichman JH. Facilitating access to Cross-border supplies of patented pharmaceuticals: the case of the COVID-19 pandemic. J Int Econ Law 2020; 23(3): 535-61.
[http://dx.doi.org/10.1093/jiel/jgaa022]

[99] Kayode-Afolayan SD, Ahuekwe EF, Nwinyi OC. Impacts of pharmaceutical effluents on aquatic ecosystems. Sci Am 2022; 17: e01288.

[100] Pandey A, Rai N, Tripathi SM, Mishra S. Pharmaceutical waste: risks & challenges faced by aquatic ecosystem. AIJR Proceedings. 2023 Dec 29:147-57.

[101] Zenker A, Cicero MR, Prestinaci F, Bottoni P, Carere M. Bioaccumulation and biomagnification potential of pharmaceuticals with a focus to the aquatic environment. J Environ Manage 2014; 133: 378-87.
[http://dx.doi.org/10.1016/j.jenvman.2013.12.017] [PMID: 24419205]

[102] Sabir S, Akhtar MF, Saleem A. Endocrine disruption as an adverse effect of non-endocrine targeting pharmaceuticals. Environ Sci Pollut Res Int 2019; 26(2): 1277-86.
[http://dx.doi.org/10.1007/s11356-018-3774-4] [PMID: 30467752]

[103] Rayan RA. Pharmaceutical effluent evokes superbugs in the environment: A call to action. Biosafety and Health 2023; 5(6): 363-71.
[http://dx.doi.org/10.1016/j.bsheal.2023.10.005] [PMID: 40078743]

[104] Kock A, Glanville HC, Law AC, Stanton T, Carter LJ, Taylor JC. Emerging challenges of the impacts of pharmaceuticals on aquatic ecosystems: A diatom perspective. Sci Total Environ 2023; 878: 162939.
[http://dx.doi.org/10.1016/j.scitotenv.2023.162939] [PMID: 36934940]

[105] Neergheen-Bhujun V, Awan AT, Baran Y, *et al.* Biodiversity, drug discovery, and the future of global health: Introducing the biodiversity to biomedicine consortium, a call to action. J Glob Health 2017; 7(2): 020304.
[http://dx.doi.org/10.7189/jogh.07.020304] [PMID: 29302312]

[106] Rojas-Reyes JJ, Rivera-Cadavid L, Peña-Orozco DL. Disruptions in the food supply chain: A literature review. Heliyon 2024; 10(14): e34730.
[http://dx.doi.org/10.1016/j.heliyon.2024.e34730] [PMID: 39149054]

[107] Pinto I, Simões M, Gomes IB. An overview of the impact of pharmaceuticals on aquatic microbial communities. Antibiotics (Basel) 2022; 11(12): 1700.
[http://dx.doi.org/10.3390/antibiotics11121700] [PMID: 36551357]

[108] Nguyen MK, Lin C, Nguyen HL, *et al.* Occurrence, fate, and potential risk of pharmaceutical pollutants in agriculture: Challenges and environmentally friendly solutions. Sci Total Environ 2023; 899: 165323.
[http://dx.doi.org/10.1016/j.scitotenv.2023.165323] [PMID: 37422238]

[109] Ortúzar M, Esterhuizen M, Olicón-Hernández DR, González-López J, Aranda E. Pharmaceutical Pollution in Aquatic Environments: A Concise Review of Environmental Impacts and Bioremediation Systems. Front Microbiol 2022; 13: 869332.
[http://dx.doi.org/10.3389/fmicb.2022.869332] [PMID: 35558129]

[110] Shore RF, Taggart MA, Smits J, Mateo R, Richards NL, Fryday S. Detection and drivers of exposure and effects of pharmaceuticals in higher vertebrates. Philos Trans R Soc Lond B Biol Sci 2014; 369(1656): 20130570.
[http://dx.doi.org/10.1098/rstb.2013.0570] [PMID: 25405960]

[111] Gworek B, Kijeńska M, Wrzosek J, Graniewska M. Pharmaceuticals in the soil and plant environment: a review. Water Air Soil Pollut 2021; 232(4): 145.
[http://dx.doi.org/10.1007/s11270-020-04954-8]

[112] Akinnawo SO. Eutrophication: Causes, consequences, physical, chemical and biological techniques for mitigation strategies. Environmental Challenges 2023; 12: 100733.
[http://dx.doi.org/10.1016/j.envc.2023.100733]

[113] Kotchen M, Kallaos J, Wheeler K, Wong C, Zahller M. Pharmaceuticals in wastewater: Behavior, preferences, and willingness to pay for a disposal program. J Environ Manage 2009; 90(3): 1476-82.
[http://dx.doi.org/10.1016/j.jenvman.2008.10.002] [PMID: 19028416]

[114] US Food and Drug Administration. How to dispose of unused medicines [Internet]. Silver Spring (MD): FDA; 2012 [updated 2024. Available from: https://www.fda.gov/consumers/consumer-updates/where-and-how-dispose-unused-medicines

[115] Smith CA, Skibinski K, Livingston M. The US Environmental Protection Agency Focus on Compliant Pharmaceutical Waste Management Now Includes Long-term Care. Sr Care Pharm 2022; 37(10): 488-94.
[http://dx.doi.org/10.4140/TCP.n.2022.488] [PMID: 36171663]

[116] Vidalis A, Dumoulin O, Godbole M, Proenca CC. The role and value of real-world evidence in health technology decision-making in france, germany, italy, spain, and the uk: insights on external control arms. Int J Technol Assess Health Care 2025; 41(1): e25.

[117] Han J, He S, Lichtfouse E. Waves of pharmaceutical waste. Environ Chem Lett 2023; 21(3): 1251-5.
[http://dx.doi.org/10.1007/s10311-022-01491-0] [PMID: 35975196]

[118] Sahu P. Policies and Legal Aspects of Environmental Management. In: Sikdar P K, Ed. Environmental Management: Issues and Concerns in Developing Countries. Cham: Springer 2021; pp. 381-99.
[http://dx.doi.org/10.1007/978-3-030-62529-0_17]

[119] Pollack JB, Carey IQ, Xu VY. Regulation of Products with PFAS. Env't L Rep 2024; 54: 10148.

[120] Sabbatucci M, Ashiru-Oredope D, Barbier L, *et al.* Tracking progress on antimicrobial resistance by the quadripartite country self-assessment survey (TrACSS) in G7 countries, 2017–2023: opportunities and gaps. Pharmacol Res 2024; 204: 107188.
[http://dx.doi.org/10.1016/j.phrs.2024.107188] [PMID: 38705262]

[121] Bain R, Johnston R, Mitis F, Chatterley C, Slaymaker T. Establishing sustainable development goal baselines for household drinking water, sanitation and hygiene services. Water 2018; 10(12): 1711.
[http://dx.doi.org/10.3390/w10121711]

[122] Wess RA. Update of EMA's guideline on the environmental risk assessment (ERA) of medicinal products for human use. Ther Innov Regul Sci 2021; 55(2): 309-23. [http://dx.doi.org/10.1007/s43441-020-00216-1] [PMID: 32996106]

[123] Zwiener C, Gremm T J, Frimmel F H. Pharmaceutical Residues in the Aquatic Environment and Their Significance for Drinking Water Production. In: Kümmerer K, Ed. Pharmaceuticals in the Environment: Sources, Fate, Effects and Risks. Berlin: Springer 2001; pp. 81-9. [http://dx.doi.org/10.1007/978-3-662-04634-0_9]

[124] Honkonen T, Khan S A. Chemicals and waste governance beyond 2020: exploring pathways for a coherent global regime. Copenhagen: Nordic Council of Ministers 2017.

[125] Ly R, Shojaei A. Decentralized autonomous organization in built environments: Applications, potential and limitations. Inf Syst E-Bus Manag 2025; 23(2): 577-622.

[126] Ibáñez-Cruz AJ, Vergara-Florián AM, Algoner WC. Hospital solid waste management strategies to prevent healthcare-associated infections from occupational exposure to bloodborne pathogens and improve occupational safety. Front Public Health 2025; 13: 1499463.

[127] Smith CA, Skibinski K, Livingston M. Response: Update on pharmaceutical waste disposal regulations–strategies for success. Am J Health Syst Pharm 2020; 77(21): 1720-1. [http://dx.doi.org/10.1093/ajhp/zxaa227] [PMID: 32778896]

[128] Malnes D, Tyka M, Golovko O. Övervakning för bevakningslistan 2022-2023. Uppsala: Sveriges Lantbruksuniversitet 2024.

[129] Organization World Health. Global analysis of healthcare waste in the context of COVID-19: status, impacts and recommendations. World Health Organization 2022.

[130] Kümmerer K, Dionysiou DD, Olsson O, Fatta-Kassinos D. A path to clean water. Science 2018; 361(6399): 222-4. [http://dx.doi.org/10.1126/science.aau2405] [PMID: 30026210]

[131] Gupta PP, Bankar NJ, Mishra VH, Sanghavi S, Badge AK. The Efficient Disposal of Biomedical Waste Is Critical to Public Health: Insights from the Central Pollution Control Board Guidelines in India. Cureus 2023; 15(10): e47303. [http://dx.doi.org/10.7759/cureus.47303] [PMID: 38022120]

[132] Organization World Health. 2021. Compendium of WHO and other UN guidance on health and environment [Internet]. Geneva: World Health Organization; 2024. Available from: https://www.who.int/tools/compendium-on-health-and-environment

[133] Richman C, Castensson S. Impact of waste pharmaceuticals: an environmental hazard or greenwash? Pharm J 2008; 280(7494): 335-6.

[134] Chakraborty S, Loutatidou S, Palmisano G, *et al.* Photocatalytic hollow fiber membranes for the degradation of pharmaceutical compounds in wastewater. J Environ Chem Eng 2017; 5(5): 5014-24. [http://dx.doi.org/10.1016/j.jece.2017.09.038]

[135] Sarkar KK, Majee S, Pathak U, Mandal DD, Mandal T. Design and development of an integrated treatment system for pharmaceutical waste with toxicological study. Desalination Water Treat 2019; 164: 75-85. [http://dx.doi.org/10.5004/dwt.2019.24341]

[136] Yusuf Y, Fitriani FY. Preliminary study on enzymatic degradation of model of pharmaceutical waste by laccase from *trametes* sp. J Crit Rev 2020; 7(1): 205-8.

[137] Shi X, Leong KY, Ng HY. Anaerobic treatment of pharmaceutical wastewater: A critical review. Bioresour Technol 2017; 245(Pt A): 1238-44. [http://dx.doi.org/10.1016/j.biortech.2017.08.150] [PMID: 28899679]

[138] Davarnejad R, Zangene K, Fazlali A R, Behfar R. Ibuprofen removal from a pharmaceutical wastewater using electro-Fenton process: an efficient technique (research note). Int J Eng 2017;

30(11): 1639-46.

[139] Smith CA. Managing pharmaceutical waste. J Pharm Soc Wis 2002; 5: 17-22.

[140] Vijayalakshmi M K, Showbharnikhaa S, Snega K, *et al.* Pharmaceutical waste management: review article. Journal of Pharma Insights and Research 2023; 1(2): 166-73.

CHAPTER 3

Classification of Hazardous *vs.* Non-Hazardous Pharmaceutical Waste

Akhalesh Kumar[1,*], **Mukul Yadav**[1], **Rakhi Mishra**[2], **Ravi Shekhar**[1] and **Anjali Chouhan**[1]

[1] *Department of Pharmacy, Institute of Pharmacy & Paramedical Sciences, Dr. Bhimrao Ambedkar University, Agra, Uttar Pradesh, India*

[2] *Department of Pharmacy, Noida Institute of Engineering and Technology (Pharmacy Institute), Greater Noida, Uttar Pradesh, India*

Abstract: Pharmaceutical discard management is essential to protecting the environment and public health. Improper disposal of pharmaceutical waste can pose risks to public health, expose people to harmful compounds, and cause ecological damage. This paper divides pharmaceutical waste into hazardous and non-hazardous categories, highlighting the significance of proper disposal procedures. This study aims to examine the standards for differentiating between hazardous and non-hazardous pharmaceutical waste, as well as the consequences of improper waste disposal. Chemotherapy agents and regulated compounds are examples of hazardous pharmaceutical waste, which include materials that are toxic, contagious, or environmentally hazardous. Materials that do not present serious risks, such as unused vitamins and over-the-counter medications, are classified as non-hazardous trash. The current literature and regulatory recommendations from organizations like the EPA and WHO were reviewed using a qualitative approach. The study pinpoints important classification criteria, such as physical characteristics, chemical makeup, and legal requirements. The results demonstrate that incorrect classification can lead to contaminated environments and higher medical expenses. Clear rules and adherence to best practices for both hazardous and non-hazardous items are necessary for the efficient handling of pharmaceutical waste. Improved safety in hospital settings, reduced environmental contamination, and more effective waste management systems are among the future benefits of better classification. To reduce dangers and advance sustainable pharmaceutical waste management practices globally, more research and more stringent enforcement of waste disposal regulations are necessary.

Keywords: Chemotherapy agents, Environmentally hazardous, Hazardous, Non-hazardous.

* **Corresponding author Akhalesh Kumar:** Department of Pharmacy, Institute of Pharmacy & Paramedical Sciences, Dr. Bhimrao Ambedkar University, Agra, Uttar Pradesh, India; E-mail: akhleshbaghel121@gmail.com

Suman Gautam, Jai Narayan Mishra, Preeti Mishra, Preeti Verma & Sudhanshu Mishra (Eds.)

INTRODUCTION

Medicines that are thrown away, unused, or expired, as well as objects that come into contact with them, are all considered pharmaceutical waste. Pharmaceutical trash can come from homes, clinics, hospitals, pharmacies, and healthcare facilities [1]. The environment, animals, and human health can all be seriously endangered by improper disposal of these items. To guarantee safe disposal and lessen the influence on the environment, this trash must be properly classified [2].

To safeguard the environment and public health, medicinal waste management is crucial. Because inappropriate handling and disposal of pharmaceutical waste can be dangerous, there are strict standards governing its classification and disposal. Hazardous or non-hazardous waste are the two main classifications into which pharmaceutical waste falls. The purpose of this chapter is to examine the complexities of pharmaceutical waste classification, with particular attention to the distinctions between hazardous and non-hazardous pharmaceutical waste, the classification criteria, and the importance of appropriate disposal procedures [3].

It can be challenging to know what to do with the many types of hazardous and non-hazardous waste that industries produce. The 7.6 billion tons of industrial trash produced annually in the US must be disposed of somewhere. However, what kinds of garbage are there, and how should they be handled? This guide covers the distinction between hazardous and non-hazardous waste, the many forms of hazardous waste, examples of each category, how to identify whether your company generates hazardous waste, and advice on what to do about it [4].

Pharmaceutical waste is divided into hazardous and non-hazardous categories (Fig. **1**) to help select appropriate disposal methods and ensure compliance with environmental laws. Because hazardous pharmaceutical waste is poisonous, corrosive, flammable, or reactive, it directly endangers both human well-being and the environment. Non-hazardous pharmaceutical excess is less dangerous, but it still needs to be properly disposed of [5].

HAZARDOUS PHARMACEUTICAL WASTE

The term "hazardous pharmaceutical waste" describes pharmaceutical materials or products whose chemical makeup makes them hazardous to the environment or human health. Medications and toxic, flammable, corrosive, or reactive compounds are examples of these. To avoid exposure, contamination, and injury, hazardous pharmaceutical waste needs to be handled, stored, and disposed of carefully [6].

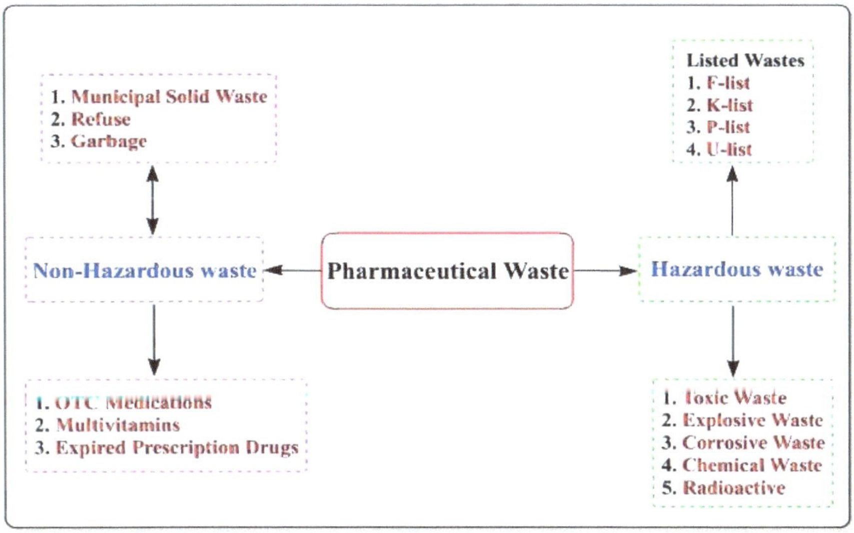

Fig. (1). Types of hazardous waste besides non-hazardous waste.

Hazardous pharmaceutical waste is any pharmaceutical material that meets the requirements established by regulatory agencies for hazardous waste.

Waste items generated during pharmaceutical manufacturing, research, and clinical settings, as well as unused or terminated medicines, can all be classified as hazardous pharmaceutical waste. Harmful waste is defined as waste that poses a substantial risk to human well-being or the environment if inappropriately disposed of. A material is categorized as dangerous waste by the EPA if it is on a particular list of hazardous discarded materials or if it possesses the known characteristics of hazardous waste. Hazardous waste is governed by the Resource Conservation and Recovery Act (RCRA) [7].

KEY CHARACTERISTICS OF HAZARDOUS PHARMACEUTICAL WASTES

Toxicity:

Substances that can cause long-term health problems or environmental impact when consumed, breathed, or absorbed by the body. Because of their mutagenic or carcinogenic qualities, toxic medications, including chemotherapeutic medicines, are frequently regarded as dangerous. When toxic waste is consumed or absorbed by living things, it can cause harm. Toxic wastes are found in many hazardous pharmaceutical wastes. Chloroform, Mercury, cadmium, arsenic, selenium, chromium, barium, m-cresol, lindane, mercury, or silver are commonly found in toxic medications [8].

Flammability:

Flammability can undoubtedly catch fire under specific circumstances. If exposed to heat or an ignition source, some pharmaceutical compounds can be readily ignited and present a fire hazard. Examples include solvents and other combustible substances used in laboratory or pharmaceutical manufacturing operations. Generally speaking, flammable wastes include non-liquids that can catch fire, compressed gases and oxidizers that can catch fire, and liquids having flashpoints lower than 60 degrees Celsius. Ignitable pharmaceutical medicines frequently have gel bases or contain more than 24% alcohol [9].

Corrosiveness:

Corrosiveness may injure biological tissues or components. Waste that can destroy other materials or seriously harm biological tissue. This group includes pharmaceuticals that are extremely alkaline or acidic. The pH of corrosive wastes is typically extremely high. Any liquid that can harm steel, including those with a pH of less than 2 or more than 12.5, is usually corrosive. Strong acids and bases are typically employed as compounding ingredients in corrosive medications [10].

Reactivity:

Substances, when exposed to certain conditions such as heat, pressure, or moisture may explode, ignite, or release toxic gases. Some pharmaceutical waste, particularly volatile compounds, can exhibit reactive behavior under these conditions. Reactive wastes can react with water, become unstable in normal circumstances, release harmful gases, or explode when heated [11].

EXAMPLES OF HAZARDOUS PHARMACEUTICAL WASTE

- Chemotherapy Agents
    - Because of their high toxicity and use in cancer treatments, they must be disposed of carefully. If not disposed of inappropriately, these extremely hazardous medications can have a major, undesirable impact on both human health and the environment. Cyclophosphamide, methotrexate, and doxorubicin are typical examples (Fig. **2**) [12].
- Controlled Substances:
    - If not disposed of appropriately, these can be addictive and have a high potential for abuse. Similar to opioids, some barbiturates and sedatives are misused or disposed of inappropriately, and certain regulated substances, like opioids, can be detrimental to human health. These are frequently governed by regulations about the disposal of hazardous and pharmaceutical waste [13].

- Mercury-containing pharmaceutical
  - Mercury is toxic to both humans and the environment: some older thermometers, certain antiseptics, and vaccines [14].
- Heavy Metals
  - Because heavy metals are poisonous, they pose a significant danger. Such as some antacids and thimerosal, because of their toxicity and propensity to bio-accumulate in the environment, pharmaceutical items containing heavy metals like lead or mercury are considered hazardous waste [15].
- Expired or damaged drugs with toxic effects
  - Some anesthetics or antibiotics can become hazardous or reactive if they are stored incorrectly or expire. After their expiration, several medications may become more hazardous or toxic due to changes in their chemical makeup [16].

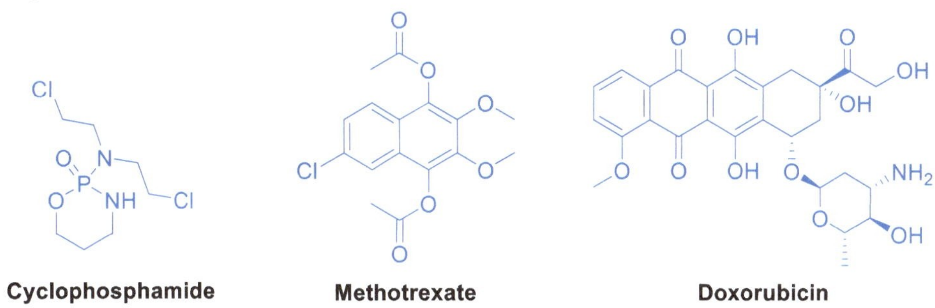

Fig. (2). Examples of chemotherapy agents.

DIFFERENT TYPES OF PHARMACEUTICAL WASTES

Solid Pharmaceutical Waste

Used goods that contain pharmaceutical residues are typically included in solid pharmaceutical waste:

- Sharp substances, such as needles, scalpels, and syringes.
- Items such as masks, gloves, bandages, IV bags, and tubing that are contaminated.
- Substances that include either non-hazardous or hazardous compounds.
- Drug distribution tools such as auto-injectors, inhalers, and nebulizers.
- Empty containers such as blister packs, pill bottles, liquid medicine vessels, and ointment tubes [17].

Liquid Pharmaceutical Waste

As pharmaceutical production facilities carry out specific processing activities, liquid pharmaceutical waste accumulates. Sludge from organic processing and tank-washing solvents are two examples of these wastes. Unused liquid medications may be categorized as pharmaceutical waste, but in certain places, like Michigan, they are considered liquid industrial wastes and are governed by distinct laws [18].

TYPES OF HAZARDOUS WASTE IN THE PHARMACEUTICAL INDUSTRY

Every kind of hazardous waste created by the pharmaceutical sector is subject to RCRA regulations.

Certain hazardous wastes are classified into specific chemical lists under the RCRA. Additionally, it classifies hazardous wastes according to their unique qualities. Below, let us talk about a few of those wastes [19].

List of Hazardous Pharmaceuticals Discarded

Numerous pharmaceutical wastes are listed on particular RCRA hazardous waste lists. Various wastes are categorized by different alphabet letters on these lists. For example, some hazardous pharmaceutical waste types are listed on the RCRA's F and K lists. Hazardous wastes from specific manufacturing and industrial activities are listed on the F list [20]. These wastes are not industry-specific; rather, they belong to the following categories:

- Chlorinated aliphatic hydrocarbon production wastes
- Waste products from various sources
- Dioxin-containing wastes
- Wastewater treatment sludges from petroleum refineries,
- Leachate from various sources
- Spent solvents (Fig. **3**)
- Spent wood preservers

The majority of F-listed wastes in the pharmaceutical industry originate from solvent processes carried out in diagnostic labs. Spent non-halogenated chemical solvents, such as these, are examples of pertinent hazardous compounds on the F list:

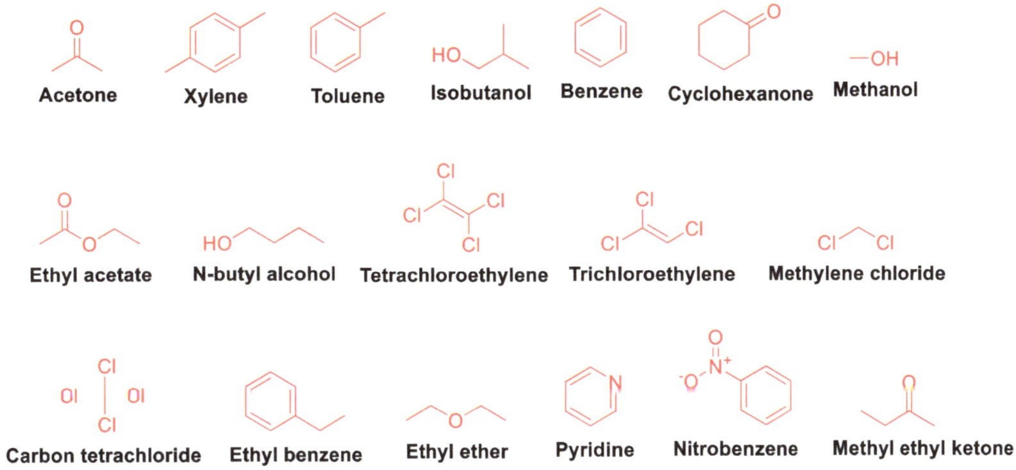

Fig. (3). Chemical structure of spent solvent wastes.

- Spent solvent wastes
  - Acetone
  - Xylene
  - Toluene
  - Isobutanol
  - Benzene
  - Cyclohexanone
  - Methanol
  - Ethyl acetate
  - N-butyl alcohol
  - Tetrachloroethylene
  - Trichloroethylene
  - Methylene chloride
  - Carbon tetrachloride
  - Ethyl benzene
  - Ethyl ether
  - Pyridine
  - Nitrobenzene
  - Methyl ethyl ketone

Some chlorinated fluorocarbons are examples of spent solvent wastes. These spent halogenated solvents are utilized in degreasing. Still, bottoms from spent solvent recovery and spent solvent combinations are likewise eligible, as are all spent solvent elucidations containing 10 percent or more of any of these compounds.

• Electroplating and added metal finishing waste

Spent cyanide bath plating elucidations, as well as any plating steam bath solutions and residues from procedures involving the use of cyanides, are among the wastes associated with electroplating and other metal-finishing processes. They also consist of wastewater treatment sludges from aluminum's chemical coating.

• Dioxin, class of chemical-containing wastes

Wastes from the manufacturing of tetra-, tri-, and pentachlorophenol or their analogs, typically pesticides, are among those that include dioxin. This group also includes wastes from the synthesis of penta-, tetra, and hexachlorobenzene (Fig. **4**) [21].

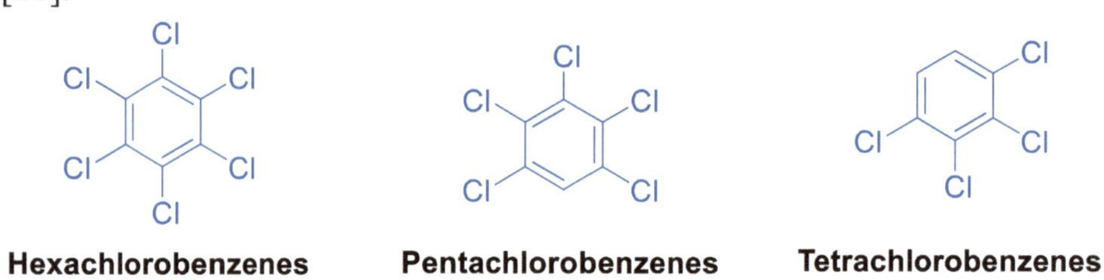

Fig. (4). Examples of dioxin-containing wastes.

• Waste from the manufacture of aliphatic hydrocarbons

Perchloroethylene and trichloroethylene (Fig. **5**) are two examples of chlorinated aliphatic hydrocarbons that are frequently utilized as solvents in dry spring cleaning and other manufacturing. Distillation deposits, heavy ends, tars, reactor clean-out wildernesses, condensed light ends, wasted filters, and filter aids, or spent desiccant waste are among their hazardous wastes.

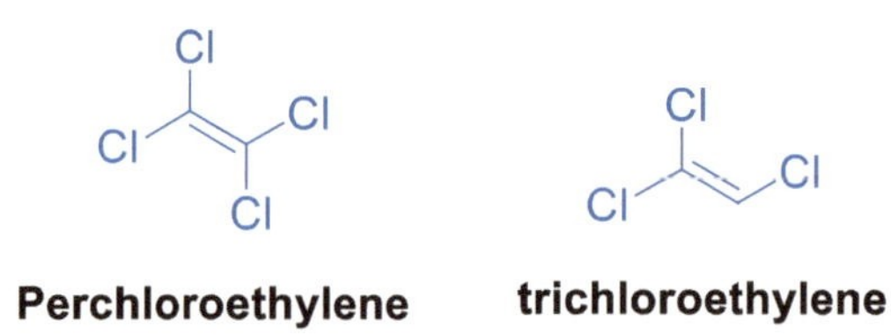

Fig. (5). Examples of aliphatic hydrocarbons.

COMMON WASTES ON THE CLASS K LIST

Unlike those on the F list, the hazardous wastes on the class K list originate from certain industrialized and manufacturing sectors. The 13 categories listed below correspond to the sources of the various waste types on the K list:

1. Preservation of wood
2. Manufacturing of organic compounds
3. Production of pesticides
4. Refinement of petroleum
5. Production of veterinary medications
6. Production of inorganic pigments
7. The manufacture of inorganic chemicals
8. Manufacturing of explosives
9. Production of steel and iron
10. Primary manufacturing of aluminum
11. Processing secondary leads
12. Formulation of ink
13. Making coke from coal

The following are some examples of typical dangerous items found on the K-class list:

- The bottom-sediment sludge from wastewater used for wood preservation contains the insecticide and disinfectant pentachlorophenol or creosote.
- Sludge from wastewater treatment is used in the manufacture of pigments with various colors.
- Side cuts or distillation bases from the conversion of ethylene to acetaldehyde.
- Heavy ends commencing the fractionation column in the manufacturing of ethyl chloride, which is frequently used as a topical anesthetic.
- Still bottoms on or after the distillation of benzyl chloride.
- Aqueous spent chemical antimony catalyst waste from the creation of fluoromethane, which is frequently employed in the manufacturing of semiconductors or electronic devices.
- Heavy ends from distillation in the manufacture of vinyl chloride or ethylene dichloride.
- Bottoms come from the distillation of nitrobenzene.
- Centrifuge or distillation residues from the manufacturing of toluene diisocyanate, which is frequently used in adhesives, coatings, sealants, and foam for furniture, bedding, and carpet underlay.
- Heavy ends and column undersides from the joint synthesis of the industrial solvents perchloroethylene or trichloroethylene.
- Salts are produced as byproducts during the manufacturing of the arsenic-based herbicides cacodylic acid and MSMA.
- Sludge from wastewater treatment is used to produce chlordane or creosote, or toluene reclamation distillation is used to produce the insecticide disulfoton.
- The filter cake is produced when diethylphosphorodithioic acid is filtered to create phorate, a popular insecticide.

The production of organic compounds and veterinary medications is among the hazardous wastes from specific manufacturing and industrial sectors listed on the K list. These wastes are source-specific, unlike those on the F list [22]. The following are a few instances of dangerous compounds on the K list:

- Sludges from wastewater treatment processes are used to make veterinary medications that contain arsenic or organoarsenic compounds.

ACUTE HAZARDOUS PHARMACEUTICAL WASTE

Furthermore, acute hazardous pharmaceutical waste encompasses a wide range of pharmaceutical waste categories. Acute hazardous waste, even in extremely small amounts, is poisonous. Chemicals on the EPA's P list can be found in acute hazardous pharmaceutical wastes. Commercial and pure versions of unused compounds are listed in the P and U classes. Commercial chemical compounds that contain acute hazardous (Fig. **6**) wilds are listed on the P list, whereas those that do not are listed on the U list. These wastes must contain compounds that are either the only active component in a particular product or 100% pure [23]. The following are a few instances of dangerous medications on the P list at quantities more than 0.3%,

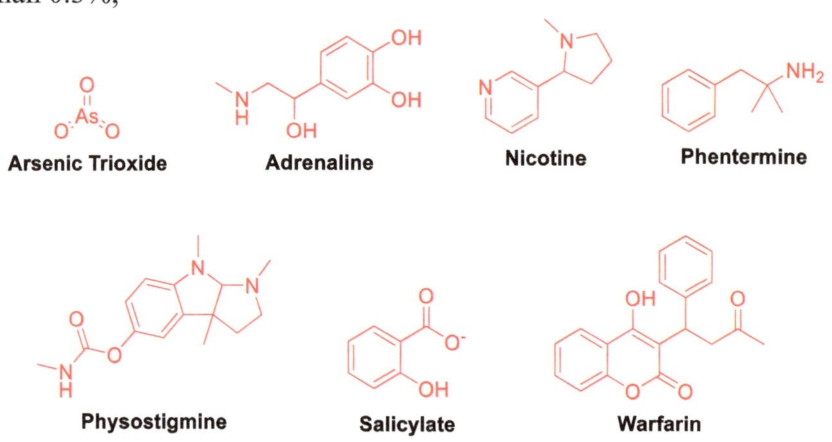

Fig. (6). Chemical structure of acute hazardous pharmaceutical waste.

- Arsenic Trioxide
- Adrenaline
- Nicotine
- Phentermine
- Physostigmine
- Salicylate
- Warfarin

Some chemotherapy agents (Fig. **7**) can result in serious birth abnormalities; these are instances of dangerous pharmaceuticals on the class of U list:

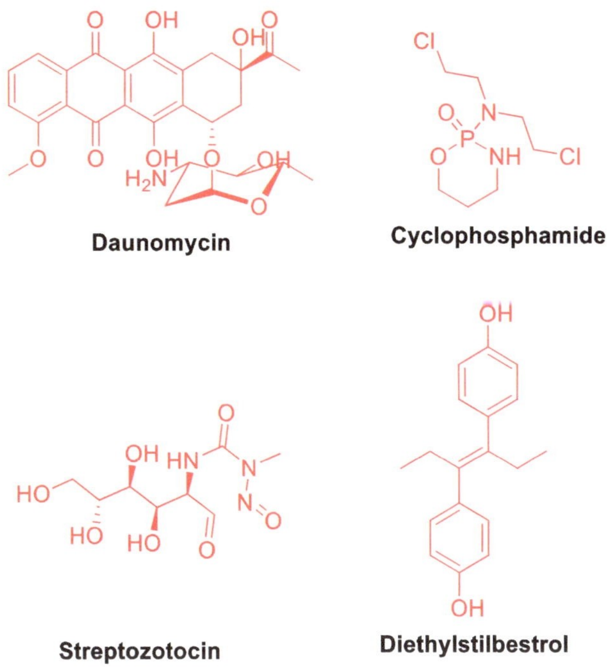

Fig. (7). Some chemotherapy agents.

- Daunomycin
- Cyclophosphamide
- Diethylstilbestrol (DES)
- Melissan
- Streptozotocin

COMMON WASTES IN THE CLASS OF P LIST

The P list's hazardous wastes (Fig. **8**) are categorized as acute hazardous unwanted because, even in small amounts or under the right conditions, they are toxic to people [24]. The following are a few instances of the numerous acute hazardous pollutants in the class of P list:

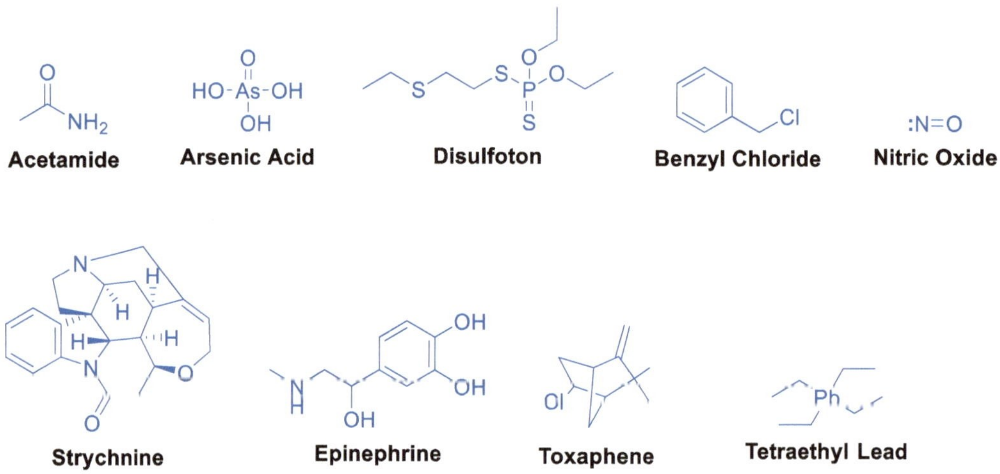

Fig. (8). Examples of common P-list waste.

- Acetamide and Allyl Alcohol
- Arsenic Acid,
- Cyanides of Barium,
- Calcium (Ca)
- Copper (Cu)
- Hydrogen (H)
- Potassium (K)
- Silver (Ag)
- Sodium (Na)
- Zinc (Zn)
- Powdered Beryllium
- Disulfoton
- Benzyl Chloride
- Fluorine (F)
- Nicotine and Salts
- Nitric Oxide
- Nitrogen Oxide or Dioxide
- Strychnine and Its Salts
- Epinephrine
- Toxaphene
- Thalic Oxide
- Tetraethyl Lead

COMMON WASTES IN THE CLASS OF U LIST

The following are some typical hazardous materials found on the U list (Fig. **9**):

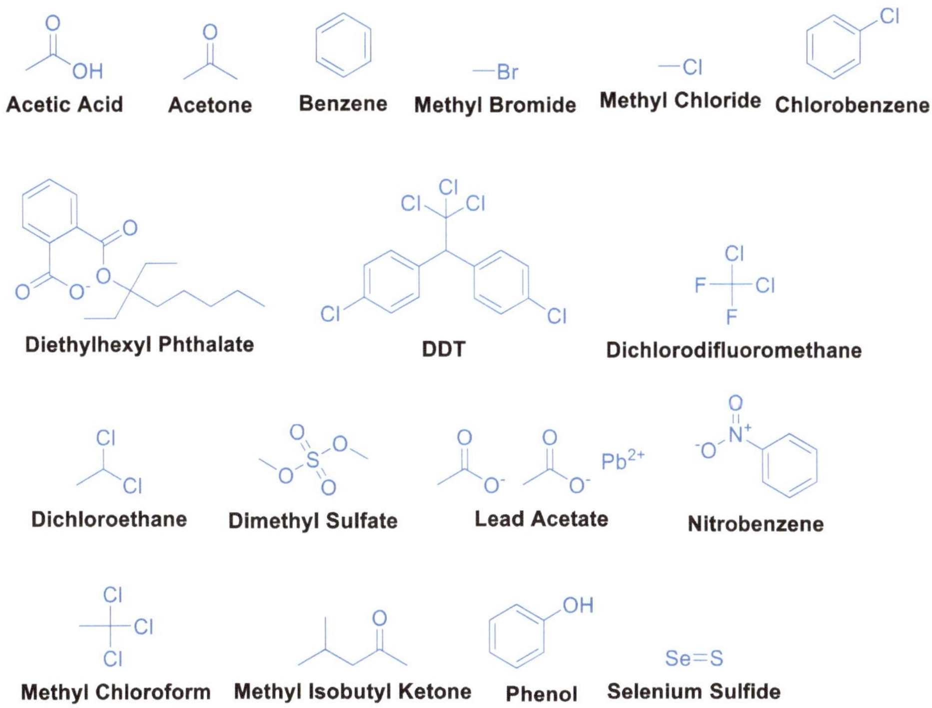

Fig. (9). Chemical structure of common U-list waste.

- Acetic Acid
- Acetone
- Benzene
- Methyl Bromide
- Diethylhexyl Phthalate
- Chlorobenzene
- DDT
- Creosote
- Methyl Chloride
- Chloroform
- Dichlorodifluoromethane
- Dichloroethane
- Ethyl Ether
- Ethyl Acetate
- Dimethyl Sulfate
- Formaldehyde
- Hydrogen Fluoride (HF)
- Isobutyl Alcohol
- Mercury

- Methyl Alcohol
- Lead Acetate
- Nitrobenzene
- Methyl Chloroform
- Methyl Isobutyl Ketone
- Benzene Pentachloro
- Phenol
- Pyridine
- Selenium Sulfide
- Tetra-chloroethylene
- Toluene
- Uracil Mustard
- Xylene.

CLASSIFICATIONS OF HAZARDOUS WASTE ORIGINATORS

The EPA created three groups of generators for hazardous waste, which are defined as those that produce waste in varying amounts and are classified or described in part 261 of chapter 40 of the Code of Federal Regulations (CFR):

- **Large Quantity Originators (LQO):**

LQOs produce more than one kilogram of acutely hazardous waste or 1,000 kg of hazardous waste each month.

- **Small Quantity Originators (SQOs):** SQOs produce more than 100 kilograms of hazardous waste each month, but less than 1,000 kilograms.
- **Very Small Quantity Originators (VSQOs):** One kilogram or less of acutely hazardous waste or 100 kilograms or a smaller amount of hazardous waste per month is produced. The majority of states are permitted to administer the RCRA program, and state-generating categories may differ from federal categories [25].

Who Panel on How Pharmaceutical Waste Is Willing?

The primary regulatory agency that controls how pharmaceutical waste is disposed of is the U.S. Environmental Protection Agency (EPA) [26]. Other regulatory organizations include the following:

(A) DEA (Drug Enforcement Agency)
(B) Occupational Safety and Health Administration (OSHA)
(C) Joint Commission (JC)

(D) Department of Transportation (DOT)
(C) Fish and Wildlife Services (FWS)

DISPOSAL OF HAZARDOUS PHARMACEUTICAL WASTE

The appropriate management, treatment, and disposal of pharmaceuticals or pharmaceutical by-products that endanger human well-being, the environment, or both is known as hazardous pharmaceutical waste disposal. Products that contain toxic, flammable, or infectious materials, as well as medications that are contaminated, expired, or unused, are considered hazardous pharmaceutical waste. Inappropriate disposal can lead to environmental contamination, unintentional poisoning, or the development of drug-resistant diseases. Pharmaceutical waste is usually categorized into specific groups (such as sharps, cytotoxic drugs, or controlled substances) and handled in accordance with rules established by organizations such as the Food and Drug Administration (FDA) and the Environmental Protection Agency (EPA) to ensure safe disposal. Among the disposal techniques are:

- **Chemical Neutralization:** Some drugs and their byproduct can be neutralized through chemical reactions, converting them into less harmful substances before disposal.
- **Landfill**: In cases where pharmaceutical waste is not categorized as hazardous, it may be safely disposed of in an appropriate landfill; however, this is not advised for toxic substances.
- **Incineration:** The most popular and secure method for destroying hazardous pharmaceutical waste, incinerators are built to withstand high temperatures, guaranteeing that dangerous substances are destroyed.
- **Reverse Distribution**: Some pharmacies or manufacturers offer take-back programs for unused medications, allowing them to be safely returned and disposed of [27].

ACCOUNTABILITIES OF A HAZARDOUS WASTE ORIGINATOR

Producers of hazardous waste are liable for the hazardous materials they generate and for any costs associated with subsequent releases. Cradle-to-grave liability was established by the EPA for all industries that produce hazardous waste. Under RCRA, this obligation extends to all producers of hazardous waste. Cradle-to-grave accountability holds generators accountable for their hazardous products from the moment of creation through disposal, assisting facilities in selecting appropriate storage, treatment, and disposal practices for the hazardous waste they generate. The cradle-to-grave liability of each hazardous waste generator includes joint and several liability. As a result, all parties who have ever dumped waste into a landfill are liable for cleaning expenses if hazardous wastes that have been land-disposed or land-filled are discharged [28].

Among the rules governing generators are:

- Whether an EPA identification number is required.
- Extra reporting and exceptions.
- Prerequisites for transportation.
- Limitations on land disposal.
- Reducing waste.
- Closing the facility.
- Manifest.
- Type of facility.
- Maintaining records.
- The biennial report.
- Emissions from the air.
- Personnel training.
- Time limits for accumulation.
- Preventive measures and readiness.
- Emergency protocols and contingency plans.
- The potential gathering of hazardous waste.

NON-HAZARDOUS PHARMACEUTICAL WASTE

Discarded drugs and materials that do not meet the definition of hazardous waste are considered non-hazardous pharmaceutical waste. While there may still be some risk to the environment or public well-being from non-hazardous pharmaceutical waste, this risk is usually less than that of hazardous pharmaceutical waste. Non-hazardous, medication waste must nevertheless be disposed of properly to prevent contamination and harm to the environment. Despite our extensive discussion of hazardous pharmaceutical wildernesses, the majority of pharmaceutical wastes are classified as non-hazardous. Only 5% to 15% of hazardous waste is typically produced by healthcare facilities. So what exactly is non-hazardous trash, and why should it be given extra attention? From the perspective of pharmaceutical waste, the word "non-hazardous" is somewhat misleading. It does not unavoidably apply to waste that is completely harmless if it gets into the environment; rather, it discusses waste that is not regulated by the RCRA. Even "non-hazardous" trash may have negative impacts on the surroundings and human fitness. Therefore, even though pharmaceutical waste is theoretically non-hazardous, it still needs to be handled carefully and disposed of according to certain safe protocols.

The following are a few instances of non-hazardous pharmaceuticals that are unwanted:

- Over-the-counter drugs, in some places, include over-the-counter nicotine replacement treatments.
- OSHA considers certain medications as harmful, even though the RCRA does not classify them as class P or class U listed wastes, in which the specified substances are not the only active constituent, hormones, antibiotics, contraceptives, or endocrine-disrupting composites.

Rebelliously, non-hazardous excess does not directly endanger the environment or human health, but due to the probable hazards, it cannot be disposed of in a trash can or sewer line. Because it is not naturally poisonous, the majority of waste generated in the US, including plastics, paper, metals, glass, *etc.*, is classified as harmless waste. Although rubbish and other solid materials are encompassed in the RCRA's definition of solid non-hazardous waste, additional materials such as semisolids, slurries, liquids, or gas canisters are also regarded as solid waste. It is challenging to create accurate estimates of the amount of non-hazardous garbage produced annually in the United States (US) since non-hazardous waste is not as closely monitored as hazardous waste. Nonetheless, industrial analysts estimate that at seven billion tons or more, manufacturing non-hazardous waste is by far the greatest class of garbage generated each year. Large volumes of harmless waste, frequently in the form of wastewater, have historically been produced by the paper and pulp, mining, chemical, and metal sectors [29].

Pharmaceutical materials that do not pose a risk to human health or the environment and do not necessitate special processing are referred to as non-hazardous pharmaceutical waste. Usually, disposing of this trash without taking extra care is safe.

Important Features:

- **Non-toxic:** Does not endanger human health.
- **Non-flammable:** Doesn't burn readily.
- **Non-corrosive:** Able to preserve materials and tissues.
- **Non-reactive:** Is incapable of triggering hazardous chemical reactions.

Examples Include

- Prescription drugs that have expired, such as antibiotics or painkillers.
- OTC medications, such as aspirin and ibuprofen.
- Medical supplies that have not been used, such as syringes or bandages.
- Supplements or vitamins: Past-due tablets or powders.

NON-HAZARDOUS WASTE DISPOSAL METHODS

Because there are so many distinct kinds of garbage and different laws governing them, there are many ways to dispose of non-hazardous waste. While smaller firms are more likely to hire private disposal providers, larger manufacturing operations may have their own disposal grounds. The employees there can offer you advice on the best solutions for your site and will be well-versed in the assemblage, conveyance, and disposal of non-hazardous trash.

Landfills: Ordinary landfills are safe for disposal.

Incineration: Burning at a high temperature in a controlled environment. Returning unwanted medications to pharmacies for appropriate disposal is known as a take-back program. Even with non-hazardous garbage, proper disposal avoids abuse and environmental damage [30].

COMMON EXAMPLES OF NON-HAZARDOUS WASTE

Here are a few typical types of non-hazardous waste:

- **Unused and expired non-prescription pharmaceuticals:** If disposed of appropriately, over-the-counter (OTC) medicines, such as antihistamines, cold remedies, and pain relievers like acetaminophen and ibuprofen, are regarded as non-hazardous.
- **Vitamins and supplements**: Although they are typically regarded as non-hazardous waste, they still need to be disposed of in accordance with local laws to prevent environmental pollution.
- **Prescription pharmaceuticals that are not under control**: Unless otherwise noted, drugs such as antibiotics, antihypertensives, and non-controlled painkillers (such as acetaminophen) may be regarded as non-hazardous.
- **Agricultural waste:** Certain kinds of agricultural waste are not dangerous. Although chemical waste may be categorized as hazardous trash, organic chemical waste, such as animal dung, urine, or bedding, is not.
- **Batteries:** If batteries are thrown in the trash, they may harm the environment since they contain heavy metals, including lead, nickel, and cadmium. The Mercury Containing and Rechargeable Battery Management Act of 1996 established mercury-unrestricted alkaline batteries as the norm, meaning that the majority of batteries do not contain mercury. Mercury is currently only allowed in button cell batteries or mercuric oxide batteries.
- **Debris from construction:** Debris from construction and demolition is likewise classified as non-hazardous trash. Instead of being thrown in the closest trash, many building materials, including glass, wood, concrete, bricks, asphalt, plastics, gypsum from drywall, solvents, and metal components, must be

disposed of correctly. The same is true of fallen trees, branches, boulders, and earth from clearing and excavation sites, as well as repurposed construction elements like doors, windows, and plumbing fixtures. The majority of non-hazardous construction waste is dumped in landfills that have been specifically designated for that purpose.

- **Industrial waste:** Most companies generate significant volumes of non-hazardous waste, even though some of it is toxic. Although they may not be environmentally harmful, substances such as lactic acid, sugars, carbonates, and bromides still need to be properly managed to prevent contamination.
- **Medical garbage:** Old equipment and uncontaminated animal tissue make up over 85% of medical waste, even though some of it is categorized as hazardous. Medical waste is produced by healthcare facilities, medical investigation institutes, veterinary hospitals, and medical laboratories [31].

DIFFERENCE BETWEEN HAZARDOUS AND NON-HAZARDOUS PHARMACEUTICAL WASTE

Understanding the key differences between hazardous and non-hazardous pharmaceutical waste (Table **1**) is crucial to effective waste management. These differences impact the disposal methods, costs, and environmental consequences associated with each type of waste [32].

Table 1. Differences between hazardous and non-hazardous wastes.

S. No	Criteria	Hazardous	Non-Hazardous
1	**Toxicity**	High toxicity, harmful to human health and the environment.	Low toxicity and generally considered safe.
2	**Corrosivity**	Highly corrosive and can damage tissues or materials.	Low toxicity and generally considered safe.
3	**Reactivity**	Can react dangerously under certain conditions (heat, pressure).	No significant reactivity.
4	**Flammability**	Flammable and risk of ignition under certain conditions.	Non-flammable.
5	**Examples**	Chemotherapy drugs, controlled substances, and heavy metals	OTC medications, vitamins, and non-controlled prescription drugs.

THE ROLE OF HEALTH PROVIDERS IN PHARMACEUTICAL WASTE MANAGEMENT

The appropriate handling and discarding of pharmaceutical waste depend on pharmacists, doctors, nurses, and other medical personnel. These professionals are usually responsible for correctly sorting pharmaceutical waste, classifying it into hazardous and non-hazardous categories, and ensuring that it is disposed of in compliance with regulatory regulations [33].

TRAINING AND AWARENESS

For pharmaceutical waste to be properly classified, healthcare personnel must participate in appropriate training and awareness campaigns. The features of hazardous pharmaceutical waste, the significance of following rules, and safe disposal techniques should all be covered in these courses.

WASTE SEGREGATION

Healthcare services should put in place strict waste segregation procedures to keep hazardous and non-hazardous pharmaceutical waste separate. This reduces the risk of cross-contamination and ensures that trash is handled and disposed of in compliance with applicable laws [34].

CONCLUSION

Pharmaceutical waste must be categorized as hazardous or non-hazardous to protect the environment and community health. Because of its poisonous, corrosive, reactive, or combustible properties, hazardous pharmaceutical waste poses serious risks and must be disposed of using specific techniques. Although less toxic, non-hazardous pharmaceutical waste still needs to be handled carefully to prevent misuse and environmental pollution. To ensure that pharmaceutical waste is properly identified and disposed of safely and in an environmentally responsible manner, healthcare providers, regulatory bodies, and waste management specialists must collaborate. The hazards associated with pharmaceutical waste can be reduced through sustained efforts in awareness-raising, education, and regulatory compliance, thereby creating a safer and healthier environment.

REFERENCES

[1] Rogowska J, Zimmermann A. Household pharmaceutical waste disposal as a global problem—a review. Int J Environ Res Public Health 2022; 19(23): 15798. [http://dx.doi.org/10.3390/ijerph192315798] [PMID: 36497873]

[2] Hossain MS, Santhanam A, Norulaini NN, Omar AM. Clinical solid waste management practices and its impact on human health and environment–A review. Waste Manag 2011; 31(4): 754-766. [http://dx.doi.org/10.1016/j.wasman.2010.11.008]

[3] Vijayalakshmi MK, Showbharnikhaa S, Snega K, Nadhiya J, Akshaya T, Muthu Kaviya M. Pharmaceutical waste management. J Pharma Insights Res 2023; 1(2): 166-73.

[4] Krones J S, Chertow M R, Li X. Making up for lost time (and space): Quantifying non-hazardous industrial waste generation in the US. J Ind Ecol 2024; 28(1): 15-30.

[5] Sapkota B, Pariatamby A. Pharmaceutical waste management system – Are the current techniques sustainable, eco-friendly and circular? A review. Waste Manag 2023; 168: 83-97. [http://dx.doi.org/10.1016/j.wasman.2023.05.052] [PMID: 37285639]

[6] Power LA, Coyne JW. ASHP guidelines on handling hazardous drugs. Am J Health Syst Pharm 2018; 75(24): 1996-2031. [http://dx.doi.org/10.2146/ajhp180564] [PMID: 30327293]

[7] Wagner TP. The complete guide to the hazardous waste regulations: RCRA, TSCA, HMTA, OSHA, and Superfund. John Wiley & Sons. 1999.

[8] Ayaz M, Nawaz A, Ahmad S, *et al.* Underlying anticancer mechanisms and synergistic combinations of phytochemicals with cancer chemotherapeutics: potential benefits and risks. J Food Qual 2022; 2022(1): 1-15. [http://dx.doi.org/10.1155/2022/1189034]

[9] Liu S. Combustion, reactive hazard, and bioprocess safety. In: Liu S, Ed. Bioprocess Engineering. Kinetics, Sustainability, and Reactor Design. 3rd ed.. Amsterdam: Elsevier 2020; pp. 719-72. [http://dx.doi.org/10.1016/B978-0-12-821012-3.00016-6]

[10] El-Shamy AM, Mouneir SM. Medicinal materials as eco-friendly corrosion inhibitors for industrial applications: A review. J Bio Tribocorros 2023; 9(1): 3. [http://dx.doi.org/10.1007/s40735-022-00714-9]

[11] Pohanish R P. Sittig's Handbook of Toxic and Hazardous Chemicals and Carcinogens. 7th ed.. Oxford: William Andrew 2019; p. 3060.

[12] Hamed KM, Dighriri IM, Baomar AF, *et al.* Overview of methotrexate toxicity: a comprehensive literature review. Cureus 2022; 14(9): e29518. [http://dx.doi.org/10.7759/cureus.29518] [PMID: 36312688]

[13] Ifeadi C N, Agodi F. Misuse and abuse of prescription drugs: an overview. Disseminating scholarly research across the globe. Fayetteville: International Institute for African Scholars 2024; pp. 27-35.

[14] Basu M. Impact of Mercury and Its Toxicity on Health and Environment: A General Perspective. In: Kumar N, Ed. Mercury Toxicity. Singapore: Springer 2023; pp. 61-80. [http://dx.doi.org/10.1007/978-981-99-7719-2_4]

[15] Balali-Mood M, Naseri K, Tahergorabi Z, Khazdair MR, Sadeghi M. Toxic mechanisms of five heavy metals: mercury, lead, chromium, cadmium, and arsenic. Front Pharmacol 2021; 12: 643972. [http://dx.doi.org/10.3389/fphar.2021.643972] [PMID: 33927623]

[16] Baraldi E, Ciabuschi F, Fratocchi L. The pros and cons of reshoring to address the problems of shortages in global pharmaceutical value chains: the case of antibiotics. J Glob Oper Strateg Sourc 2023; 16(3): 618-40. [http://dx.doi.org/10.1108/JGOSS-11-2021-0092]

[17] Environmental cleaning and infection prevention and control in health care facilities in low-and middle-income countries: modules and resources. World Health Organization 2023.

[18] Wang L K, Wang M H S, Shammas N K, Wang P. Waste Treatment in the Pharmaceutical Biotechnology Industry Using Green Environmental Technologies. In: Wang L K, Wang M H S, Hung Y T, Eds. Waste Treatment in the Biotechnology, Agricultural and Food Industries. Cham: Springer 2022; pp. 33-85. [http://dx.doi.org/10.1007/978-3-031-03591-3_2]

[19] Pandey A, Rai N, Tripathi S M, Mishra S. Pharmaceutical waste: risks & challenges faced by aquatic ecosystem AIJR Proceedings 2023; 147-57.

[20] Ozymy J, Ozymy MJ. Beyond Midnight Dumping: Exploring the Prosecution of Companies for Environmental Crimes under the US Resource Conservation and Recovery Act (RCRA). JL Bus & Ethics 2023; 29: 57.

[21] Beigh S. A Phytochemicals Approach towards the Role of Dioxins in Disease Progression Targeting Various Pathways: Insights. Indian J Pharm Educ Res 2024; 58(3s): s732-56. [http://dx.doi.org/10.5530/ijper.58.3s.76]

[22] Fu H, Chen Y, Liu T, Zhu X, Yang Y, Song H. Research on hazardous waste removal management: identification of the hazardous characteristics of fluid catalytic cracking spent catalysts. Molecules 2021; 26(8): 2289. [http://dx.doi.org/10.3390/molecules26082289] [PMID: 33920910]

[23] Chauhan K, Khare S, Rathore S S, Tiwari S, Singh A. Hazardous Waste: Chemical Identification and Safe Disposal. In: Singh A, Tiwari S, Eds. Waste Management for Smart Cities. Singapore: Springer Nature Singapore 2024; pp. 81-104.

[24] Watts R J, Teel A L, Gardner C M. Hazardous Wastes: Assessment and Remediation. 2nd ed.. Hoboken: John Wiley & Sons 2023; p. 688.

[25] Singh G, Yadav P K S. Hazardous Waste Characteristics and Standard Management Approaches. In: Saleh H M, Hassan A I, Eds. Hazardous Waste Management: An Overview of Advanced and Cost-Effective Solutions. Amsterdam: Elsevier 2022; pp. 145-64. [http://dx.doi.org/10.1016/B978-0-12-824344-2.00008-2]

[26] Smith CA, Skibinski K, Livingston M. The US Environmental Protection Agency Focus on Compliant Pharmaceutical Waste Management Now Includes Long-term Care. Sr Care Pharm 2022; 37(10): 488-94. [http://dx.doi.org/10.4140/TCP.n.2022.488] [PMID: 36171663]

[27] Cirstea I, Nemeth T S, Tit D M, *et al.* From policy to practice: community pharmacists' self-reported counseling role in pharmaceutical waste management Healthcare 2026; 14(3): 386. [http://dx.doi.org/10.3390/healthcare14030386]

[28] Hassan A I, Saleh H M. Toxicity and Hazardous Waste Regulations. In: Saleh H M, Hassan A I, Eds. Hazardous Waste Management. Amsterdam: Elsevier 2022; pp. 165-82.

[29] Mohammed SA, Kahissay MH, Hailu AD. Pharmaceuticals wastage and pharmaceuticals waste management in public health facilities of Dessie town, North East Ethiopia. PLoS One 2021; 16(10): e0259160. [http://dx.doi.org/10.1371/journal.pone.0259160] [PMID: 34710189]

[30] Li J, Lin F, Li K, *et al.* A critical review on energy recovery and non-hazardous disposal of oily sludge from petroleum industry by pyrolysis. J Hazard Mater 2021; 406: 124706. [http://dx.doi.org/10.1016/j.jhazmat.2020.124706] [PMID: 33418275]

[31] Banerjee T, Nair A P, Smitha M S. Hazardous waste management: lessons from developed countries. In: Pichtel J, Ed. Waste Management and Resource Recycling in the Developing World. Amsterdam: Elsevier 2023; pp. 487-504. [http://dx.doi.org/10.1016/B978-0-323-90463-6.00001-4]

[32] Herliana E, Qainvincena F. Evaluation of hazardous and toxic wastes management by a pharmaceutical company in Bandung, Indonesia. IOP Conf Ser: Earth Environ Sci 2025; 1438(1): 012077.

[33] Letho Z, Yangdon T, Lhamo C, *et al.* Awareness and practice of medical waste management among healthcare providers in National Referral Hospital. PLoS One 2021; 16(1): e0243817. [http://dx.doi.org/10.1371/journal.pone.0243817] [PMID: 33406119]

[34] Chisholm JM, Zamani R, Negm AM, *et al.* Sustainable waste management of medical waste in African developing countries: A narrative review. Waste Manag Res 2021; 39(9): 1149-63. [http://dx.doi.org/10.1177/0734242X211029175] [PMID: 34218734]

CHAPTER 4

Physical and Chemical Processes Involved in Recycling Pharmaceutical Waste

Prottay Dutta[1], **Sakshi Verma**[1,*], **Jeet Kumar Ghosh**[1], **Nripendra Singh**[2] and **Ashruti Hor**[3]

[1] *Department of Pharmacy, Usha Martin University, Ranchi, Jharkhand, India*

[2] *Department of Pharmacy, Veer Bahadur Singh Purvanchal University, Jaunpur, Uttar Pradesh, India*

[3] *Department of Pharmacy, Netaji Subhas University, Jamshedpur, Jharkhand, India*

Abstract: Pharmaceutical industries are essential for the survival of any contemporary society, as their products are crucial to the health and well-being of the general public. However, the waste generated by these industries has become a significant concern due to its detrimental effects on ecosystems and human health. This issue is particularly pronounced in many developing nations, where pharmaceutical waste is often carelessly dumped into the environment, resulting in inadequate handling or treatment. Pharmaceuticals can enter the environment through various pathways, including the discharge of treated wastewater, leakage from landfills, sewer lines, runoff from animal waste, and the application of manure fertilizers to agricultural land. Pharmaceutical waste contains high concentrations of organic matter, microbial toxicants, salt, and non-biodegradable substances. Due to limited resources, it is essential to develop methodologies for treating pharmaceutical waste. The current approaches to the treatment and disposal of pharmaceutical waste are the main subject of this review, which aims to classify the treatment techniques into clearly defined categories. It highlights the related benefits and drawbacks of both established and new approaches, as well as the difficulties in resolving the latter.

Given the wide range of contaminants and the low success rates of current technologies, it is evident that no single traditional method can adequately address the risks associated with pharmaceutical waste discharges. On the other hand, some more contemporary technologies, such as membrane-integrated hybrid technologies, are starting to outperform traditional ones. However, confidence in scaling up these novel technologies remains low and must be significantly bolstered through pilot-scale research using real pharmaceutical waste rather than synthetic alternatives. The suggestions from the analysis will aid in the recycling and treatment of pharmaceutical waste generated by the pharmaceutical sector.

* **Corresponding author Sakshi Verma:** Department of Pharmacy, Usha Martin University, Ranchi, Jharkhand, India; E-mail: vermasakshi933@gmail.com

Suman Gautam, Jai Narayan Mishra, Preeti Mishra, Preeti Verma & Sudhanshu Mishra (Eds.)

Keywords: Environment, Hybrid technologies, Pharmaceutical waste, Recycling, Waste management.

INTRODUCTION

Pharmaceutical waste (PW) is primarily collected at its point of origin and is often disposed of comprehensively as part of healthcare waste (HCW). Pharmaceutical waste, as stated by the World Health Organization (WHO), is a healthcare product labeled beyond its service date or a product that no longer meets medical needs and that also contains polluting substances [1]. Therefore, the distinct chemical properties and persistent hazards of PWs make them individually nano or micro-spiked from other healthcare waste materials, and they need their own distinctive 'Hazardous Waste Pharmaceuticals' colored tag or different 'PHRM code' to identify in the healthcare waste management process [2]. The four-character PHRM code established by the United States Environmental Protection Agency (USEPA) Code of Federal Regulations (CFR), 40 CFR part 266, subpart P, was designed by HCFs to do off-site sending of non-creditable hazardous PWs under the shipping permit. The four-character 'PHRM' code replaced the previous six-character 'PHARMS' code, per USEPA December 19th circular [3]. Pharmaceutical products have a network of chemical ingredients, comprising active pharmaceutical ingredients and numerous excipients. PWs with hazardous properties also meet all USEPA hazardous drug criteria, in addition to their corrosiveness, reactivity, and toxicity [4].

With advancements in medical technology, population growth, and improved healthcare systems, global medicine usage has become widespread. Doctors predict that new medicine brands will account for over $165 billion of this amount, driving medical expense growth at an annual rate of 2–5 percent to reach $1.1 trillion by 2024. In 2019, patients worldwide completed 1.8 trillion days of therapy, averaging 234 days per person. Wasted or expiring medicines, also known as CUE medicine, are disposed of at $790 per ton in the USA and $£450 per ton in the UK [5]. Every year, in the UK, patients take medicines without a physician's prescription or without authorization from the National Health Service, resulting in wasted medicines valued at over £300 million [6]. The United States stated that an assessment of two-thirds of the prescriptions provided to patients found that their medication would remain unused. Due to limited documentation on medicine use and disposal patterns in low- and middle-income countries (LMICs), researchers are, in some senses, able to relate to findings from high-income countries. The German health sector is expecting pharmaceuticals to grow at a range of 40% to 70% in the next three decades. The two problems caused by medicine use in human and animal populations, relate to this. It is anticipated that global veterinary antibiotic use for disease treatment, farming, or growth promotion will rise by 67% by 2030. Pharmaceutical use can also be increased by overprescribing in hospitals and clinics, consumer self-medication, early termination or change of treatment due to misdiagnosis, and other causes, whether medically justified or not [7].

PHARMACEUTICAL WASTE

Roughly, the pharmaceutical industry wastewater can be classified according to its sources as: a) municipal wastewater; b) spent liquors from the fermentation process; c); chemical wastes; d) condenser wastes from evaporation, and e) floor and laboratory washing waste. During the biotechnological production of pharmaceutical chemicals, such as buffers, chelators, and antibiotics, used as ancillary substances, these substances are discharged into the water biotope, resulting in the accumulation of harmful chemicals in soil and water. Though estimated to be as low as 15-20%, recent studies confirm that 20-35% of medicines used in hospitals are potentially bioaccumulative. Consequently, the pseudo-persistence and ecotoxicological impacts of continuously discharged pharmaceutically active compounds (PhACs)—the primary harmful constituents—must also be considered. Most PhACs are complex molecules that are polar in nature, having molecular weights in the range of 200 to 1000 Da. Due to their specific biological activity, they are widely used in drug applications [8]. Pharmaceutical waste can be divided into two categories to facilitate the identification of available treatment methods and the development of systematic policies for environmentally friendly, minimal waste discharge.

a) Secondary wastes from medicinal companies and the treatment and recycling plants; and b) the medical wastes from hospitals and the domestic sector contaminate the sewage systems significantly. The second type of waste is sources that cause active pharmaceutical residues to enter public sewers and, thus, municipal wastewater treatment plants, which are often poorly equipped to handle these specific types of waste [9].

Some guidelines on the management of PWs produced by pharmaceutical industries, hospitals, clinics, research laboratories, and domestic sources suggest that the solid and semi-solid PWs should be treated by incineration/pyrolysis, encapsulation, and amortization or engineered landfill, respectively, whereas the liquid PWs should be treated in a wastewater treatment plant (WWTP) [10]. However, there are some controversies on the applicability of the said guidelines in the management of pharmaceutical waste (PWM). Discrepancies in recommendations for techniques such as incineration, encapsulation, and sanitary landfilling—where one guideline or study endorses them while others label them as "partially recommended" or "not recommended"—may arise because these assessments are often based on subjective perceptions of practitioners and experts [11]. The recycling of pharmaceutical waste is essential to minimize environmental pollution and recover valuable materials. This process involves both physical and chemical methods to safely separate, neutralize, and repurpose pharmaceutical components.

The Recycling Process Involves

Collection of Waste Accoutrements

The first step in recycling involves collecting waste from major sources such as residential areas, apartments, drop off centers, and community centers. After collection, the waste is separated into categories like plastics, glass, metals, and biodegradable materials. These sorted materials are then transported to recycling facilities, where they are processed as raw materials. The final stage involves transporting and accumulating these materials at the recycling plant [12].

Separation of Waste Material

The next step in the recycling process is the separation of collected waste—such as plastics, glass, metals, and biodegradable materials—into distinct categories based on material type [13].

Filtration, Extraction & Purification

In some cases, pharmaceutical waste is dissolved in solvents or water with the active ingredients separated from the excipients. Solid impurities of the liquid waste are removed by filtration for treatment. Distillation or solvent extraction can be used to extract some valuable compounds, such as active pharmaceutical ingredients (APIs) from waste. Recoverable usable substances can be further purified employing chromatography or crystallization [14].

Drawing and Drying

A crucial step in the recycling process is the thorough cleaning of sorted waste to ensure it can be recycled and reclaimed effectively. Once cleaned, the material is dried and prepared for further recycling.

Manufacturing of the New Product

After drying, the next step is manufacturing the final product. Production is based on the availability of processed raw materials, resulting in a variety of goods made from recycled waste such as paper, soft drink containers, glass, steel barrels, plastic containers, laundry detergents, paper bags, plastic cups, and other disposable items.Quilting and dealing make up the final process of product recycling. The products manufactured are packed duly with markers and canons. Additionally, it carries the requests of noncommercial and retail trade to the dealer [15].

Physical Processes Involved in Pharmaceutical Waste Treatment

Recycling pharmaceutical waste involves a number of physical processes that safely recover and use materials while minimizing the environmental impact. These processes ensure that pharmaceutical waste is handled properly, both as hazardous and non-hazardous waste. The physical processes that are key to this reversibility observed are as follows:

Incineration and landfilling: Incineration, open burning, and landfilling are common methods for sludge disposal. Incineration-based processes can be categorized into two groups: low-temperature thermal disposal technologies and high-temperature thermal disposal technologies. Such incineration may or may not include air pollution controls. Simple incineration often refers to open-air burning, where ash disposal is poorly managed, and no measures are taken to prevent the spread of pathogens. Before going to incineration or other disposal options, pharmaceutical wastes are often combusted with other, more diverse categories of pharmaceutical waste. From an environmental point of view, this may be extremely dangerous. Studies [16, 17] demonstrate that the incineration facilities must be located away from populated areas. Medical waste has often been disposed of *via* landfilling. However, there is no foolproof method to prevent water contamination from landfill leachates, nor is there a technique that fully neutralizes the toxic effects of hazardous compounds and their chain reactions in the presence of other wastes. The pharmaceutical residues in leachate from landfills are endocrine-disrupting and bioaccumulate, making them dangerous. Positive removal rates at various wastewater plants do not result in the effective degradation of pharmaceuticals. Therefore, the studies [18] are significant in showing the disadvantages of using ordinary landfills to treat hazardous wastes. For the analysis of the environmental consequences of leachate release from a municipal solid waste landfill containing household hazardous waste, an important study has modeled waste behavior in landfills using LandSim (Landfill Performance Simulation). Although replacing ordinary landfills with sanitary landfills offers some safeguards against potential threats, they remain insufficient to handle the enormous global volume of medical waste. Since incineration merely transfers pollutants from water to air and disperses them into the broader environment, it cannot be considered environmentally friendly. The major objection to thermal incineration is that dioxin is released into the atmosphere during incineration. Immediately after the severe acute respiratory syndrome epidemic in 2003 in China, the National authorities in China promptly planned and set up dedicated centralized medical waste disposal facilities mainly based on non–incineration methods. Nevertheless, *in situ*ations involving medical waste with extremely high infectious potential and danger, incineration often remains the most viable solution when no alternative methods can adequately ensure safety under those conditions. Therefore, thermal incineration processes need to be followed by a downstream air pollution control device, such as an adsorber, scrubber, or electrostatic precipitator, to keep dioxin concentrations below 0.1 ng/m3. Therefore, research efforts are essential to develop eco-friendly alternatives to replace incineration. As far as landfilling is concerned, the practice cannot really be termed a scientific approach, unless the sludge is well stabilized to prevent the leakage of harmful components that usually pollute surface and groundwater resources. While somewhat costly, only sanitary landfilling should be permitted, after the effective stabilization of harmful compounds [19].

Microwaving: One such waste treatment method is microwaving, a process that uses electromagnetic wave frequency to generate heat within waste materials, thereby enabling disinfection. Specific types of waste consist of biomedical and some pharmaceutical waste. The objectives of microwaving for waste treatment are to sterilize or disinfect the waste by elevating its temperature to a level high enough to inactivate microorganisms (bacteria and viruses) [20].

Sterilization by Autoclaving: This is a form of treatment involving sterilization by steam. It is a commonly used method for the treatment of biomedical waste like pharmaceutical waste. The waste is treated in combination with high-pressure steam and heat to achieve the conditions of temperature and pressure required for the effective killing of microorganisms, including bacteria, viruses, and spores. Glassware, surgical instruments, laboratory equipment, and certain pharmaceutical waste (such as used vials and syringes) may be suitable for autoclaving. Basically, the autoclave is used to reduce the microbial load of these waste materials before disposal to prevent further contamination [21].

Encapsulation solidification: Technology in hazardous waste management physically immobilizes hazardous waste to prevent contact with leaching agents (*e.g.*, water). The technology aims to coat the waste with inert materials such as polybutadiene, sulfur polymer, high-density polyethylene, and optionally other similar materials. The goal of this treatment method is to minimize the environmental impact of waste and reduce its hazard level to an acceptable point. Burial or storage is used for sharps and mercury-contaminated hazardous waste. The encapsulated material exhibits high corrosion resistance in acidic and saline environments [22].

Shredding: This is a waste management method in which the waste materials are shredded mechanically into more manageable, smaller pieces and disposed of in designated landfills. Usually, this approach is used for non-hazardous and non-biomedical waste. Shredding effectively reduces waste volume by breaking down debris into smaller fragments, facilitating compaction, simplifying transportation, and optimizing landfill space utilization. Application shredding is typical for a wide range of materials, such as paper, cardboard, plastics, textiles, and other nonhazardous solid waste [23].

Plasma pyrolysis: Plasma pyrolysis is an advanced waste treatment technology that utilizes plasma—an intensely ionized gas generated at temperatures exceeding 3000 °C *via* an electric arc or other energy source in the presence of air or steam. This creates a highly energized state of matter composed of ions, electrons, and excited neutral particles, which thermally decompose organic compounds in waste materials. This process is also known as plasma gasification or plasma arc gasification. This combination of physical processes also facilitates pharmaceutical waste recycling to minimize pollution and recover valuable materials as well as to dispose of hazardous substances safely [24].

Chemical Processes

Chemical processes for recycling pharmaceutical waste involve breaking down harmful compounds into useful substances for recovery, thereby preventing environmentally damaging disposal. This section discusses the key chemical processes used in pharmaceutical waste recycling, as outlined in the following subsections.

Neutralization

Neutralization is the process of balancing the pH of pharmaceutical waste, particularly acidic and alkaline streams. It is essential to perform this step to prevent dangerous reactions and ensure safe handling. Alkaline substances such as sodium hydroxide (NaOH) or calcium carbonate ($CaCO_3$) are used to treat acidic waste such as hydrochloric acid and sulfuric acid. Acids such as hydrochloric acid (HCl) or sulphuric acid (H_2SO_4) are used to neutralize alkaline waste such as sodium hydroxide solution. This reaction makes water and salts easier to dispose of or recycle [25].

Oxidation and Reduction (Redox Reactions)

The oxidation and reduction reactions cause the breakdown of complex pharmaceutical compounds into simpler and harmless forms. Process-related detoxification is particularly useful for treating pharmaceutical waste.

Pharmaceutical compounds are broken down by reacting with strong oxidizing agents such as hydrogen peroxide (H_2O_2), ozone (O_3), or chlorine (Cl_2). Sodium bisulfite ($NaHSO_3$) or iron (Fe) is used as a reducing agent to reduce some oxidized pharmaceutical waste materials. Acetylcysteine is often used to detoxify heavy metals and chemical residues [26].

Precipitation

Dissolved pharmaceutical waste components, such as heavy metals or some toxic compounds, are precipitated and removed by converting into an insoluble solid form. Chemical agents, such as sodium sulfide (Na_2S) or calcium hydroxide ($Ca(OH)_2$), are added to the waste solution. This process produces solid precipitates that can be filtered out and disposed of safely [27].

Chemical Immobilization

Chemical immobilization converts hazardous pharmaceutical waste into stable nonleachable compounds in order to prevent environmental contamination. The waste is immobilized using immobilizing agents such as silicates, phosphates, or cement. These agents form a solid matrix that encapsulates toxic substances, preventing them from leaching into soil and groundwater [28].

Iron reduction method (Fe-C Fe-C process, iron microelectrolysis technology with ferric and carbon, also called zero-valent method). Cast iron scrap and activated carbon or coke are used as the electrolytic materials. Electric erosion is carried out under acidic conditions to form numerous fine galvanic cells within the iron filings and between the iron filings and the carbon powder. This generates a sufficient amount of highly reductive active hydrogen, which is capable of decomposing macromolecular organic matter. Fe2+ generates Fe(OH)3 flocs, which have an adsorption effect, under aeration conditions. The Fe–C process is, therefore, an oxidation-reduction, adsorption, complexation, and electrofloculation method that alters the form and structure of contaminants to leach out refractory substances and promote biodegradability. The main advantages of adsorption are its simple process, low operating costs, and wide applicability. However, iron sludge accumulation and the potential need for active regeneration are notable drawbacks [29].

Advanced Oxidation Processes

Treatments based on a class of Advanced Oxidation Processes (AOPs) include near-ultraviolet (UV) or solar-visible irradiated heterogeneous and homogeneous photocatalysis, electrolysis, supercritical water oxidation, ozonation, and ultrasound oxidation. Other examples are wet air oxidation (WAO), electrochemical oxidation, and Fenton's treatment. Ionizing radiation and treatment subject to microwaves and pulsed plasma are the emerging processes. AOPs can leverage certain features of oxidizing agents to degrade PhACs. The literature [30] shows that such AOPs can be very effective, especially for the treatment of persistent pollutants or drugs such as carbamazepine. The mechanisms of degradation may differ from treatment to treatment. For example, the lytic activity of ozone in an ozone-based advanced oxidation process is employed simultaneously to digest and remove personal care products in wastewater. Furthermore, in Fenton's method (iron-catalyzed hydrogen peroxide oxidation), the degradation and mineralization of PhACs by photocatalysis and the stabilization power of Fenton's reagent are used in the removal of PhACs. In some studies [31], the effectiveness of ozonation in treating effluents from waste treatment plants containing bio-refractory and/or toxic organic pollutants, including pharmaceutically active compounds (PhACs), has been well established. Fenton's treatment significantly improves the biodegradability of pharmaceutical wastewater, often increasing the BOD/COD ratio by 3-5 times. This enhancement facilitates the removal of wastes in subsequent downstream biological treatment processes. It is generally observed that Fenton's process alone can reduce the COD of wastewater by approximately 50%, and this reduction can be further increased to about 98% with the addition of downstream processes such as aerobic biological degradation. In this way, the cost of the treatment may also rise. Finally, bio-degradation-resistant elusive contaminants in the secondary effluents have also been oxidized using an ultraviolet hydrogen peroxide (UV/H2O2) combination. The pharmaceutical residues in laboratory wastes were proven to be degraded by Fenton and photo-assisted Fenton's oxidation. The data indicated that Fenton's treatment not only stabilized organic matter such as PhACs but also made them subsequently removable through oxidation and coagulation. TiO2 nanofibers not only degrade the environmentally persistent residues such as carbamazepine but also improve dewatering. A UV dose of 923 mJ cm−2 has been found to remove about 90% of selected pharmaceuticals, such as carbamazepine, through an individual process named the UV/H2O2 process. In some cases, removal rates close to 100% have been reported for certain compounds—for example, through advanced oxidation, irradiation techniques, or a combination of both. However, most studies reporting such high removal efficiencies for selected compounds have been conducted under ideal conditions using synthetic wastewater. In general, irradiation or AOP alone is not found to be particularly effective, and many intermediates are formed during the process, which may even be more environmentally harmful than the original contaminant. The critical importance of radiation dose, along with maximally controlled techniques and comprehensive facilities for the analysis of formed intermediates, must be emphasized. Nevertheless, it is worth noting that the adopted AOPs have very limited downstream applicability and are not yet established as effective techniques for waste volume minimization or complete pharmaceutical compound removal, leaving associated hazards largely unaddressed [32].

Wet air oxidation (WAO): F. J. Zimmer Mann in 1958 put forward a WAO application for the papermaking black liquid treatment. This method uses air or oxygen as an oxidant and decomposes organic matter at high temperatures (150-350°c) and high pressure (0.5-20 Mpa). Typically, WAO is applied in the advanced treatment of wastewater. This method has a wide range of applications, high COD removal efficiency (up to 90% under appropriate conditions), relatively low energy consumption, minimal secondary pollution, and is easy to manage [33].

The Fenton reagent: It is the combination of hydrogen peroxide with ferrous salt. The strong oxidant hydroxyl radicals (•OH), which possess superoxidizing potential to oxidize organic species in the wastewater, can be generated from hydrogen peroxide in the presence of ferrous salt. OH exhibits non-selectivity and strong oxidizing power (E_0 = 2.8eV), enabling it to degrade a wide range of contaminants [9]. Consequently, the Fenton process is well-suited for treating wastewater with high concentrations of persistent, toxic compounds, or as a pretreatment step prior to biological treatment. Although Fenton oxidation has the advantages of simple equipment, mild reaction conditions, and easy operation, it uses a wide range and a large number of iron ions contained in the effluent for further treatment [34].

Ozone: Ozone is a strong oxidant with a redox potential of 2.07 V, the highest among commonly used chemical oxidants. It is also a highly effective disinfectant and sterilizing agent. The oxidation process involves two primary mechanisms: direct reaction and indirect reaction. In direct reaction, ozone is transformed into pollutants employing strong oxidation. Ozone decomposes in water indirectly, giving • OH, which is highly reactive and then oxidizes contaminants in wastewater. However, ozone can induce open-loop and chain scission, converting macromolecular organic compounds into smaller, biodegradable organic molecules, thereby enhancing the biodegradability of wastewater [35]. For this reason, ozonation shows high potential for pretreating highly concentrated, hard-to-degrade wastewater, as well as for advanced treatment of biotreated effluent containing resistant and stable organic compounds. The advantages of this method include fast reaction rates, high efficiency, minimal sludge production, and no secondary pollution [36].

SCWO (supercritical water oxidation): SCWO is a chemical reaction of dissolved oxygen in organic pollutants at supercritical water. Complete mixing of organic matter, air, and supercritical water was achieved at 24 MPa pressure and 400 °C, resulting in a homogeneous phase. Under these conditions, organic compounds undergo spontaneous oxidation. As the reaction temperature grows higher, the organic matter is rapidly oxidized into 99.9 percent or simpler, non-toxic small molecules within a certain period for decontamination. Organic matter can be completely oxidized through SCWO, which offers high oxidation efficiency and avoids secondary pollution. However, this method requires high operating conditions and is consequently costly [37].

Photocatalytic oxidation: The catalysts employed for photochemical degradation processes in photocatalytic oxidation processes are n-type semiconductors like TiO2, SrO2, WO3, SnO2, *etc*. Upon irradiation with ultraviolet light, these catalysts generate electron-hole pairs (h^+–e^-) that migrate to the semiconductor surface, inducing a strong oxidation effect that produces hydroxyl radicals (•OH), which subsequently oxidize contaminants in the wastewater. Photocatalytic oxidation, with its strong oxidizing power, absence of secondary pollution, and mild reaction conditions, is an effective method for treating refractory organic wastewater. As a result, it offers broad application prospects. A key research priority is the development of photocatalysts that are low-cost and highly stable [38].

Ultrasonic oxidation: Ultrasonic oxidation of organic matter in wastewater is a physicochemical degradation process driven by ultrasonic cavitation. This process encompasses three main mechanisms: free radical oxidation, pyrolysis, and supercritical water oxidation. The effect of ultrasonic degradation of organic pollutants in wastewater is affected by many factors. The most important factors are the nature of organic matter, ultrasound frequency, sound power, solution temperature, and pH, as well as ultrasonic time [39].

Electrochemical methods utilize electrochemical reactions to remove toxic and harmful pollutants from water. This approach represents an emerging technique in the field of water treatment.-In an electrochemical reaction, oxidation occurs at the anode, where reactants lose electrons, while reduction occurs at the cathode, where reactants gain electrons. The removal of refractory organic matter is primarily achieved through oxidation at the anode. Some conventional electrochemical wastewater treatment processes include electrolytic recovery, electrochemical oxidation, electrolytic air flotation, electrodialysis, and micro-electrolysis. The electrochemical method is also known as an “environmentally friendly” process, giving it a significant advantage over other treatment methods. For example, this electrochemical process operates at normal temperature and pressure, offers high efficiency, can be used alone or integrated with other methods, requires minimal space, avoids secondary pollution, and is highly automated. Future development of electrochemical reactors will focus primarily on optimizing electrochemical reactions, particularly at the anode [40].

Irradiation treatment: One effective removal method involves gamma-ray or ionizing irradiation, which has proven highly successful in eliminating various pharmaceutical compounds, including antibiotics, hormones, X-ray contrast agents, antineoplastic drugs, and anti-inflammatory drugs. An important advantage of ionizing irradiation is its ability to achieve near-complete (close to 100%) removal of precipitated contaminants. However, extreme care must be taken to ensure the correct effective radiation dose is applied during treatment. At low doses (*e.g.*, 0.1–0.4 kGy), numerous intermediate by-products are formed. These intermediates are often difficult to detect, and some may be more harmful than the original PhACs. However, a dose of radiation above 1 kGy is needed for complete degradation, while there is a potential risk of forming additional harmful intermediates. LambdaMax can be even more effective when combined treatment is applied with H2O2 or TiO2 and with gamma irradiation [41]. At high radiation doses, a high degree of efficiency and organic pharmaceutical ingredients have been removed from various pharmaceutical waste streams by means of irradiation techniques. Nevertheless, no comprehensive, scalable treatment scheme based on irradiation technology has been successfully implemented to date.

Physicochemical Methods

These wastewaters, containing various toxic concentrations, are treated through physicochemical methods such as ion exchange, adsorption, coagulation-flocculation, froth flotation, precipitation, chemical reduction, and electrochemical processes. These methods are often applied in combination and at different stages, starting from initial production [38]. These integrated processes are applicable only where direct physical or chemical treatment methods are unsuitable due to poor efficiency in removing dissolved COD or risks associated with temperature increases from adding complex chemicals. In such cases, conjugate methods have proven effective [42]. The results indicate that the COD removal efficiency by processes like precipitation–air flotation is higher than that of the coagulation–precipitation process (4), but the operating costs of the former are almost 25% higher than the latter. Based on a comparison of the relative potential of ferric chloride, calcium hydroxide, and calcium oxide and chloride to remove phosphorus from a predominantly phosphorus-bearing wastewater, flocculant removal rates are dependent on concentration and pH [43]. The pharmaceuticals are treatment-specific and are diverse in nature. For example, studies on fluoroquinolone removal mechanisms have shown that adsorption onto sludge and/or flocs is more effective than biodegradation. The major treatment categories are subdivided in the sections below, with a focus on referencing key breakthroughs [44].

Adsorption Process

The removal of persistent PhACs can be preferentially accomplished through adsorption. Selected problematic compounds can be eliminated from treated pharmaceutical wastewater using adsorbents, making the effluent suitable for discharge into water bodies. It has been demonstrated that adsorbents derived from plant-based sources are easy to fabricate and environmentally friendly [45]. Nevertheless, it is relevant to question whether burning tree trunks to produce adsorbents for treating large volumes of pharmaceutical wastewater is justified. Most successful demonstrations have been conducted in batch mode. For large-scale continuous industrial applications, the high treatment cost is largely due to the frequent need to regenerate or replace exhausted adsorbents. Additionally, adsorption processes require explicit knowledge of the waste composition to be effective, as Pharmaceuticals and Personal Care Products (PPCPs) exhibit widely varying adsorption potentials influenced by complex functional group interactions and pH dependence [46]. In the last few years, research has been directed towards the incorporation of zeolites for the removal of selected compounds/ micropollutants, which are poorly removed by conventional activated carbon-based adsorbents. Thus, it is possible to use zeolites to remove highly effective compounds such as metformin and lincomycin. Such successful doping opens new avenues for methodical development, leveraging the chemical structure of zeolites to our advantage. Compounds with a Stokes diameter compatible with the silica-alumina zeolite lattice can be removed very effectively. In recent years, the integration of magnetic particles and nanotechnology into adsorption processes has gained significant attention. The use of nanoparticles, nanotubes, and related components as adsorbents greatly increases surface area, tensile strength, and material resistance, leading to substantially higher adsorption efficiency. Counteracting pH sensitivity, high chemical leaching, and other impediments are additional advantages of these materials. Nanoclays (organically modified layered silicates) and nano-scale particles are potent adsorbents of pharmaceuticals [47] due to their high surface area at the nanoscale. Carbon nanotubes have already established as a better substitute for common adsorbents for the removal of pharmaceutical compounds such as 1,2-dichlorobenzene, trihalomethanes, and microcystins. Compounds can be adsorbed from both aqueous and gaseous systems on the surface of the magnetic particles [48]. Magnetic nanocomposite adsorbents with high selectivity and biocompatibility can be obtained when these are combined with nanocomposite materials. However, very few researchers support these findings as a source of pharmaceutical waste. Therefore, although we have evidence that nanocomposite materials are able to remove dangerous levels of heavy metals, such as lead or chromium, these medical compound removal indices need further investigation. However, given the need for replacement and/or regeneration of adsorbent materials in continuous operations, zeolite-based and nanocomposite-based adsorbents represent a promising new generation of materials for pharmaceutical wastewater remediation [49]. While adsorption is more attractive than many conventional techniques for treating small wastewater volumes, its application in large-scale continuous plants remains less feasible. An additional challenge is the disposal of spent adsorbents loaded with toxic contaminants [50].

Coagulation and Precipitation

Coagulation and precipitation processes serve as an effective pre-treatment step in increasing the biodegradability of wastewater through the removal of oil and grease, suspended particulate matter, and specific compounds. Coagulation is a unit operation that removes colloids from water and wastewater. Its principal mode of action is destabilizing colloidal particles by charge neutralization and promoting collisions between neutralized particles, resulting in cohesion [51]. The use of coagulants reduces COD loading at a relatively low cost and helps stabilize leaching-prone components. A comparative analysis of commonly available coagulants, such as lime, alum, ferrous sulfate, and ferric chloride, has shown that ferric chloride removes BOD5 and COD to the greatest extent. Ferric chloride produces compact sludge with a good settleability as reflected in its low sludge volume index of 76 ± 29 mL/g TSS [52]. However, in integrated coagulation-dissolved air flotation experiments, alum demonstrated higher COD removal (77.5 ± 3.2%) as compared to ferric chloride (71.6 ± 2.9%) and ferrous sulfate (67.7 ± 3.7%). However, the removal efficiencies of all the coagulants mentioned above are sensitive to pH changes in the medium, while the effectiveness is largely subject to the specific compounds present. For instance, Cheng *et al.* [56] obtained a poor COD removal rate of 17.2% using polyaluminum chloride at a dosage of 0.5 g/L on concentrated effluents from a triazine manufacturing facility [53]. The drawbacks and special features of some treatment processes are presented in Table **1**. Coagulation-precipitation can only be used to reduce the load on the downstream secondary treatment unit.

Table 1. Features and limitations of different treatment options.

Technology	Features	Limitations	References
Precipitation	Suitable for large-scale operations and can treat high salt content waste.	Efficiency depends on the solid-liquid separation step.	[52]

(Table 1) cont.....

Technology	Features	Limitations	References
Sedimentation	Primary treatment: removes floating and settleable solids.	A large quantity of reagents are needed.	
Coagulation and flocculation	Can be used for building a compact treatment plant for further purification of treated water.	Preliminary chemical Coagulation and flocculation are generally not used.	[53]
Ion Exchange	Good chemical, thermal and radiation stability, ensuring high selectivity.	Blockage problems need regeneration.	[54]
Evaporation	Well-established technology, high volume reduction factor.	Process limitations include foaming, corrosion.	-
Solvent Extraction	Suitable for a variety of radionuclides. Selectivity enables the removal and recycling of actinides.	High capital costs generate aqueous and organic secondary waste.	-

Electro-coagulation

Electro-coagulation is the conventional coagulation process with the addition of electric current that leads to the formation of hydroxide ions, which form a large surface area for adsorption of organic ions and colloidal particles from the substrate, and then deposited as insoluble flocks by electro-floatation. Improvements in electro-coagulation for pharmaceutical wastewater treatment have made it a popular choice, as the process utilizes alternative energy sources to drive the reactions. The application of an electric potential dissolves the anode, releasing active coagulant precursors in the electrocoagulation process. Researchers applied this method to real pharmaceutical wastewater, achieving a significant 72% reduction in COD loadings. Simultaneously, the BOD/COD ratio improved from 0.18 to 0.3. This approach demonstrates notable energy efficiency, high treatment capacity within a short timeframe, and a substantial enhancement in wastewater biodegradability [56]. It has been observed that when comparing basic electrocoagulation with its hybrid variants in terms of COD removal efficiency, the order of effectiveness is as follows:

peroxi-electrocoagulation > peroxi-photoelectrocoagulation > photoelectro-coagulation > electrocoagulation. Additionally, it leads to a progressive increase in COD remediation costs — particularly in Fenton's process, where hydrogen peroxide, the most expensive reagent, accounts for the majority of these expenses. This is a critical consideration, as the pH of the medium influences the conversion of higher-oxidation-state cations, the surface charge of coagulating species, and the COD removal efficiency, which peaks at a pH value specific to the underlying mechanism, whether adsorption or precipitation. Thus, pH needs careful monitoring. Since batch-mode systems may require further development and testing to achieve robustness, the technology remains immature. The need for multiple simultaneous, optimally coordinated reactions complicates process control, posing a significant challenge. Furthermore, a longer retention time indicated that, in the future, improved performance of integrated processes such as electrocoagulation and TiO2 photoassisted treatment, or biodegradability enhancement oxidation of the electrocoagulation byproducts, can be expected from this technique. Before the high electricity and electrode costs associated with the process can be justified, the possibility that flocks and coagulated species might turn out to be recalcitrant or engage in subsequent ecotoxic or stabilizing behavior that prevents the leaching of hazardous components must be explicitly addressed. Therefore, electrocoagulation is a rapid coagulation process driven by electricity [57 - 61]. This step can be skipped for studies that do not require text filtering, as it serves only as a pre-treatment. It is sensitive to pH, and the control of the simultaneous reaction is very difficult. Yet, a system for large-scale successful demonstration has to be developed [58].

Flotation

It is an effective solid-liquid and liquid-liquid separation method that utilizes numerous micro-bubbles to adhere to and concentrate impurities in water, lifting them to the surface for removal. The flotation process can be divided according to different ways to produce micro-bubbles, including electro-flotation, induced air flotation, and dissolved air flotation. The flotation process is commonly used to separate small particles with densities less than or close to that of water. Its advantages include lower investment and energy costs, a simple process, and easy maintenance [59].

Recent Methods of Membrane Separation

Detailed studies have shown that these emerging membrane-based systems can be compact, eco-friendly, flexible, economically viable, and easy to install, operate, and maintain. High selectivity of the applied membranes ensures such plants are characterized by a high degree of separation, while concentration polarization and membrane fouling must be combated with an appropriate module to allow sustainable operation of the plant. Quite a few such studies have demonstrated the reusability of water recovered after membrane-based filtration. It has been observed that a novel approach integrating a second reverse osmosis (RO) recovery unit with two-stage nanofiltration (NF) units can form a complete system eligible for Leadership in Energy and Environmental Design (LEED) certification as a water treatment plant. Thus, the present research on membrane technology utilization for the treatment of pharmaceutical wastewater directly revealed demonstrable proof of success and manifold benefits. Membrane processes have a high separation potential, and they may be a very effective tool in separating the organic loading and all obnoxious persistent causes. These modules feature relatively low maintenance costs, high flux, and strong environmental friendliness, making them a suitable technology. One such process is nanofiltration (NF), which can serve as a secondary treatment to remove residual medicinal drugs from municipal sludge and industrial effluents [60]. Table **2** gives the relative characteristics of different membrane processes. In the first part, the treatment of waste concentrates from pressure-driven membrane processes—particularly from RO—has been studied to some extent. Quite a few studies have been conducted in this field to develop techniques to treat secondary RO concentrates. A recent study shows that nanofiltration-forward osmosis can be an effective method for treating complex and hazardous pharmaceutical wastewater. This study presents a novel approach to pharmaceutical waste treatment, proposing new policy recommendations for industrial wastewater management, particularly relevant for rapidly growing economies with large populations. A novel design for the treatment scheme has successfully recovered reusable water from pharmaceutical wastewater, which largely overcomes the difficulties of internal and external concentration polarization of forward osmosis. Dynamic mathematical modeling of such integrated processes is necessary for industrial scale-up. Therefore, the Visual Basic software tools [61] have also been developed to facilitate the monitoring of the plant performance using a graphical interface in the well-known Microsoft Excel® environment for proper control and monitoring of such a membrane-integrated advanced treatment plant. Such plants, however, need to be efficient and economical for commercialization. Because of these studies, which augment the operational strategy, the development, accompanied by techno-economic analysis of such, needs to be considered.

Table 2. The relative characteristics of different membrane processes.

Process	Membrane	Transfer Mode	Pressure (atm)	References
Microfiltration	Porous Isotropic	Sieving and adsorption	500- 10,000	[56]
Ultrafiltration	Porous Asymmetric	Sieving and preferential	100- 2,000	[62]
Nanofiltration	Finely porous Asymmetric or composite	Sieving or electrostatic hydration or diffusive	20- 200	[63]
Reverse Osmosis	Non- porous Asymmetric or composite	Diffusive	10-100	[64]

Forward Osmosis (FO) and Membrane Distillation (MD) have been adapted to reduce the waste volume generated by the RO process and to recover water and other components from the RO concentrates. Furthermore, the required energy in such hybrid processes is greatly reduced. A critical oversight is the lack of discussion regarding the final concentrated effluents from FO processes and their subsequent handling. Treatment alone is insufficient without a comprehensive waste management strategy that addresses the disposal or reuse of these concentrates. However, the ecological danger from the active pharmaceutical compounds is still present and remains the risk of reaction of these compounds with other agents disposed of in the landfills. However, the disposal and effective management of the solid residues can be done by stabilizing the sludge and drying it before disposing it of [62]. The potential to emerge as the most sustainable technologies could be realized if final disposal is effectively managed. Unlike conventional or emerging technologies, tailor-made membranes offer the potential to completely separate toxic contaminants from water without adverse environmental impacts—a capability currently unmatched by existing or foreseeable alternatives in separation and purification [63].

Membrane-integrated Hybrid Technology

A membrane bioreactor is a powerful piece of equipment for the treatment of pharmaceutical wastewater in a consolidated form and municipal sludge. It offers significant advantages over conventional treatment processes, including superior sludge retention, greater compactness, the ability to handle fluctuating pollution loads, and consistent production of high-quality treated water at a reasonable cost. COD removal efficiency in membrane bioreactors has been shown to exceed 95% in a pilot-scale study. Hence, it is a particularly lucrative option for treating medicinal wastes, which are characterized by very high COD loadings [64]. Due to the effectiveness of the additives and some specific treatments, *e.g.*, electrocoagulation and advanced oxidation, as well as the treatment schemes where membrane bioreactors are integrated with some conventional techniques for a certain class of pharmaceuticals, the results have been highly successful [65]. Membrane bioreactors have an entire segment of research directed in this area, which includes possible integration of these with other existing processes or with new schemes like an integrative fungal bioreactor and Submerged membrane electro-bioreactor (SMEBR). Fig. (**1**) exhibits a membrane-bioreactor, while Fig. (**2**) shows a more compact design [66]. The combination of integrated membrane bioreactors and TiO_2 photocatalysis was investigated for the removal of non-degradable pharmaceuticals, such as carbamazepine, from simulated industrial pharmaceutical effluent. A recycling ratio of 4:1 (recycled material to discarded material) results in a 95% removal rate for carbamazepine. The respirometric tests indicated that the products of oxidation are mainly biodegradable and do not harm microbial activity, besides the elimination of effluent COD and the enhancement of sludge yield. However, in a few studies, the conventional physical processes, such as adsorption, can be integrated with bioreactors by selectively removing some adsorbents and transferring the bulk to the bioreactors, or by segmenting and treating the inorganic constituents in the adsorption chamber and inorganic

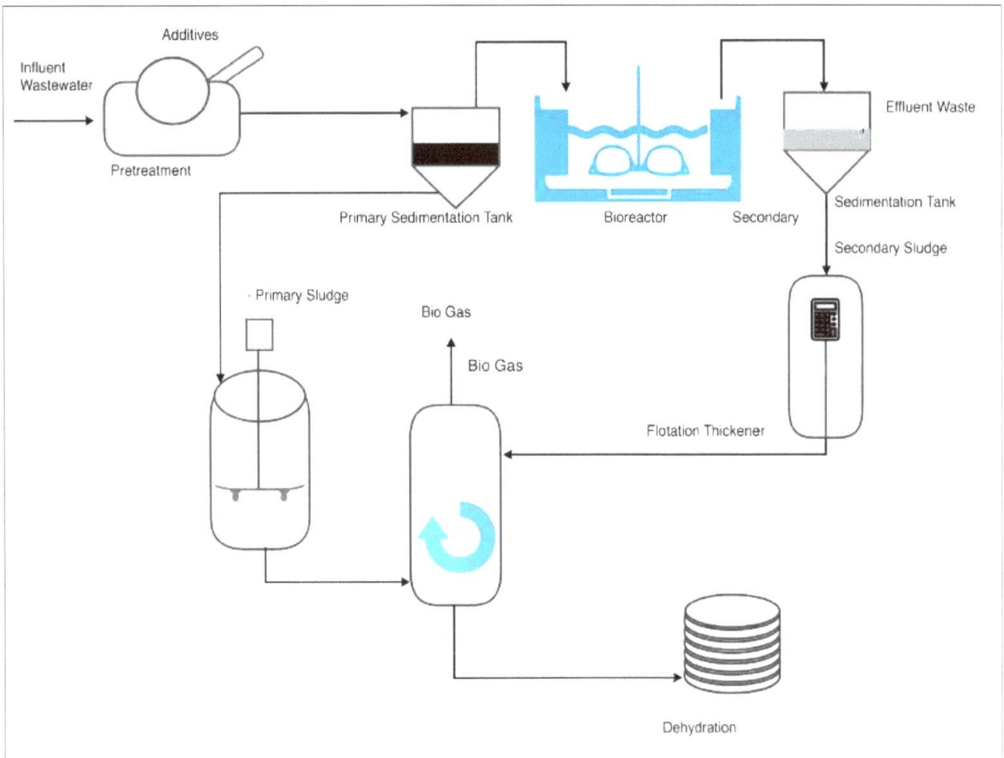

Fig. (1). Bioreactor treatment scheme [65].

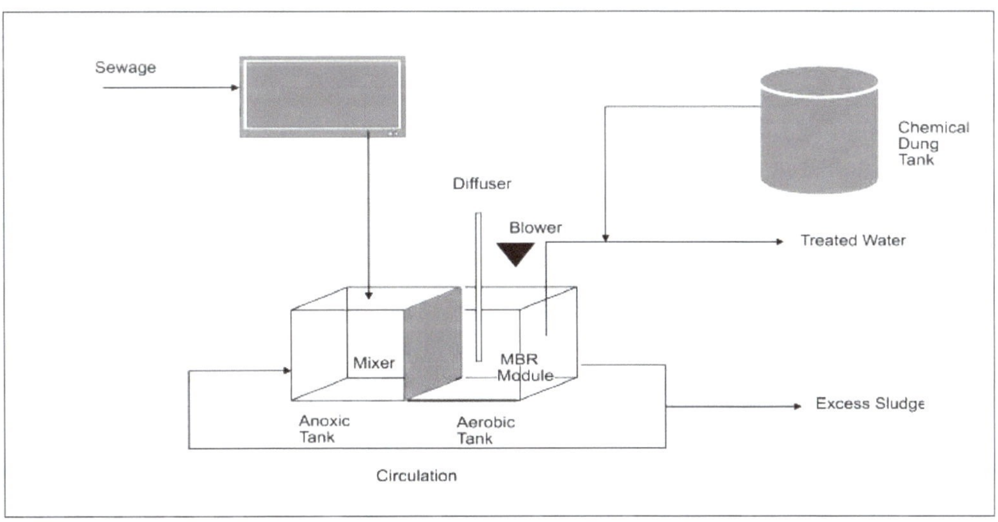

Fig. (2). A compact bioreactor module [66].

constituents in the reactor chamber [67]. While many of these systems are highly innovative, their effectiveness has not yet been demonstrated on a large scale or in continuous real-world operations. In Fig. (**3**) [68], some membrane-integrated hybrid treatment schemes are shown.

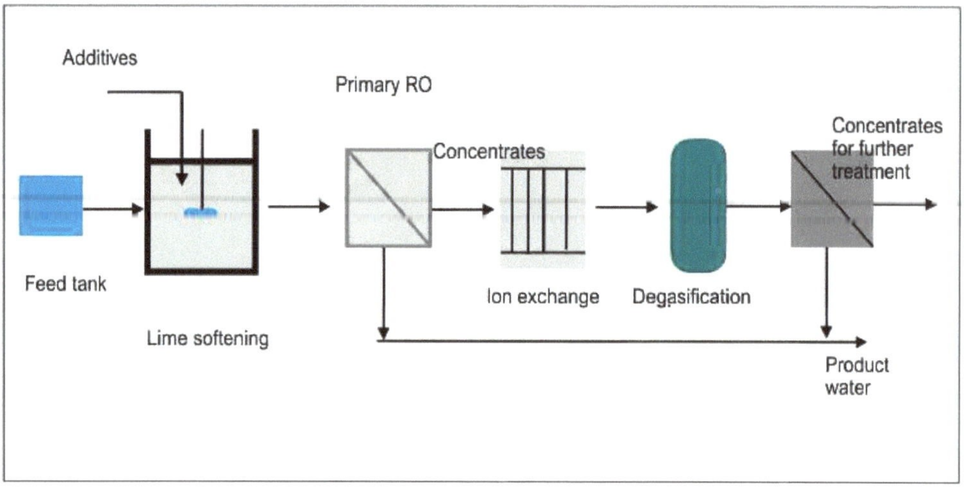

Fig. (3). A membrane–integrated hybrid treatment scheme [68].

By adding a membrane-integrated hybrid treatment scheme, not only can hazardous wastewater be converted into reusable water, but it can also potentially improve the plant's financial performance by recovering valuable byproducts. The recovery of struvite from hazardous wastewater using Fenton's method integrated with downstream membrane separation has been regarded as a classic example. The proposal of a novel approach for hazardous process wastewater treatment highlights that judicious selection and logical sequencing of unit operations can make treatment plants financially viable. By effectively processing poor-quality, toxic, or hazardous wastewaters, otherwise non-revenue-generating units can become financially attractive [69].

FUTURE TRENDS AND INNOVATIONS ADVANCEMENTS

Hybrid Technology on the Integration of Thermophilic Processes with Membrane Bioreactor

Thermophilic processes significantly improve organic matter removal yields, making them particularly suitable for treating waters containing toxic compounds or high salinity [70, 71]. The integrated thermophilic processes with the membrane reactor eliminate the disadvantage of poor sludge sedimentation by the inability of concerned particles in suspension to form flocks. The thermophilic aerobic membrane reactor enables processes capable of working with higher concentrations of biomass (greater than 50 kg TSS/m3) and thus, significantly reduces the reactor and the aeration tank volumes for dealing with high-strength liquid residues (rich in organic matter – COD, nutrients, and salinity) directly from the pharmaceutical industry. While thermophilic membrane bioreactors offer a compact design, they face challenges such as very low sludge production rates and the need for biomass acclimatization. These limitations must be addressed before the process can be considered competitive. In general, in the field of separation and purification, membranes do vary widely in terms of the degree of purification. Tailor-made membranes, which can be fabricated today with varied compatible materials of relatively high selectivity, reasonably high flux, and durability, can be promised [72]. A major issue, membrane fouling—which obstructs purification—has been largely resolved through improved designs for fouling-resistant membrane modules. If the most precise separation step always requires pre-filtration using microfiltration or ultrafiltration, the goal of minimizing frequent membrane cleaning or replacement will not be achieved. The great reduction in the filtration load of the fouling-sensitive membranes can be achieved through the integration of conventional coagulation-precipitation. However, the advent of a new generation of membranes—featuring excellent selectivity, high flux, long-term durability, fouling resistance, temperature stability, and chemical solvent compatibility—along with the development of fouling-free modules, has created new opportunities to meet these requirements, even at large scales. However, current scale-up confidence remains limited, preventing the direct transfer of membrane-integrated hybrid technologies to field deployment. This necessitates further pilot-scale studies and techno-economic analyses before the full-scale deployment of sustainable technology can be achieved to protect the integrity of surface water resources [73].

Zero Discharge Approach: Green Pharmacy and Biopharmaceuticals

Invariably, the best strategy in any waste management approach is the zero-discharge approach. The concept aims to eliminate waste generation during the manufacturing process, thereby ensuring it is environmentally sustainable ("green"). Even though it is extremely difficult to practically reach zero discharge, the production processes can be made as green as possible, resulting in the generation of only small amounts of waste. The green chemistry approach or green pharmacy approach is one such approach. In this concept, the product monitors its entire life cycle, and the product is made as innocuous as possible [74]. Production routes are selected to be carried out in fewer steps, requiring less energy and material, while minimizing undesired by-products. Any by-products generated should be readily biodegradable. The use of this approach makes the entire production process eco-friendly. Another green suggestion for production involves the production of biopharmaceuticals with biotechnology. They comprise biocatalysts, including enzymes and microorganisms isolated in the production of pharmacologically valuable materials. In addition to being environmentally friendly, they also bring an economic advantage over synthetic catalysts [75]. The greatest direct effect is anticipated on the management of pharmaceutical waste. Bio-catalytic processes can now be used to develop many of the obnoxiously persistent active pharmaceutical compounds that permeate most of the waste treatment plants into potentially biodegradable forms. Green Pharmacy has already started providing synthesis services for small-molecule APIs such as simvastatin, atorvastatin, pregabalin, paroxetine, and levetiracetam. Consequently, high conversion (>99%) and purity (>98%) of simvastatin and high throughput (200 g/L·day) and high yield (90–95%) with excellent stereo control [98% enantiomeric excess and 97% diastereomeric excess [76] can be obtained during biotransformation synthesis of atorvastatin. This technique is highly valuable as it truncates the process steps for atorvastatin, bypassing two of the most energy-intensive stages. This eliminates significant energy consumption and reduces waste by saving solvents and raw materials. It is estimated that such material saving is hundreds of metric tons per year. When we apply this technique, the use of hazardous reactions, for example, in the case of levetiracetam, where the conventional alkylation is replaced by a benign SN 2 reaction with a cheap pyrrolidinone, is eliminated. Notwithstanding the differences in opinion over the biodegradability of biopharmaceuticals, one thing is for sure: when there is less use of energy, materials, and a lesser generation of waste, the risk of pharmaceutical waste is avoided [77]. Membranes are used to concentrate waste to such a high level that it can be disposed of as solid material in minimal volumes. Currently, pharmaceutical manufacturers may not find the green chemistry approach to be economically attractive; however, in the long run, it will be beneficial to the various stakeholders and the environment. To accelerate the commissioning of green plants, green production processes must be investigated on a larger scale to build confidence in scale-up. Process intensification due to green production yields environmentally friendly production and offers operational flexibility with even lower workforce, material, energy, and capital requirements, promising higher profit margins [78]. However, recent publications have focused on modeling, economic analysis, and design aspects of novel advanced water treatment plants, with major emphasis on innovative developments. Incremental technological improvements are insufficient to address massive environmental pollution problems; novel solutions are essential [79].

CONCLUSION

The pharmaceutical industry is one of the world's largest and most prominent sectors. However, the worsening pollution caused by pharmaceutical waste today underscores the need for a sustainable treatment process. A range of different treatment technologies should be adopted to meet the discharge standard. The continuous accumulation, toxicity, persistence, and development of microorganismal strains resistant to drugs constitute a threat to the ecosystem due to the pharmaceutically active compounds. The result is often a treated waste that still contains pharmaceutically active compounds, demonstrating the inadequacy of existing treatment technologies. However, thermal incineration of highly hazardous medical waste has been adopted in 90% of cases, and has never been environmentally justified due to the release of toxins and the indirect transfer of obnoxious substances from one phase of the environment to another. However, it is very difficult to determine whether there are thousands of APIs in the water environment and what impact they have on the ecotoxicological effects. Therefore, targeted attention should be given to the most widely used and most accumulated pharmaceuticals. Over the decades, extensive research on pharmaceutical waste treatment has been conducted. However, the vast majority of these studies relied solely on synthetic solutions in lab-scale experiments, resulting in low scale-up confidence due to the absence of techno-economic feasibility analyses. However, the problem continues to persist and, in fact, worsens with the growing population and the generation of pharmaceuticals, with concomitant discharge of hazardous waste from these production plants; a change in this strategy of waste management is therefore indispensable. The most environmentally desired approach for producing pharmaceuticals seems to be a green chemistry, and the biological transformation of the waste pharmaceutical ingredients into harmless substances. Long-term environmental desirability, technology efficiency, social acceptability, and economic viability will determine the selected technology. Research and development efforts towards new treatment schemes will continue. The current state of the art necessitates that, alongside the hundreds of available lab-scale treatment options, those technologies demonstrating strong potential for high-efficiency separation and purification at affordable costs must be urgently advanced to pilot-scale studies. These studies must comprehensively address all relevant techno-economic challenges. This will pave the way for implementing some sustainable technologies until more mature solutions emerge. However, the optimal long-term strategy remains transitioning to green production technologies.

REFERENCES

[1] Vijayalakshmi MK, Showbharnikhaa S, Snega K, Nadhiya J, Akshaya T, Muthu Kaviya M. Pharmaceutical waste management. J Pharma Insights Res 2023; 1(2): 166-73.

[2] Sreekanth K, Vishal GN, Raghunandan HV, Nitin KU. A review on managing of pharmaceutical waste in industry. Int J Pharm Tech Res 2014; 6(3): 899-907.

[3] Veal L. United States environmental protection agency. US Environmental Protection Agency (EPA)(2005) National Management Measures to Control Non-Point Source Pollution for Urban Areas. 2021 Jun 7.

[4] US Environmental Protection Agency. Hospital surface disinfectant and deodorizer. EPA Reg. No. 3862-104. Washington (DC): EPA; 2020.

[5] Giakoumakis G, Politi D, Sidiras D. Medical waste treatment technologies for energy, fuels, and materials production: A review. Energies 2021; 14(23): 8065.
[http://dx.doi.org/10.3390/en14238065]

[6] Trueman P, Lowson K, Blighe A. Evaluation of the scale, causes and costs of waste medicines: final report. York: York Health Economics Consortium and School of Pharmacy, University of London; 2010.

[7] Wettstein DJ, Boes S. Effectiveness of national pricing policies for patent-protected pharmaceuticals in the OECD: a systematic literature review. Appl Health Econ Health Policy 2019; 17(2): 143-62.
[http://dx.doi.org/10.1007/s40258-018-0437-z] [PMID: 30367350]

[8] MacDonald K, Taylor M, Gardiner K, Gunn T, Singleton J. An observational cross-sectional study of pharmaceuticalwaste disposal practices in Australian medical imagingdepartments: A comparison of community versus hospitalpractice. Radiography. 2024; 30: 1342-1348.
[http://dx.doi.org/10.1016/j.radi.2024.07.009]

[9] Ahmed B, Rizvi A, Khan MS. Microbial biosorption: a sustainable approach for metal removal and environmental remediation. Int J Environ Sci Technol. 2025; 22: 13245-13276.
[http://dx.doi.org/10.1007/s13762-025-06611-1]

[10] Castensson S. Pharmaceutical waste In: Kümmerer K Ed Pharmaceuticals in the environment: Sources, fate, effects and risks. Berlin, Heidelberg: Springer 2008; pp. 489-99.
[http://dx.doi.org/10.1007/978-3-540-74664-5_31]

[11] Attrah M, Elmanadely A, Akter D, Rene ER. A review on medical waste management: treatment, recycling, and disposal options. Environments (Basel) 2022; 9(11): 146.
[http://dx.doi.org/10.3390/environments9110146]

[12] Gupta R, Sati B, Gupta A. Treatment and Recycling of Wastewater from Pharmaceutical Industry. In: Singh R, Singh R, Eds. Advances in Biological Treatment of Industrial Waste Water and Their Recycling for a Sustainable Future. Singapore: Springer 2019; pp. 247-68.
[http://dx.doi.org/10.1007/978-981-13-1468-1_9]

[13] Sapkota B, Pariatamby A. Pharmaceutical waste management system – Are the current techniques sustainable, eco-friendly and circular? A review. Waste Manag 2023; 168: 83-97.
[http://dx.doi.org/10.1016/j.wasman.2023.05.052] [PMID: 37285639]

[14] Dalal SP, Dalal P, Motiani R, Solanki V. Experimental investigation on recycling of waste pharmaceutical blister powder as partial replacement of fine aggregate in concrete. Resour Conserv Recycl Adv 2022; 14: 200076.
[http://dx.doi.org/10.1016/j.rcradv.2022.200076]

[15] Toh MR, Chew L. Turning waste medicines to cost savings: A pilot study on the feasibility of medication recycling as a solution to drug wastage. Palliat Med 2017; 31(1): 35-41.
[http://dx.doi.org/10.1177/0269216316639798] [PMID: 27430975]

[16] Azzahra L, Saptarini NM. Pharmaceutical Industrial Waste Regulation in Five Countries in Asia. Indones J Pharm 2021; 3(1): 9.
[http://dx.doi.org/10.24198/idjp.v3i1.33383]

[17] Kakaraparthy R, Palivela N, Reddy Karri L G. Chemotherapeutic Challenge: A Case of Acute Kidney

Injury During Breast Cancer Management. Indian Journal of Pharmacy Practice 2025; 19(1): 116-9. [http://dx.doi.org/10.5530/ijopp.9.1.2]

[18] Rajbongshi S, Shah YD, Sajib AU. Pharmaceutical waste management: a review. Eur J Biomed Pharm Sci 2016; 3(12): 192-206.

[19] Jaseem M, Kumar P, John RM. An overview of waste management in pharmaceutical industry. Pharma Innov 2017; 6(3, Part C): 158.

[20] Zhou J, Wu H, Shi L, *et al.* Sustainable on-farm strategy for the disposal of antibiotic fermentation residue: co-benefits for resource recovery and resistance mitigation. J Hazard Mater 2023; 446130705 [http://dx.doi.org/10.1016/j.jhazmat.2022.130705]

[21] Nikolić B, Nikolić N, Milošević A, Milošević-Georgiev A. Opportunities for sustainable waste management in the pharmaceutical industry declaration of competing interest. Arh Farm (Belgr) 2024; 74(6): 832-51.
[http://dx.doi.org/10.5937/arhfarm74-52016]

[22] Bungau S, Tit D, Fodor K, *et al.* Aspects regarding the pharmaceutical waste management in Romania. Sustainability (Basel) 2018; 10(8): 2788.
[http://dx.doi.org/10.3390/su10082788]

[23] Pandit P, Misal R, Pawar G, Davkar S. Approaches of pharmaceutical waste management and handling. Systematic Reviews in Pharmacy 2024; 15(8): 251-6.

[24] Pal P. Treatment and disposal of pharmaceutical wastewater: toward the sustainable strategy. Separ Purif Rev 2018; 47(3): 179-98.
[http://dx.doi.org/10.1080/15422119.2017.1354888]

[25] Kumar D, Malviya R, Singh DP. Innovative Techniques for Pharmaceutical Waste Management: Enhancing Drug Recovery and Environmental Sustainability. Curr Green Chem 2025; 12(2): 138-45. [http://dx.doi.org/10.2174/0122133461322762240926072018]

[26] Brechtelsbauer E, Shah S. Update on pharmaceutical waste disposal regulations: Strategies for success. Am J Health Syst Pharm 2020; 77(7): 574-82.
[http://dx.doi.org/10.1093/ajhp/zxz360] [PMID: 32050015]

[27] Ojha S, Tripathi S M, Vishwakarma P K, Mishra S. Pharmaceuticals in the water: emerging concerns and innovative remediation solutions Curr Green Chem 2024 Mar 01; 11(1): 50-62.

[28] Mohammed SA, Kahissay MH, Hailu AD. Pharmaceuticals wastage and pharmaceuticals waste management in public health facilities of Dessie town, North East Ethiopia. PLoS One 2021; 16(10): e0259160.
[http://dx.doi.org/10.1371/journal.pone.0259160] [PMID: 34710189]

[29] Ariffin M. Regulatory Gaps in Pharmaceutical Waste Management: A Case Study of Malaysia. International Journal of Research and Innovation in Social Science 2024; VIII(X): 813-20. [http://dx.doi.org/10.47772/IJRISS.2024.8100066]

[30] Jani M, Kumari S. Pharmaceutical Wastewater and Environmental Contamination: Challenges, Innovations, and Future Direction. PEXACY Int J Pharm Sci 2024; 3(1): 79-98.

[31] Khatoon Z, Orozco-Mosqueda MC, Santoyo G. Microbial contributions to heavy metal phytoremediation in agricultural soils: a review. Microorganisms. 2024; 12(10): 1945. [http://dx.doi.org/10.3390/microorganisms12101945]

[32] Fakhri B MS, Ghassemi Barghi N, Moradnia Mehdikhanmahaleh M, *et al.* Pharmaceutical wastewater toxicity: An ignored threat to the public health. Sustainable Environment 2024; 10(1): 2322821. [http://dx.doi.org/10.1080/27658511.2024.2322821]

[33] Agarwal S, Saha H, Kaushik S, Patil VM, Verma S. Critical Review of Biomedical Waste Management for Future Pandemics: Pharmaceutical Perspective. J Chem Health Saf 2024; 31(6): 444-67.

[http://dx.doi.org/10.1021/acs.chas.4c00067]

[34] Ai X, Zhang X, Tian Y, Lu M, Wang W. Research status, key technologies and development trends of pharmaceutical waste salt treatment technology: A review. Waste Manag Res: The J Sus Circular Eco 2025; 43(10): 1525-47.

[35] Akwalu EK. Green Supply Chain Management Practices and Sustainability of Pharmaceutical Firms: A Systematic Literature Review. Afr Multidiscip J Res 2024; 9(II): 92-107.

[36] Hosseini-Motlagh SM, Jazinaninejad M, Nami N. Coordinating a socially concerned reverse supply chain for pharmaceutical waste management considering government role. Environ Dev Sustain 2022; 24(2): 1852-77.
[http://dx.doi.org/10.1007/s10668-021-01511-z]

[37] Mahmoodzadeh F, Navidjouy N, Jafari SJ, Soltani F, Rezai H. Infectious, Chemical, and Pharmaceutical Waste Management: A Case Study from Northwest Iran. J Health Syst Res 2025; 21(1): 107-12.

[38] Sapkota B, Pariatamby A. Pharmaceutical waste management legislations: Where do ASEAN countries stand in harmonization? A review of regulatory documents. Waste Manag 2025; 195: 107-28.
[http://dx.doi.org/10.1016/j.wasman.2025.01.039] [PMID: 39908624]

[39] Sági G, Suresh D P, Takács E, Wojnárovits L. Pharmaceutical Waste Management by Ionizing Technology. In: Shayanfar S, Pillai S D, Eds. Ionizing Radiation Technologies: Managing and Extracting Value from Wastes. Hoboken (NJ): Wiley 2022; pp. 301-24.
[http://dx.doi.org/10.1002/9781119488583.ch14]

[40] Rogowska J, Zimmermann A. Household pharmaceutical waste disposal as a global problem—a review. Int J Environ Res Public Health 2022; 19(23): 15798.
[http://dx.doi.org/10.3390/ijerph192315798] [PMID: 36497873]

[41] Alshemari A, Breen L, Quinn G, Sivarajah U. Can we create a circular pharmaceutical supply chain (CPSC) to reduce medicines waste? Pharmacy (Basel) 2020; 8(4): 221.
[http://dx.doi.org/10.3390/pharmacy8040221] [PMID: 33218038]

[42] Tushir R, Das S, Chauhan A, *et al.* Exponential Global Health Hazards of Pharmaceutical Pollution and Its Preventive Measures: A Comprehensive Review. J Environ Health Sustain Dev 2025; 10(1): 2499-520.
[http://dx.doi.org/10.18502/jehsd.v10i1.18298]

[43] Almeida MAR, Wilson AMMM, Peterlini MAS. Evaluating pharmaceutical waste disposal in pediatric units. Rev Esc Enferm USP 2016; 50(6): 922-8.
[http://dx.doi.org/10.1590/s0080-623420160000700007] [PMID: 28198956]

[44] Kawade H M, Kokare D M. Development Strategies for Pharmaceutical Waste Management: In View of Healthcare Perspectives. In: Raut N A, Kokare D M, Dhoble S J, Eds. 360-Degree Waste Management, Volume 2: Biomedical, Pharmaceutical, Industrial Waste, and Remediation. Amsterdam: Elsevier 2023; pp. 97-121.
[http://dx.doi.org/10.1016/B978-0-323-90909-9.00006-X]

[45] Shetty A, Gupta G. Design Methodologies for Eco-friendly Pharmaceutical Waste Management - A Review. In: Singh H, Garg P, Kaur I, Eds. Proceedings of the 1st International Conference on Sustainable Waste Management through Design: ICSWMD 2018. Cham: Springer 2019; pp. 624-33.
[http://dx.doi.org/10.1007/978-3-030-02707-0_66]

[46] Das AK, Islam MN, Billah MM, Sarker A. COVID-19 pandemic and healthcare solid waste management strategy – A mini-review. Sci Total Environ 2021; 778: 146220.
[http://dx.doi.org/10.1016/j.scitotenv.2021.146220] [PMID: 33711590]

[47] Toma A, Crişan O. Green pharmacy - a narrative review. Clujul Med 2018; 91(4): 391-8.
[PMID: 30564014]

[48] Hasan MM, Rahman MH. Assessment of healthcare waste management paradigms and its suitable treatment alternative: a case study. J Environ Public Health 2018; 2018(1): 1-14.
[http://dx.doi.org/10.1155/2018/6879751] [PMID: 30151013]

[49] Manojlović J, Jovanović V, Georgiev AM, Tesink JG, Arsić T, Marinković V. Pharmaceutical waste management in pharmacies at the primary level of health care in Serbia-situation analysis. Indian Journal of Pharmaceutical Education and Research 2015; 49(2): 106-11.
[http://dx.doi.org/10.5530/ijper.49.2.5]

[50] Khan BA, Cheng L, Khan AA, Ahmed H. Healthcare waste management in Asian developing countries: A mini review. Waste Manag Res 2019; 37(9): 863-75.
[http://dx.doi.org/10.1177/0734242X19857470] [PMID: 31266407]

[51] Upadhyay S, Sinha A. Waste Management in Indian Pharmaceutical Industries. In: Yadav S, Negm A M, Yadava R N, Eds. Environmental Management in India: Waste to Wealth. Cham: Springer 2022; pp. 89-112.
[http://dx.doi.org/10.1007/978-3-030-93897-0_5]

[52] Kumar R, Pal P. Assessing the feasibility of N and P recovery by struvite precipitation from nutrient-rich wastewater: a review. Environ Sci Pollut Res Int 2015; 22(22): 17453-64.
[http://dx.doi.org/10.1007/s11356-015-5450-2] [PMID: 26408116]

[53] Lucas MS, Peres JA, Li Puma G. Advanced oxidation processes for water and wastewater treatment. Water 2021; 13(9): 1309.
[http://dx.doi.org/10.3390/w13091309]

[54] Başaran Dindaş G, Çalışkan Y, Çelebi EE, Tekbaş M, Bektaş N, Yatmaz HC. Treatment of pharmaceutical wastewater by combination of electrocoagulation, electro-fenton and photocatalytic oxidation processes. J Environ Chem Eng 2020; 8(3): 103777.
[http://dx.doi.org/10.1016/j.jece.2020.103777]

[55] Alam R, Sheob M, Saeed B, *et al.* Use of electrocoagulation for treatment of pharmaceutical compounds in water/wastewater: A review exploring opportunities and challenges. Water 2021; 13(15): 2105.
[http://dx.doi.org/10.3390/w13152105]

[56] Zhang Y, Liu J, Wang X, *et al.* Advances in microbial remediation of heavy metal-contaminated soils: mechanisms, synergistic technologies, field applications and future perspectives. Toxics. 2025; 13(12): 1069.
[http://dx.doi.org/10.3390/toxics13121069]

[57] Islam MM, Saxena N, Sharma D. Phytoremediation as a green and sustainable prospective method for heavy metal contamination: a review. RSC Sustain. 2024; 2: 1269-1288.
[http://dx.doi.org/10.1039/D3SU00440F]

[58] Kaur H, Hippargi G, Pophali G R, Bansiwal A K. Treatment methods for removal of pharmaceuticals and personal care products from domestic wastewater. In: Prasad M N V, Vithanage M, Kapley A, Eds. Pharmaceuticals and Personal Care Products: Waste Management and Treatment Technology. Kidlington: Elsevier 2019; pp. 129-50.
[http://dx.doi.org/10.1016/B978-0-12-816189-0.00006-8]

[59] Cheng H, Xu W, Liu J, Wang H, He Y, Chen G. Pretreatment of wastewater from triazine manufacturing by coagulation, electrolysis, and internal microelectrolysis. J Hazard Mater 2007; 146(1-2): 385-92.
[http://dx.doi.org/10.1016/j.jhazmat.2006.12.038] [PMID: 17229523]

[60] Imad EM, Asim AE, Tasneem JM, Wadha MM, Bhagavathula AS. Management of post-consumer pharmaceutical waste: an overview. SOJ Pharm Pharm Sci 2017; 4(5): 1-5.

[61] Trumbulović L, Pavlović M, Radulović D, Petrov M, Andrić L. Pharmaceutical waste managment. In: Marković Z, Ed. XII International Symposium on Recycling Technologies and Sustainable

Development. 2017 Sep 13-15; Bor, Serbia. Bor: University of Belgrade, Technical Faculty in Bor 2017; pp. 270-7.

[62] Pandis PK, Kalogirou C, Kanellou E, *et al.* Key points of advanced oxidation processes (AOPs) for wastewater, organic pollutants and pharmaceutical waste treatment: A mini review. ChemEngineering 2022; 6(1): 8.
[http://dx.doi.org/10.3390/chemengineering6010008]

[63] Fazal S, Zhang B, Zhong Z, Gao L, Lu X. Membrane separation technology on pharmaceutical wastewater by using MBR (Membrane Bioreactor). J Environ Prot (Irvine Calif) 2015; 6(4): 299-307.
[http://dx.doi.org/10.4236/jep.2015.64030]

[64] Fonseca Couto C, Lange LC, Santos Amaral MC. A critical review on membrane separation processes applied to remove pharmaceutically active compounds from water and wastewater. J Water Process Eng 2018; 26: 156-75.
[http://dx.doi.org/10.1016/j.jwpe.2018.10.010]

[65] Thakur AK, Kumar R, Kumar A, *et al.* Pharmaceutical waste-water treatment *via* advanced oxidation based integrated processes: An engineering and economic perspective. J Water Process Eng 2023; 54: 103977.
[http://dx.doi.org/10.1016/j.jwpe.2023.103977]

[66] Calisto V, Ferreira CIA, Oliveira JABP, Otero M, Esteves VI. Adsorptive removal of pharmaceuticals from water by commercial and waste-based carbons. J Environ Manage 2015; 152: 83-90.
[http://dx.doi.org/10.1016/j.jenvman.2015.01.019] [PMID: 25617872]

[67] Ferrer-Polonio E, Fernández-Navarro J, Iborra-Clar MI, Alcaina-Miranda MI, Mendoza-Roca JA. Removal of pharmaceutical compounds commonly-found in wastewater through a hybrid biological and adsorption process. J Environ Manage 2020; 263: 110368.
[http://dx.doi.org/10.1016/j.jenvman.2020.110368] [PMID: 32883474]

[68] Mamo J, García-Galán MJ, Stefani M, *et al.* Fate of pharmaceuticals and their transformation products in integrated membrane systems for wastewater reclamation. Chem Eng J 2018; 331: 450-61.
[http://dx.doi.org/10.1016/j.cej.2017.08.050]

[69] Eniola JO, Kumar R, Barakat MA, Rashid J. A review on conventional and advanced hybrid technologies for pharmaceutical wastewater treatment. J Clean Prod 2022; 356: 131826.
[http://dx.doi.org/10.1016/j.jclepro.2022.131826]

[70] Ghazal H, Koumaki E, Hoslett J, *et al.* Insights into current physical, chemical and hybrid technologies used for the treatment of wastewater contaminated with pharmaceuticals. J Clean Prod 2022; 361: 132079.
[http://dx.doi.org/10.1016/j.jclepro.2022.132079]

[71] Abdelhaleem A, Aziz F, Alalm MG, Mahmoud AE. Hybrid Treatment Technologies for the Removal of Pharmaceuticals in Wastewater InEnvironmental Nexus Approach. CRC Press 2024; pp. 20-40.

[72] Hassan ZU, Rehman M, Ali S. Heavy metal pollution and transformation in soil: a comprehensive review of natural bioremediation strategies. J Umm Al-Qura Univ Appl Sci. 2025; 11: 528-544.
[http://dx.doi.org/10.1007/s43994-025-00241-6]

[73] Sun W, Ma G, Sun Y, *et al.* Effective treatment of high phosphorus pharmaceutical wastewater by chemical precipitation. Can J Chem Eng 2017; 95(8): 1585-93.
[http://dx.doi.org/10.1002/cjce.22799]

[74] Rashed IGAA, Afify HA, Ahmed AEM, Ayoub MAES. Optimization of chemical precipitation to improve the primary treatment of wastewater. Desalination Water Treat 2013; 51(37-39): 7048-56.
[http://dx.doi.org/10.1080/19443994.2013.792147]

[75] Lykouras M, Isari E A, Grilla E, Kokkinos P, Kalavrouziotis I K. The Role of Biochar and Earthworms in Pharmaceutical Remediation of Contaminated Soil: A Systematic Review Environ Process 2026 Mar; 13(1): 2.

[76] Zaied BK, Rashid M, Nasrullah M, Zularisam AW, Pant D, Singh L. A comprehensive review on contaminants removal from pharmaceutical wastewater by electrocoagulation process. Sci Total Environ 2020; 726: 138095.
[http://dx.doi.org/10.1016/j.scitotenv.2020.138095] [PMID: 32481207]

[77] Das TK, Ed. Toward zero discharge: innovative methodology and technologies for process pollution prevention. John Wiley & Sons 2005.

[78] Badawi AK, Hassan R. Optimizing sludge extract reuse from physico-chemical processes for zero-waste discharge: A critical review. Desalination Water Treat 2024; 319: 100527.
[http://dx.doi.org/10.1016/j.dwt.2024.100527]

[79] Sharma R, Prakash N, Kumari S, *et al.* From Challenges to Opportunities: Exploring Minimum Liquid Discharge and Zero Liquid Discharge Strategies for Wastewater Management and Resource Recovery. Role of Science and Technology for Sustainable Future. Singapore: Springer Nature 2025; pp. 371-94.

CHAPTER 5

Novel Recycling Technologies for Pharmaceutical Waste

Rakesh Swain[1], **Ankita Moharana**[2,*], **Swagatam Sahoo**[3], **Sujit Kumar Martha**[4] and **Snigdha Rani Behera**[2]

[1] *School of Pharmaceutical Sciences, Siksha O Anusandhan Deemed to be University, Bhubaneswar, Odisha, India*

[2] *School of Pharmacy, ARKA JAIN University, Jamshedpur, Jharkhand, India*

[3] *School of Pharmacy, DRIEMS University, Tangi, Tangi, Cuttack, Odisha, India*

[4] *Department of Pharmaceutical Analysis, Jeypore College of Pharmacy, Jeypore, Odisha, India*

Abstract: Innovative recycling techniques should focus on pharmaceutical waste since sustainable environmental practices have become a major global issue. Pharmaceuticals pose substantial dangers to both the environment and public health because improper disposal of these substances remains widespread. Standard pharmaceutical waste disposal practices, such as landfilling and incineration, are inefficient for both waste management and sustainability. Modern recycling technologies offer genuine solutions to control pharmaceutical waste while promoting sustainability initiatives. The purpose of these technological methods is to extract important compounds, including excipients alongside active pharmaceutical ingredients (APIs) and additional bioactive components from discarded medications. Modern methods of solvent extraction, chemical reprocessing and biocatalytic breakdown processes separate pharmaceutical waste into reusable components. The research addresses the development of membrane filtration and adsorption technologies as advanced filtration techniques to recover valuable resources while achieving purification. Companies are exploring the development of waste monitoring systems that combine waste identification along with recycling methods through advanced AI and IoT technologies. Innovative recycling methods convert waste materials into useful resources, helping reduce environmental degradation from pharmaceutical waste while establishing circular economic systems. A comprehensive discussion of modern pharmaceutical waste recycling methods appears in this section, followed by a review of both existing possibilities and future expectations within this nascent discipline.

Keywords: Active pharmaceutical ingredients, Environmental sustainability, Pharmaceutical waste, Recycling technologies, Waste management.

[*] **Corresponding author Ankita Moharana:** School of Pharmacy, ARKA JAIN University, Jamshedpur, Jharkhand, India; E-mail: ankitamoharana333@gmail.com

Suman Gautam, Jai Narayan Mishra, Preeti Mishra, Preeti Verma & Sudhanshu Mishra (Eds.)

INTRODUCTION

The term pharmaceutical waste includes expired medications, unused medications and unwanted pharmaceutical items, including chemicals and non-pharmaceutical materials that have lost their use because they have either expired or gone unused or are unwanted by users. Multiple areas, including healthcare institutions, clinics and pharmacies, and domestic spaces, generate this type of waste. Poor pharmaceutical waste management produces multiple environmental threats, such as water contamination and ecological damage, because it allows drugs to affect wildlife and creates drug-resistant microorganisms [1].

Handling pharmaceutical waste is a vital practice because it safeguards human health while protecting the environment from harmful effects. A series of procedures exists to properly identify hazardous pharmaceuticals before safely separating them for disposal, which follows governmental regulations. The growing pharmaceutical industry poses significant challenges for effective pharmaceutical waste management. Strategies that focus on pharmaceutical waste management need to become standard practice because they reduce the environmental impacts while making medicine use both safe and sustainable [2].

Standard waste management methods for pharmaceuticals aim to reduce both environmental pollution and public health risks. The disposal process applies to medications across three categories: expired products, unused materials and substances contaminated with contamination, and production scraps. The following list contains the most typical techniques used for pharmaceutical waste management.

INCINERATION

Incineration is one of the most reliable methods for healthcare facilities to dispose of hazardous pharmaceutical waste, expired drugs, cytotoxic (chemotherapy) waste, and controlled substances by burning them at high temperatures for safe decomposition into nontoxic byproducts.

Pre-Incineration Steps

A separation process arranges hazardous pharmaceutical waste (such as chemotherapy drugs along with antibiotics) separately from all other waste streams. The waste undergoes proper packaging in burnable sealed containers while abstaining from using PVC containers because they release dioxins during the process [2]. The collected waste travels to professional facilities for sanctioned incineration services.

Incineration Stages

The incineration process occurs in distinct temperature-dependent stages, each serving a critical function in waste treatment (Table **1**).

Table 1. Different stages of incineration [3].

Stage	Temperature	Process
Drying & Ignition	200–400°C	Moisture evaporates; waste starts burning.
Primary Combustion	850–1,000°C	Organic compounds break down into gases and ash.
Secondary Combustion	1,100–1,200°C	Toxic gases (*e.g.*, dioxins) are further oxidized.
Flue Gas Treatment	≥ 1200°C	Scrubbing removes acidic gases (HCl, SO_2), and filters capture particulate matter.
Ash Disposal	1200–1600°C	Residual ash (non-hazardous) is landfilled or used in construction.

Types of Incinerators for Pharmaceutical Waste

Table **2** compares four primary incinerator types used for pharmaceutical waste treatment, outlining their optimal applications, advantages, and disadvantages.

Table 2. Different types of incinerators [4].

Type	Best For	Advantages	Disadvantages
Rotary Kiln	Hazardous, liquid, solid waste	High efficiency, handles diverse waste	High cost, complex maintenance
Static Hearth	Small-scale medical waste	Simple operation	Lower temperature range
Fluidized Bed	Powder/liquid waste	Uniform burning, low emissions	Not for large, solid items
Pyrolysis/Gasification	Advanced treatment	Energy recovery, fewer emissions	Expensive, limited availability

Advantages of Incineration

- **Complete Destruction:** Eliminates toxic drugs (*e.g.*, chemotherapy agents, opioids).
- **Volume Reduction:** Converts waste into sterile ash (90% less volume).
- **Pathogen Elimination:** Kills bacteria, viruses, and prions.
- **Energy Recovery:** Some plants convert heat into electricity (Waste-to-Energy).

Disadvantages & Risks

- **Air Pollution:** If temperatures <850°C, may release:

Dioxins/Furans (from burning PVC plastics).

Heavy Metals (*e.g.*, mercury in some drugs).

High Cost: Requires advanced scrubbers and filters.

Public Opposition: Concerns over emissions and health impacts.

Alternatives to Incineration

- Autoclaving (for non-hazardous waste).
- Chemical Neutralization (for liquid lab waste).
- Plasma Arc Gasification (emerging zero-emission tech).

LANDFILL DISPOSAL

- Landfill disposal has been widely used in the past, but is now recognized as environmentally harmful and increasingly regulated [5]. Here is an overview of landfill disposal for pharmaceutical waste and its associated concerns:

Process:

- Unused or expired medications are discarded into municipal solid waste (MSW) landfills.
- In some cases, pharmaceuticals are first rendered "unusable" (*e.g.*, mixed with inert materials) to discourage diversion.
- Waste may be sent to secured landfills with liners and leachate collection systems to reduce environmental contamination [5].

Types of Pharmaceutical Waste Suitable for Landfills:

- Non-hazardous medications (*e.g.*, certain over-the-counter drugs).
- Some regulated medical waste (if treated and deemed safe).

Environmental and Health Concerns

- **Leachate Contamination:** Landfills produce leachate (liquid waste) that can seep into groundwater, potentially carrying active pharmaceutical ingredients (APIs).
- **Ecosystem Impact:** Trace pharmaceuticals have been detected in water supplies, affecting aquatic life and potentially entering the human food chain.

- **Antibiotic Resistance:** Improper disposal of antibiotics may contribute to the spread of antimicrobial resistance (AMR).
- **Regulatory Restrictions:** Many countries now ban or restrict landfill disposal of pharmaceuticals due to environmental risks (*e.g.*, the EU's Waste Framework Directive, U.S. EPA guidelines).

Alternatives to Landfill Disposal

- Due to these concerns, modern pharmaceutical waste management favors:
- Incineration (high-temperature destruction, especially for hazardous drugs).
- Chemical Neutralization (for certain liquid pharmaceuticals).
- Take-Back Programs (pharmacy or manufacturer-led collection).
- Reverse Distribution (returning unused drugs for credit or proper disposal).
- Biological Treatment (experimental methods like biodegradation)

CHEMICAL TREATMENT

- Chemical treatment is a conventional pharmaceutical waste management technique that involves using chemical reactions to neutralize, degrade, or immobilize hazardous components in pharmaceutical waste [6]. This method is often used for liquid pharmaceutical waste (*e.g.*, expired syrups, chemotherapy drugs, antibiotics) but can also treat certain solid forms.

Types of Chemical Treatment Methods

- Oxidation (Advanced Oxidation Processes - AOPs)
  - Uses strong oxidizing agents (*e.g.*, hydrogen peroxide, ozone, Fenton's reagent) to break down pharmaceutical compounds.
  - Effective against antibiotics, hormones, and cytotoxic drugs.
  - Example: Ozonation destroys persistent organic pollutants in wastewater.
- Hydrolysis (Alkaline or Acidic Hydrolysis)
  - Uses high pH (alkaline) or low pH (acidic) conditions to break down drugs into less harmful byproducts.
  - Common for penicillin-based antibiotics and beta-lactam drugs.
  - Example: Sodium hydroxide (NaOH) treatment degrades amoxicillin.
- Chemical Precipitation
  - Adds reagents (*e.g.*, alum, ferric chloride) to form insoluble complexes, removing heavy metals and certain drugs from liquid waste [7].
  - Used in hospital wastewater treatment.
- Neutralization
  - Adjusts the pH of acidic or alkaline pharmaceutical waste to make it safer for disposal.
  - Example: Neutralizing chemotherapy waste (*e.g.*, cyclophosphamide

solutions) before disposal.

- Chlorination (Less Common Due to Byproduct Risks)
  - Uses chlorine-based compounds to disinfect and degrade pharmaceuticals.
  - It can produce toxic byproducts (*e.g.*, trihalomethanes), so its use is declining.
- Advantages of Chemical Treatment
  - Effective for liquid waste (*e.g.*, IV solutions, syrups, chemotherapy residues).
  - Can break down hazardous compounds (*e.g.*, cytotoxic drugs, hormones).
  - Faster than biological methods for certain drugs.
  - Can be combined with physical treatments (*e.g.*, filtration, adsorption).
- Disadvantages & Risks
  - **Toxic byproducts**: Some treatments produce harmful residues (*e.g.*, chlorinated compounds).
  - **High operational costs**: Requires specialized chemicals and monitoring.
  - **Not universal**: Some pharmaceuticals resist degradation (*e.g.*, certain endocrine disruptors).
  - **Regulatory compliance needed**: Improper handling can lead to environmental contamination.
- Current Status and Alternatives
  - Chemical treatment is still used but often combined with other methods (*e.g.*, incineration, adsorption).
  - Advanced Oxidation Processes (AOPs) are gaining popularity for persistent pollutants.
  - Take-back programs and incineration are preferred for high-risk drugs (*e.g.*, opioids, chemotherapy agents).

AUTOCLAVING (STEAM STERILIZATION)

- Autoclaving (steam sterilization) is a conventional thermal treatment method used primarily for infectious medical waste but sometimes applied to certain types of pharmaceutical waste, particularly when combined with other disposal methods [8].

Process: High-pressure saturated steam (typically 121°C at 15 psi for 15–60 minutes) penetrates waste, killing microorganisms and degrading some organic compounds.

Suitable for

- Contaminated packaging (*e.g.*, vials, blister packs with residual drugs).
- Non-hazardous pharmaceutical waste (*e.g.*, expired oral tablets, empty IV bags).
- Sharps waste (needles, syringes) if properly containerized [9].

Not suitable for

- Hazardous drugs (*e.g.*, chemotherapy agents, cytotoxic waste).
- Controlled substances (*e.g.*, opioids, which require DEA-approved destruction).
- Thermally stable compounds (some antibiotics, hormones).

Advantages of Autoclaving

- **Effective sterilization**: Destroys pathogens, reducing infection risk.
- **Environmentally safer than incineration**: No direct air emissions (unlike burning).
- **Cost-effective for large volumes**: Cheaper than incineration for non-hazardous waste.
- **Volume reduction**: Some compaction is possible post-treatment.
    - Disadvantages & Limitations
- **Does not destroy chemical hazards**: Pharmaceuticals may remain active after autoclaving.
- **Limited to certain waste types**: Not approved for hazardous or regulated drugs.
- **Moisture residue**: Treated waste may require drying before landfill disposal.
- **Regulatory restrictions**: Some countries prohibit autoclaving for pharmaceutical waste due to incomplete degradation.

Current Use in Pharmaceutical Waste Management

- Mostly used for secondary waste (*e.g.*, containers, PPE contaminated with non-hazardous drugs).
- Often combined with shredding to render waste unrecognizable before landfill disposal.
- An alternative to incineration, where emissions regulations are strict.
    - Best Practices for Autoclaving Pharmaceutical Waste
- **Segregate waste** – Only autoclave non-hazardous, non-regulated pharmaceuticals.
- **Validate sterilization** – Use biological indicators (*e.g.*, *Geobacillus stearothermophilus* spores) to ensure effectiveness.
- **Follow local regulations** – Some jurisdictions require additional treatment (*e.g.*, chemical neutralization) before disposal.
- **Avoid autoclaving hazardous drugs** – Cytotoxic, hormonal, and narcotic waste should be incinerated or chemically treated.

RETURN-TO-PHARMACY OR TAKE-BACK PROGRAMS

- Return-to-Pharmacy (RtP) or Drug Take-Back Programs are community-based initiatives that allow consumers to return unused or expired medications to designated collection points (*e.g.*, pharmacies, hospitals, or authorized facilities) for safe disposal. These programs aim to reduce improper disposal (*e.g.*, flushing, trash dumping) and prevent drug misuse, environmental contamination, and accidental poisoning [10].

Process:

a. Collection Points

- Pharmacies (*e.g.*, Walgreens, CVS in the U.S.)
- Hospitals & Clinics (often for controlled substances)
- Police Stations (for narcotics disposal)
- Mobile Collection Events (periodic community drives)

b. Accepted Waste Types

- Expired or unused medications (pills, capsules, patches)
- Over-the-counter (OTC) drugs
- Controlled substances (*e.g.*, opioids, if DEA-compliant)
- Veterinary medications

c. Exclusions (varies by program)

- Sharps (needles, syringes – require separate disposal)
- Hazardous drugs (chemotherapy, mercury-containing meds)
- Illicit drugs (not accepted in most programs)

Disposal Methods After Collection

- Incineration (most common for hazardous & controlled drugs)
- High-temperature treatment (for non-hazardous waste)
- Landfill (rare, only for inert, pre-treated waste)

Advantages of Take-Back Programs

- Prevents environmental pollution (keeps drugs out of water systems)
- Reduces drug misuse & diversion (especially opioids)
- Convenient for consumers (no need for home disposal methods)
- Compliance with regulations (*e.g.*, U.S. DEA, EU Directive)
- Public awareness & education (promotes safe medication use)

Challenges & Limitations

- Limited accessibility (rural areas may lack collection points)
- Costs & logistics (funding for transportation & disposal)

- Regulatory barriers (strict rules for controlled substances)
- Consumer participation gaps (low awareness or motivation)
- Not all drugs are accepted (*e.g.*, hazardous waste may require special handling)

Pharmaceutical take-back programs offer diverse solutions to safely dispose of unused or expired medications, each with distinct operational approaches (Table 3).

Table 3. Types of take-back programs [11].

Type	Description	Examples
On-Site Pharmacy Collection	Year-round drop-off at pharmacies.	U.S. DEA-registered pharmacies
Mail-Back Programs	Prepaid envelopes for consumers to mail drugs.	Med-Project (U.S.)
Take-Back Events	Temporary collection drives (*e.g.*, National Prescription Drug Take-Back Day).	DEA-sponsored events
Hospital & Clinic Collection	For patients to return unused meds post-treatment.	EU's "Disposal of Unused Medicines" programs

Comparison with Other Methods

Table 4 evaluates four primary methods for disposing of pharmaceutical and biomedical waste, highlighting their optimal applications and key limitations.

Table 4. Comparison of biomedical waste disposal methods [12].

Method	Best For	Limitations
Autoclaving	Non-hazardous, infectious waste	Doesn't destroy drug activity
Incineration	Hazardous drugs, controlled substances	Air pollution, high cost
Chemical Treatment	Liquid waste, degradable compounds	Toxic byproducts possible
Landfill	Inert, non-leachable waste	Environmental contamination risk
Take-Back Programs	Prevents misuse, eco-friendly	Limited drug types, accessibility issues

SEWAGE DISPOSAL (LIMITED USE)

Sewage disposal is a critical component of urban and rural waste management systems, ensuring the safe treatment and disposal of wastewater to protect public health and the environment. Conventional sewage disposal methods primarily rely on centralized treatment systems, such as sewage treatment plants (STPs), septic tanks, and sewer networks, which are designed to remove contaminants before releasing water back into the environment [13].

However, these traditional approaches face significant challenges, including high operational costs, energy-intensive processes, sludge management issues, and inadequate infrastructure in developing regions. Many systems struggle with inefficiencies, leading to untreated or partially treated sewage being discharged into rivers, lakes, and oceans, causing water pollution, ecosystem damage, and public health risks [13].

As urbanization and population growth increase sewage generation, conventional methods often fall short in sustainability and scalability. Emerging solutions, such as decentralized treatment systems, resource recovery (biogas, recycled water), and nature-based technologies, are being explored to address these limitations [14].

Advantages

- Easy disposal method for households, pharmacies, and small healthcare facilities.
- No need for specialized collection or transport systems.
- Avoids expenses related to hazardous waste handling, incineration, or landfill disposal.
- Conventional wastewater treatment (*e.g.*, activated sludge) can degrade certain biodegradable pharmaceuticals.
- Some drugs adsorb to sludge or settle during primary treatment.

Disadvantages

Ineffective Removal of Persistent Drugs

- Antibiotic resistance – Low drug concentrations in water promote resistant bacteria.
- Bioaccumulation – Lipophilic drugs (*e.g.*, antidepressants) accumulate in fish and wildlife.
- Contamination of sludge & water reuse systems.
- Trace drugs in drinking water may have long-term effects (though risks are still being studied).
- Accidental exposure to cytotoxic drugs (*e.g.*, chemotherapy residues) in sewage workers.

ENCAPSULATION

Encapsulation is a widely used method for disposing of pharmaceutical waste, particularly solid medications, by immobilizing them in a stable, non-leachable matrix to prevent environmental release. This technique is commonly applied in settings where incineration or chemical treatment is not feasible [15].

Advantages of Encapsulation

- Traps pharmaceutical compounds within a solid block (*e.g.*, cement, plastic, or clay), reducing leaching into soil and water.
- Minimizes the risk of drug residues entering sewage systems or landfills.
- Does not require advanced technology—it can be done using basic materials like concrete or high-density polyethylene (HDPE).
- Lower operational costs compared to incineration or advanced oxidation.
- Encapsulated drugs are rendered inaccessible, preventing illegal retrieval and abuse (*e.g.*, opioids, sedatives).

Disadvantages of Encapsulation

- Drugs remain chemically intact; potential for long-term leakage if the matrix degrades.
- Unsuitable for liquid or injectable drugs unless first solidified.
- Requires pre-processing (*e.g.*, crushing tablets) for effective encapsulation.
- Encapsulated blocks can be bulky, increasing landfill space requirements.
- Heavy materials (*e.g.*, concrete) raise transportation costs.

CHALLENGES IN CONVENTIONAL METHODS

The current conventional pharmaceutical waste management systems, represented by incineration together with landfilling, sewage disposal, autoclaving, and encapsulation, face multiple limitations that affect their effectiveness and sustainability [16]. The commonly employed incineration process releases dioxins and heavy metals through its emissions unless it functions at proper temperatures, thus creating health hazards and environmental degradation. The energy-consuming process produces dangerous ash, which requires proper waste management[16]. The process of landfilling creates leachate problems because rainwater passes through pharmaceutical waste, until hazardous substances enter groundwater alongside the surrounding environments. Due to extended drug persistence in landfills, besides antibiotic and hormonal substances, combined with space limitations and tighter regulations, the method becomes progressively difficult to implement. The current sewage processing facilities struggle to remove pharmaceutical residue from wastewater because their equipment does not have built-in drug elimination capabilities, thus releasing active pharmaceutical compounds into aquatic environments. The present practice enables antimicrobial resistance (AMR) development while causing disruptions to aquatic endocrine systems and delivering drugs to drinking water supplies [17]. While autoclaving accomplishes sterilization, it does not break down pharmaceutical ingredients and results in the creation of microplastics from healthcare packaging materials. The drug-binding method of encapsulation prevents drug destruction but does not eliminate the potential for medications to leak from degrading packaging materials during the allocated timeframe. These limitations intensify due to ongoing environmental restrictions and public pharmaceutical awareness, and the immediate requirement for eco-friendly waste management solutions. Traditional waste management and recycling methods demonstrate insufficient capability; therefore new technologies that handle waste and recycling need immediate development [18].

NOVEL RECYCLING TECHNOLOGIES FOR PHARMACEUTICAL WASTE: A SUSTAINABLE SOLUTION TO A GROWING CRISIS

Pharmaceutical operations generate large amounts of waste, primarily consisting of expired medications, along with manufacturing residues and unused drugs from healthcare facilities and households. Incineration, landfilling, and sewage discharge remain insufficient methods because they create environmental and health hazards, so scientists have developed new waste recycling systems that convert medications into beneficial products while reducing ecological damage. Advanced approaches to pharmaceutical waste management use three techniques based on chemical decay processes and resource extraction methods, together with circular economy concepts for sustainable waste treatment [19].

Advanced Oxidation Processes (AOPs) show great promise through their use of hydroxyl radicals that perform efficient breakdown of complex pharmaceutical components into harmless substances [20]. The high efficiency degradation of persistent pharmaceutical substances like antibiotics and hormones in wastewater can be achieved through photocatalysis (TiO_2/UV) and ozonation and electrochemical oxidation techniques. Sewage treatment with AOP technologies produces almost complete degradation of contaminants, thus they do not enter into ecological systems. The method faces two significant hurdles, which need improvement regarding excessive energy utilization and production of toxic reaction products [20].

The degradation of pharmaceutical waste through enzymatic and microbial biodegradation uses modified biological systems that process pharmaceutical waste materials. White-rot fungi, along with enzymes such as peroxidase and laccase, demonstrate outstanding capability to break down antibiotics, along with painkillers. Consolidated bioelectrochemical systems integrate microbial processing of pharmaceutical waste and bioelectrochemical reactions that create renewable energy while improving degradation efficiency. The positive eco-friendly nature and economical nature of these methods experience restrictions due to limitations in their scalability, along with sensitivity to environmental conditions such as pH and temperature [21].

The process of adsorption recycling maintains increasing popularity because it efficiently extracts active pharmaceutical ingredients (APIs) from waste material. The drug molecule extraction process through selective binding occurs through advanced adsorbents, including activated carbon, together with biochar and molecularly imprinted polymers (MIPs). The wastewater treatment process employing activated carbon filters removes at least 90% of pharmaceutical compounds, but MIPs provide specific recovery possibilities for valuable substances. Achieving economic viability requires solving two primary challenges associated with adsorbent reactivation and proper management of waste products [22].

A new approach through nanotechnology brings revolutionary changes by using nano-zero-valent iron (nZVI) and magnetic nanoparticles that efficiently destroy pharmaceutical compounds. The materials present both large areas of exposure and strong chemical activity, which leads to the fast degradation of pollutants. The magnetic properties enable efficient separation methods, which also minimize operational expenses. Mandatory safety evaluations need to be conducted due to environmental sustainability concerns about nanoparticle toxicity [23].

Two advanced wastewater treatment approaches combine membrane bioreactors (MBRs) and combined AOP-adsorption systems to accomplish better performance in wastewater cleanup. The combination of biological waste treatment with ultrafiltration membranes in MBRs enables the production of effluent that contains no micropollutants. The process of recovering APIs from discarded medications becomes possible through techniques such as solvent extraction and supercritical CO_2 extraction, which subsequently decreases the necessity of extracting raw materials [24].

The plasma gasification technology operates as a modern solution for treating hazardous waste as well as materials that cannot be recycled by replacing traditional incineration methods. High-temperature plasma transforms pharmaceutical waste into syngas through its operation, as well as generating inert slag, thus creating a nearly zero-emission system. The technology demonstrates waste-to-energy conversion capability despite its high present cost, which makes it a promising choice for future applications.

LIST OF NOVEL RECYCLING TECHNOLOGIES FOR PHARMACEUTICAL WASTE

The pharmaceutical industry is adopting innovative recycling technologies to minimize waste and promote sustainability. Below is a concise overview of cutting-edge methods (Fig. **1**).

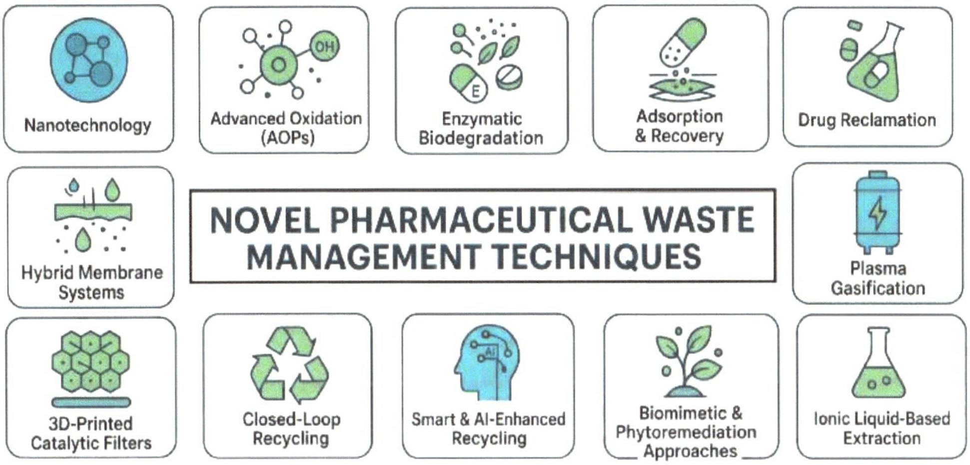

Nanotechnology
Advanced Oxidation (AOPs)
Enzymatic Biodegradation
Adsorption & Recovery
Drug Reclamation
Hybrid Membrane Systems
NOVEL PHARMACEUTICAL WASTE MANAGEMENT TECHNIQUES
Plasma Gasification
3D-Printed Catalytic Filters
Closed-Loop Recycling
Smart & AI-Enhanced Recycling
Biomimetic & Phytoremediation Approaches
Ionic Liquid-Based Extraction

Fig. (1). Novel pharmaceutical waste management techniques [25].

Advanced Oxidation Processes (AOPs)

Advanced Oxidation Processes (AOPs) represent a cutting-edge approach to pharmaceutical waste treatment, leveraging highly reactive oxygen species—particularly hydroxyl radicals (·OH)—to degrade complex drug molecules into harmless byproducts like water, CO_2, and inorganic ions [20]. These radicals, generated through chemical, photochemical, or electrochemical means, attack and break down persistent pharmaceutical compounds that conventional wastewater treatments cannot eliminate. For example, ozonation (O_3) is widely used to oxidize antibiotics like ciprofloxacin in hospital effluents, while UV/H_2O_2 systems effectively decompose endocrine disruptors such as ethinylestradiol (a contraceptive hormone). Another notable technique, photocatalysis with titanium dioxide (TiO_2/UV), has proven successful in degrading painkillers (*e.g.*, diclofenac) in surface waters by generating electron-hole pairs that initiate radical chain reactions. Electrochemical AOPs, like boron-doped diamond (BDD) electrode systems, mineralize chemotherapy drugs (*e.g.*, 5-fluorouracil) with near-complete efficiency [26]. Despite their energy intensity, AOPs are increasingly paired with renewable energy (*e.g.*, solar-driven photocatalysis) to enhance sustainability. These technologies are critical for preventing pharmaceutical pollution in aquatic ecosystems, particularly in hotspots like hospitals and drug manufacturing units, where concentrated waste streams demand robust solutions.

Key Examples

a. **Ozonation + UV**: Removes 95% of sulfamethoxazole (antibiotic) from wastewater.

b. **Electro-Fenton process**: Degrades paracetamol by combining iron catalysts and electric current.
c. **Solar photocatalysis**: Uses sunlight/TiO_2 to break down tetracycline in rural clinics.

AOPs' adaptability to diverse contaminants positions them as a cornerstone of future pharmaceutical waste recycling systems.

Enzymatic and Microbial Biodegradation

Enzymatic and microbial biodegradation offers an eco-friendly and energy-efficient approach to pharmaceutical waste treatment by harnessing natural biological processes to break down drug compounds. Specialized enzymes, such as laccases and peroxidases produced by fungi and bacteria, catalyze the oxidation of complex pharmaceuticals into simpler, non-toxic molecules. For example, the white-rot fungus Phanerochaete chrysosporium secretes ligninolytic enzymes that effectively degrade antibiotics like penicillin and tetracycline by cleaving their molecular structures. Similarly, bacterial strains such as Pseudomonas and Rhodococcus have been engineered to metabolize persistent drugs, including ibuprofen and carbamazepine, through enzymatic pathways. Another innovative approach involves bioelectrochemical systems (BES), where microbial fuel cells utilize drug-degrading bacteria to break down contaminants while simultaneously generating electricity demonstrated in the treatment of sulfamethoxazole-contaminated wastewater [27].

Key Examples

a. **Laccase-mediated degradation**: Removes 80–90% of diclofenac from hospital effluents.
b. **Pseudomonas putida:** Metabolizes estrogenic compounds in sewage sludge.
c. **Microbial fuel cells**: Degrade ciprofloxacin while producing bioelectricity.

While slower than chemical methods, these biological systems minimize secondary pollution and align with circular economy principles by avoiding harsh chemicals. Challenges like enzyme stability and microbial adaptability are being addressed through genetic engineering and immobilized enzyme technologies, making this a promising frontier for sustainable pharmaceutical waste management.

Adsorption and Recovery Technologies

Adsorption and recovery technologies provide a highly efficient and cost-effective solution for pharmaceutical waste management by capturing and concentrating active pharmaceutical ingredients (APIs) from wastewater streams for potential reuse or safe disposal. These technologies leverage porous materials with high surface areas and selective binding properties to trap drug molecules. Activated carbon, one of the most widely used adsorbents, can remove up to 90% of contaminants like antibiotics (*e.g.*, tetracycline) and analgesics (*e.g.*, acetaminophen) from hospital effluents [28]. More advanced materials, such as biochar derived from agricultural waste, offer a sustainable and low-cost alternative, effectively adsorbing hormones like 17β-estradiol. For targeted recovery, molecularly imprinted polymers (MIPs) are engineered with specific binding sites to selectively capture high-value APIs, such as recovering morphine from opioid-containing waste. Additionally, graphene oxide and carbon nanotubes exhibit exceptional adsorption capacities for complex drugs like fluoroquinolones due to their ultra-high surface area and tunable surface chemistry.

Key Examples

a. **Activated carbon filters**: Remove 85-95% of sulfamethoxazole from municipal wastewater.
b. **Biochar from rice husks**: Adsorb 80% of diclofenac in low-cost water treatment systems.
c. **MIPs for antibiotics**: Enable the selective recovery of ciprofloxacin for potential recycling.

While adsorption excels in scalability and simplicity, challenges like adsorbent regeneration and disposal of spent materials remain. Innovations in regenerable adsorbents and hybrid systems (*e.g.*, combining adsorption with AOPs) are enhancing the sustainability of these technologies, making them vital for both pollution control and resource recovery in pharmaceutical waste management [29].

Nanotechnology-Based Solutions

Nanotechnology-based solutions are revolutionizing pharmaceutical waste treatment by leveraging the unique properties of nanomaterials for enhanced degradation, adsorption, and recovery of drug contaminants. Metal nanoparticles like nano-zero-valent iron (nZVI) break down persistent pharmaceuticals through reductive processes—for instance, nZVI particles have demonstrated 95% removal of chloramphenicol (a broad-spectrum antibiotic) by cleaving its nitro groups. Magnetic nanoparticles, such as iron oxide (Fe_3O_4) coated with silica or polymers, enable rapid adsorption of drugs like tetracycline, followed by easy separation using external magnets, simplifying wastewater treatment. Silver and gold nanoparticles act as catalysts in advanced oxidation, degrading β-lactam antibiotics under visible light. Carbon-based nanomaterials, including graphene oxide nanosheets and carbon nanotubes, offer ultrahigh surface areas for adsorbing endocrine disruptors like bisphenol-A, while their functionalized derivatives can selectively trap chemotherapy drugs (*e.g.*, doxorubicin) [30].

Key Examples

a. **nZVI**: Degrades 90% of sulfamethazine in groundwater within 2 hours.
b. **Fe_3O_4@SiO_2 core-shell nanoparticles**: Remove 98% of ciprofloxacin *via* magnetic separation.
c. **TiO_2-graphene nanocomposites**: Enhance photocatalytic degradation of diclofenac by 70% under solar light.

Despite their efficacy, challenges like nanoparticle toxicity, aggregation, and high production costs persist. Research into biogenic nanoparticles (synthesized using plant extracts) and recyclable nano-catalysts aims to address these limitations, positioning nanotechnology as a transformative tool for sustainable pharmaceutical waste remediation.

Hybrid Membrane Systems

Hybrid membrane systems combine advanced filtration technologies with complementary processes like biodegradation or advanced oxidation to achieve superior removal of pharmaceutical contaminants from wastewater. These integrated systems address the limitations of standalone methods by synergizing membrane selectivity with enhanced degradation mechanisms. For example, membrane bioreactors (MBRs) couple ultrafiltration or microfiltration membranes with activated sludge treatment, achieving over 95% removal of persistent drugs like carbamazepine while producing high-quality effluent—a technology already implemented in hospitals like Germany's Charité. Nanofiltration (NF) and reverse osmosis (RO) membranes paired with activated carbon pretreatment can eliminate >99% of antibiotics (*e.g.*, sulfamethoxazole) and hormones from municipal wastewater, as demonstrated in Singapore's NEWater reclamation plants. Forward osmosis (FO) systems integrated with catalytic oxidation—such as FO-UV/H_2O_2 hybrids—simultaneously concentrate and degrade cytostatic drugs like cyclophosphamide, reducing their toxicity by 90%. Emerging innovations include electrospun nanofiber membranes embedded with TiO_2 nanoparticles, which combine physical sieving with photocatalytic degradation of beta-blockers (*e.g.*, propranolol) under sunlight [31].

Key Examples

a. **MBR-ozonation systems** in Swiss wastewater plants remove 98% of X-ray contrast media (*e.g.*, iopromide).

b. **RO-granular activated carbon (GAC) hybrids** treat pharmaceutical manufacturing effluents in India's Hyderabad region.
c. **FO-membrane distillation systems** recover clean water while concentrating APIs for disposal in US military field hospitals.

While fouling and energy demands remain a few challenges, smart membranes with self-cleaning properties (*e.g.*, graphene oxide coatings) and renewable energy integration are advancing these systems toward scalable, sustainable pharmaceutical wastewater treatment.

Drug Reclamation and Reuse

Drug reclamation and reuse technologies offer a sustainable and economically viable approach to pharmaceutical waste management by recovering active pharmaceutical ingredients (APIs) from expired, unused, or discarded medications for potential reformulation or repurposing. These processes not only reduce environmental contamination but also conserve valuable resources by minimizing the need for *de novo* drug synthesis. Solvent extraction is a widely used technique, where organic solvents selectively isolate APIs like paracetamol from expired tablets, achieving recovery rates of up to 85%. Supercritical fluid extraction (SFE), particularly using carbon dioxide ($scCO_2$), provides a green alternative for recovering heat-sensitive compounds such as antibiotics (*e.g.*, amoxicillin) without residual solvent contamination. At hospitals, a drug recycling system on site uses precipitation and crystallization toderive rescued opioids such as morphine from unused intravenous solutions to meet the imposed critical regulatory standards. Applications for paclitaxel include the chromatographic separation of oncology drugs (*e.g.*, paclitaxel) from manufacturing waste with cost savings of 30-40% in industrial production [32].

Key Examples

a. The UK's "ReMed" program recovers and freely gives unopened, unexpired medications to communities that would otherwise lack them, and saves 25% in general waste.
b. Progesterone from contraceptive pills returned to hormone therapy is extracted with supercritical CO_2 in Dutch pharmacies.
c. Selective adsorption-elution techniques in India reclaim 70% of antiretroviral drugs (*e.g.*, tenofovir) from HIV treatment waste.

However, although drug reclamation holds promise, problems in implementing it, such as those of stringent quality control, the possibility of cross-contamination, *etc.*, exist. Continuous flow extraction systems and AI-assisted purity testing have been advancing to solve these barriers, and drug reuse becomes the key to the circular pharmaceutical economy. Several regulatory frameworks, like the FDA's guidance on the drug reprocessing, address these innovations to close the global gap in drug access without harming the environment [33].

Plasma Gasification and Pyrolysis

Plasma gasification and pyrolysis are the forefront thermal technologies for the total liquid destruction of hazardous pharmaceutical waste and the utilization of energy gained from the destruction process to reduce environmental impact. In oxygen-starved environments, they carry out controlled thermal decomposition of complex drug molecules down to simpler and non-toxic compounds. Pharmaceutical waste is nearly totally destroyed through conversion to syngas (a mixture of hydrogen and carbon monoxide) and inert slag, with temperatures above 5000 degrees C and ionized gas (plasma), even for the worst (persistent) chemicals, such as chemotherapy agents (*e.g.*, cyclophosphamide). Japan's Utashinai Plasma Plant is an example: with a collection of both antibiotics and cytotoxic drugs as medical waste, it produces electricity from the syngas produced while reducing waste volume by 95%. Lower temperature pyrolysis (400–800°C) thermally decomposes drugs such as the fluoroquinolone antibiotics into bio oil, char, and combustible gases that have been demonstrated at Canadian PyroGenesis facilities to process expired medications. Two methods of accelerating waste destruction are evident in it: microwave assisted pyrolysis, which heats waste uniformly with a high conversion rate, and has been used in South Korea to degrade hormone based drugs such as ethinylestradiol with 99% conversion rate, and superheated water, which is currently being investigated in the U.S. to oxidise toxic compounds in food packaging and drug residue, with a very high destruction rate [34].

Key Examples

1. Pharmaceutical packaging waste contaminated with drug residues is gasified with the UK's Advanced Plasma Power's facility, and the clean syngas is then used for district heating.
2. Thermax pyrolysis units in India safely dispose of antiretroviral HIV drugs, recovering biochar for industrial use.
3. Portable plasma systems used by the US Army destroy opioid based medications in field hospitals to avoid diversion and environmental release.

Although these are capital-intensive technologies that can eliminate toxic residues, produce renewable energy, and meet the challenge of zero landfill mandates for the pharmaceutical industry, future waste management will be impossible without them. In recent years, innovating their sustainability and reducing their cost-effectiveness to become suitable for large-scale adoption included hybrid plasma-catalytic systems and waste-to-hydrogen conversion.

Ionic Liquid-Based Extraction

Ionic liquid-based extraction has emerged as a green and highly efficient method for recovering active pharmaceutical ingredients (APIs) from complex waste streams, leveraging the unique properties of ionic liquids (ILs)—salts that remain liquid at room temperature. These solvents exhibit exceptional thermal stability, negligible volatility, and tunable chemical properties, allowing selective extraction of specific drugs while minimizing environmental harm. For example, imidazolium-based ILs have been used to recover up to 92% of antibiotics like erythromycin from fermentation waste in pharmaceutical manufacturing, outperforming traditional organic solvents. In the treatment of hospital wastewater, choline-amino acid ILs selectively isolate cytotoxic drugs (*e.g.*, 5-fluorouracil) with 98% efficiency, as demonstrated in pilot plants in Sweden. Another breakthrough involves magnetic ionic liquids (MILs), such as trihexyltetradecylphosphonium tetrachloroferrate, which enable easy separation of NSAIDs (*e.g.*, ibuprofen) from urine samples using external magnets—a technique adopted in German recycling facilities. The US EPA's "Green Chemistry" program has endorsed IL-based systems for their ability to extract and purify opioids like oxycodone from expired medications without generating toxic byproducts[35].

Key Examples

a. **Betaine-based ILs** in French labs recover 85% of paracetamol from over-the-counter drug waste.
b. **Phosphonium ILs** selectively separate estrogenic compounds from sewage sludge in Dutch water treatment plants.
c. **MIL-assisted extraction** in China's pharmaceutical industry reclaims 90% of streptomycin from production effluents.

Despite their promise, challenges like high production costs and potential aquatic toxicity require further research into biodegradable ILs (*e.g.*, derived from amino acids) and closed-loop recycling systems. With regulatory support, IL-based extraction could revolutionize API recovery, aligning with circular economy goals while reducing reliance on hazardous solvents.

Biomimetic and Phytoremediation Approaches

Biomimetic and phytoremediation approaches harness natural and nature-inspired systems to degrade or sequester pharmaceutical contaminants in an eco-friendly and energy-efficient manner [36]. Biomimetic strategies employ synthetic catalysts that mimic natural enzymes—such as porphyrin-based catalysts replicating cytochrome P450 enzymes to break down persistent drugs like diclofenac with 80% efficiency under ambient conditions, as demonstrated in Swiss wastewater pilot projects. Phytoremediation leverages plants and their associated microbiomes to uptake, metabolize, or stabilize pharmaceuticals; for instance, constructed wetlands planted with Phragmites australis (common reed) remove 70–90% of antibiotics (*e.g.*, sulfamethoxazole) and beta-blockers from hospital effluents, a method successfully implemented in India's AIIMS hospitals. Hybrid systems combine these principles: enzyme-loaded artificial roots (inspired by plant rhizospheres) degrade estrogenic compounds in sewage, while floating treatment wetlands with Typha species absorb and metabolize antidepressants like fluoxetine, as trialed in Berlin's urban waterways.

Key Examples

a. **Laccase-mimicking polymers** degrade tetracycline in dairy farm runoff (Netherlands).
b. **Willow tree plantations** (*Salix spp.*) extract and detoxify ibuprofen from landfill leachate (Canada).
c. **Algal-bacterial consortia** in Belgium's bioreactors target chemotherapy drug residues (*e.g.*, methotrexate).

Though slower than chemical methods, these approaches offer low-cost, solar-powered solutions for decentralized treatment, especially in resource-limited settings. Innovations like genetically engineered hyperaccumulator plants and 3D-printed biomimetic scaffolds are addressing scalability challenges, making these methods vital for sustainable pharmaceutical waste management in the Anthropocene.

Smart and AI-Enhanced Recycling

Smart and AI-Enhanced Recycling is transforming pharmaceutical waste management by leveraging artificial intelligence, robotics, and IoT technologies to optimize sorting, degradation, and resource recovery processes. AI-powered computer vision systems, like those deployed in German recycling plants, use machine learning to identify and separate expired tablets by drug class (*e.g.*, opioids *vs.* antibiotics) with 95% accuracy, enabling precise downstream treatment. Predictive analytics platforms, such as IBM's Watson for Drug Repurposing, analyze chemical structures to suggest reuse pathways for recovered APIs—demonstrated with the antimalarial drug artemisinin being reformulated for cancer therapy. In India, autonomous robotic sorters equipped with near-infrared spectroscopy segregate blister packs by polymer type and drug residue, achieving 30% faster processing than manual methods [37]. The US FDA's "Digital Twin" initiative creates virtual models of waste streams to simulate plasma gasification outcomes for cytotoxic drugs, optimizing energy use by 40%. South Korea's AI-driven microreactors dynamically adjust enzymatic degradation parameters in real-time to break down variable waste compositions, improving beta-lactam antibiotic removal by 25%.

Key Examples

a. **MIT's "BioCycler" system** uses reinforcement learning to maximize API recovery yields from mixed drug waste.
b. **Singapore's SMART CENSAM labs** deploy AI-guided nanofilters that self-adjust pore sizes to capture specific contaminants like metformin.
c. **Pfizer's "Green Chemistry AI"** platform reduces solvent waste in drug recovery by predicting optimal extraction conditions.

While challenges like data security and high initial costs persist, integration with blockchain for waste tracking and edge computing for real-time monitoring is accelerating adoption. These technologies are critical for achieving zero-waste pharmaceutical manufacturing while unlocking circular economy opportunities—from automated drug redistribution to AI-designed recyclable formulations.

3D-Printed Catalytic Filters

3D-Printed catalytic filters represent a revolutionary advancement in pharmaceutical waste treatment, combining additive manufacturing with tailored catalytic properties to create highly efficient, customizable filtration systems. These precision-engineered filters are fabricated using 3D-printing techniques like stereolithography (SLA) or direct ink writing (DIW), embedding catalysts such as TiO_2 nanoparticles, metal-organic frameworks (MOFs), or enzyme-mimicking polymers within porous lattice structures. For example, researchers at MIT developed a 3D-printed graphene oxide filter doped with palladium nanoparticles, which achieves 99% degradation of chemotherapy drugs like cisplatin in hospital wastewater by maximizing surface area and catalytic exposure. In Spain, ceramic filters printed with laccase enzymes selectively break down beta-blockers (*e.g.*, propranolol) while allowing safe water molecules to pass through. The EU's "PHARM-FILTER" project employs multi-material 3D printing to create gradient-pore filters that sequentially adsorb, oxidize, and mineralize antibiotics—demonstrating 90% removal of ciprofloxacin in pilot tests at Belgian hospitals [38].

Key Examples

a. **Nano-TiO_2 printed meshes** in California degrade 85% of endocrine disruptors (*e.g.*, ethinylestradiol) under sunlight.
b. **MOF-integrated filters** at Singapore's NEWater plants recover precious metals from contrast media waste (*e.g.*, gadolinium).
c. **Enzyme-embedded cellulose filters** in India's Ayurvedic drug industry selectively detoxify herbal medicine residues.

These filters offer unmatched design flexibility, enabling pore geometry optimization for specific contaminants and scalable production *via* decentralized 3D printing. While challenges like catalyst leaching and fouling persist, innovations such as self-regenerating catalytic inks and 4D-printed shape-memory filters are pushing the boundaries of smart pharmaceutical waste remediation.

3D-Printed Catalytic Filters: Materials and Mechanisms in Depth

I. **Advanced Materials for 3D-Printed Filters**
  - **Graphene-Based Inks**:
    - **Mechanism**: High electron mobility improves photocatalytic oxidation (*e.g.*, TiO_2/graphene composites degrade 95% of tetracycline under UV).
    - **Example**: For cisplatin breakdown, MIT's filters make use of graphene-polyacrylate lattices including embedded Pd nanoparticles.
  - **Metal-Organic Frameworks (MOFs)**:
    - **Mechanism**: Ultrahigh porosity (surface areas > 10,000 m^2/g) selectively adsorbs APIs by means of host-guest interactions.
    - **Example**: In Swiss wastewater plants, HKUST-1 MOF filters grab 98% of diclofenac.
  - **Enzyme-Loaded Hydrogels**:
    - **Mechanism**: Laccase or peroxidase enzymes restrained in 3D-printed polyethylene glycol (PEG) hydrogels oxidize drugs (*e.g.*, 80% ibuprofen removal in 2 hours) [39].
    - **Example**: Spanish bioreactors custom alginate-laccase grids printed through DIW.
  - **Ceramic Nanocomposites**:
    - **Mechanism**: Al_2O_3 or SiO_2 matrices encapsulated with nZVI degrade halogenated drugs (*e.g.*, chloramphenicol) over reductive dehalogenation.
    - **Example**: ETH Zurich's Al_2O_3-nZVI filters treat antibiotic manufacturing waste.

II. **Catalytic Mechanisms**
  - **Photocatalysis**:
    - TiO_2 or ZnO nanoparticles in printed filters create hydroxyl radicals (·OH) under light, mineralizing sulfamethoxazole.

- **Example:** Singapore's solar-activated **TiO_2-resin filters* degenerate 90% of antibiotics.
- **Redox Reactions**:
  - **Fe^{3+}/Fe^{2+} cycles** in printed iron oxide filters break down nitroimidazoles (*e.g.*, metronidazole).
  - **Example:** The UK's Fenton-catalytic filters practice H_2O_2 infusion for on-demand radical generation.
- **Enzymatic Cascade**:
  - Co-printed laccase/peroxidase systems successively oxidize complex drugs (*e.g.*, sequential degradation of paracetamol to hydroquinone then CO_2).
  - **Example:** Netherlands' multi-enzyme cartridges for hospital wastewater.

III. **4D Printing Innovations**

- **Stimuli-Responsive Materials**:
  - pH-sensitive chitosan filters develop in acidic drug waste, with a cumulative catalytic surface area.
  - **Example:** India's pH-triggered MOF filters for selective estrogen adsorption [40].
- **Self-Cleaning Designs**:
  - Microfluidic channels in printed filters auto-flush collected debris by means of waste flow kinetics.
  - **Example:** Japan's "AquaRegen" filters for cytostatic drug removal.

IV. **Challenges & Solutions**

- **Catalyst Leaching**:
  - **Solution:** Atomic layer deposition (ALD) coatings (*e.g.*, Al_2O_3 shells on TiO_2 nanoparticles).
- **Fouling**:
  - **Solution:** Shark-skin-inspired anti-biofouling microtextures in printed surfaces.

Closed-Loop Pharmaceutical Recycling

Closed-Loop Pharmaceutical Recycling signifies a transformative method to sustainable drug waste management by generating circular systems where pharmaceutical waste is systematically composed, treated, and reintegrated into the production cycle as recyclable raw materials. This model diminishes environmental pollution while preserving resources and dropping manufacturing costs. For example, Pfizer's "Green Chemistry Initiative" recovers and disinfects active pharmaceutical ingredients (APIs) like sildenafil citrate (Viagra) from expired medicines, completing a 40% reduction in raw material use, complete solvent extraction, and crystallization. In India, Cipla's closed-loop program collects unused antiretroviral drugs (*e.g.*, tenofovir) from HIV clinics, reuses them into novel formulations, and redistributes them to underserved communities, cutting waste by 30%. Hospitals in Germany, such as Charité Berlin, employ on-site microreactor systems that change unused intravenous antibiotics (*e.g.*, meropenem) into stable powders for recycling, authenticated by real-time HPLC monitoring. The EU's "PharmaCycle" project links pharmacies, manufacturers, and wastewater plants, by means of supercritical CO_2 extraction to retrieve hormones from contraceptive waste for a new drug combination, indicating 90% API recovery rates [41].

Key Innovations & Examples

a. Blockchain tracked take-back programs (*e.g.*, the UK's "MedReturn") guarantee secure gathering and traceability of unused drugs.
b. Enzyme-catalyzed depolymerization in France breaks down penicillin waste into recyclable intermediates.
c. "Drug-to-Drug" factories in Canada reformulate improved oncology drugs (*e.g.*, paclitaxel) under the FDA's strict re-manufacturing guidelines.

Challenges like cross-contamination risks and regulatory hurdles are being addressed through AI-powered purity assays and good-recycling-practice (GRP) certifications. Closed-loop systems align with the UN's Sustainable Development Goals (SDG 12) and could reduce global pharmaceutical carbon emissions by 25% if scaled.

Future Outlook: Hybrid systems combining 3D-printed catalytic filters for waste pretreatment and IoT-enabled smart bins for automated organization may rapidly permit fully autonomous pharmaceutical recycling hubs.

These technologies' goal is to minimize environmental pollution, recover valuable compounds, and align with circular economy principles, offering sustainable alternatives to incineration and landfilling.

Comparison of Novel Recycling Technologies for Pharmaceutical Waste

The pharmaceutical industry is accepting innovative recycling technologies to address the limits of conventional disposal methods (*e.g.*, incineration, landfilling). Below is a comparative analysis of the most promising novel approaches based on efficiency, scalability, and environmental impact (Table **5**).

CONCLUSION: THE FUTURE OF PHARMACEUTICAL WASTE RECYCLING

Novel recycling technologies are transforming pharmaceutical waste management by evolving from linear disposal models to circular, sustainable solutions that arrange resource recovery, environmental protection, and public health. Advanced approaches like AOPs, enzymatic degradation, and nanotechnology address the limitations of conventional incineration and landfilling by allowing precise drug breakdown and API reclamation. Meanwhile, closed-loop systems, 3D-printed catalytic filters, and AI-enhanced recycling determine how innovation can transform waste into valuable inputs for new drug production.

The success of these technologies pivots on partnership across sectors:

- Governments must implement Extended Producer Responsibility (EPR) and fund green infrastructure.
- Industries should accept blockchain-tracked recycling and participate in scalable solutions like plasma gasification.
- Researchers' necessity to optimize low-cost, energy-efficient processes (*e.g.*, biogenic nanoparticles, solar-AOPs).

Table 5. Comparison of novel recycling technologies [42].

Sl No.	Technology	Mechanism	Best For	Scalability	Environmental Benefit	Key Challenges
1	Advanced Oxidation (AOPs)	Chemical degradation *via* radicals (·OH)	Antibiotics, hormones, cytotoxics	Moderate	Zero toxic residues	High energy use
2	Enzymatic Biodegradation	Microbial/enzyme breakdown	Biodegradable drugs (*e.g.*, penicillin)	Low	Low energy, no chemicals	Slow, pH-sensitive
3	Adsorption & Recovery	API capture (activated carbon, MOFs)	Wastewater treatment, API reclamation	High	Resource recovery	Regeneration needed
4	Nanotechnology	Nano-catalysts (nZVI, TiO_2)	Targeted drug removal	Limited	High precision	Toxicity concerns
5	Hybrid Membrane Systems	Filtration + oxidation/biodegradation	Hospitals, manufacturing effluents	Moderate	High-purity water output	Membrane fouling
6	Drug Reclamation	Solvent/supercritical extraction	Unused/expired medications	Low	Circular economy	Regulatory hurdles
7	Plasma Gasification	High-temperature molecular breakdown	Hazardous waste (chemo drugs)	Low	Energy recovery	High capex
8	3D-Printed Catalytic Filters	Custom-designed degradation surfaces	Point-source pollution	Emerging	Modular, adaptable	Material durability
9	Closed-Loop Recycling	API recovery → reuse in new drugs	Large-scale manufacturing waste	High	Zero-waste goal	Quality control

(Table 5) cont.....

Sl No.	Technology	Mechanism	Best For	Scalability	Environmental Benefit	Key Challenges
10	Smart & AI-Enhanced Recycling	AI-driven sorting, robotic separation, predictive analytics	Mixed waste streams (*e.g.*, packaging + APIs)	High	Optimizes efficiency; reduces human error	Data dependency; high initial tech cost
11	Biomimetic & Phytoremediation Approaches	Synthetic enzymes/materials mimicking natural systems, Plants/microbes absorb/degrade pharmaceuticals	Targeted drug degradation (*e.g.*, antibiotics, Soil/water contaminated with low-concentration drugs	Low	Carbon-negative; ecosystem restoration	Slow; limited to non-toxic compounds
12	Ionic Liquid-Based Extraction	Green solvents selectively extract APIs	High-value biologics/insulin	Lab to pilot scale	Non-toxic; reusable solvents	Expensive; low throughput

With 30% of global pharmaceuticals wasted annually, these progressions could decrease healthcare's carbon footprint by 25% while safeguarding safer water, fewer drug shortages, and cost savings. The path forward needs policy alignment, technological scaling, and public awareness—but the payoff is a sustainable, circular pharmaceutical economy that profits both people and the planet.

REFERENCES

[1] Sverdrup HU. Modelling global extraction, supply, price and depletion of the extractable geological resources with the LITHIUM model. Resour Conserv Recycling 2016; 114: 112-29. [http://dx.doi.org/10.1016/j.resconrec.2016.07.002]

[2] Kümmerer K, Ed. Pharmaceuticals in the Environment: Sources, Fate, Effects and Risks. Berlin: Springer 2001; p. 265. [http://dx.doi.org/10.1007/978-3-662-04634-0]

[3] Kamaruddin M A, Lee W S, Norashiddin F A, *et al.* Treatment and management of hazardous solid waste stream by incineration In: Wang L K, Wang M H S, Hung Y T, Shammas N K, Eds. Waste Treatment in the Biotechnology, Agricultural and Food Industries: Volume 2. Cham: Springer International Publishing 2023; pp. 285-335. [http://dx.doi.org/10.1007/978-3-031-44764-8_9]

[4] Lapworth DJ, Baran N, Stuart ME, Ward RS. Emerging organic contaminants in groundwater: A review of sources, fate and occurrence. Environ Pollut 2012; 163: 287-303. [http://dx.doi.org/10.1016/j.envpol.2011.12.034] [PMID: 22306910]

[5] Pichardo P P, Martínez-Hernández V, Meffe R, de Miguel Á, Leal M, Lillo J. Alkaline hydrolysis for beta-lactam antibiotic degradation. J Hazard Mater 2017; 321: 463-72.

[6] Kenny C, Priyadarshini A. Review of Current Healthcare Waste Management Methods and Their Effect on Global Health. Healthcare 2021; 9(3): 284. [http://dx.doi.org/10.3390/healthcare9030284]

[7] Rutala W A, Weber D J. Guideline for Disinfection and Sterilization in Healthcare Facilities, 2008. Update: May 2019. Atlanta: Centers for Disease Control and Prevention; 2019. p. 163.

[8] Roy A, Kunwar S, Bhusal U, *et al.* Bio-fabrication of trimetallic nanoparticles and their applications. Catalysts 2023; 13(2): 321. [http://dx.doi.org/10.3390/catal13020321]

[9] Francis L, Ogunbiyi O, Saththasivam J, Lawler J, Liu Z. A comprehensive review of forward osmosis and niche applications. Environ Sci Water Res Technol 2020; 6(8): 1986-2015. [http://dx.doi.org/10.1039/D0EW00181C]

[10] Sharma K, Kaushik G. Urbanization and Pharmaceutical Waste: An Upcoming Environmental Challenge. In: Kateja A, Jain R, Eds. Urban Growth and Environmental Issues in India. Singapore: Springer 2021; pp. 305-18. [http://dx.doi.org/10.1007/978-981-16-4273-9_18]

[11] Ghorbani M, Konvalina P, Walkiewicz A, *et al.* Feasibility of biochar derived from sewage sludge to promote sustainable agriculture and mitigate GHG emissions—A review. Int J Environ Res Public Health 2022; 19(19): 12983. [http://dx.doi.org/10.3390/ijerph191912983] [PMID: 36232283]

[12] de Boer S, González-Rodríguez J, Conde JJ, Moreira MT. Benchmarking tertiary water treatments for the removal of micropollutants and pathogens based on operational and sustainability criteria. J Water Process Eng 2022; 46: 102587. [http://dx.doi.org/10.1016/j.jwpe.2022.102587]

[13] Brunner G. Hydrothermal and supercritical water processes. Amsterdam: Elsevier; 2014. p. 614.

[14] Achinas S. An Overview of the Technological Applicability of Plasma Gasification Process. In: Singh P, Singh R P, Srivastava V, Eds. Contemporary Environmental Issues and Challenges in Era of Climate Change. 1st ed.. Singapore: Springer Nature 2020; pp. 261-75.

[15] Kwapis EH, Borrero J, Latty KS, Andrews HB, Phongikaroon SS, Hartig KC. Laser ablation plasmas and spectroscopy for nuclear applications. Appl Spectrosc 2024; 78(1): 9-55. [http://dx.doi.org/10.1177/00037028231211559] [PMID: 38116788]

[16] Kyzas GZ, Matis KA. Nanoadsorbents for pollutants removal: A review. J Mol Liq 2015; 203: 159-68. [http://dx.doi.org/10.1016/j.molliq.2015.01.004]

[17] Kyzas GZ, Fu J, Lazaridis NK, Bikiaris DN, Matis KA. New approaches on the removal of pharmaceuticals from wastewaters with adsorbent materials. J Mol Liq 2015; 209: 87-93. [http://dx.doi.org/10.1016/j.molliq.2015.05.025]

[18] Hu R, Zhan J, Zhao Y, *et al.* Bio-based platform chemicals synthesized from lignin biorefinery. Green Chem 2023; 25(22): 8970-9000. [http://dx.doi.org/10.1039/D3GC02927A]

[19] Pedro SNR, R Freire CS, Silvestre AJD, Freire MG. The role of ionic liquids in the pharmaceutical field: An overview of relevant applications. Int J Mol Sci 2020; 21(21): 8298. [http://dx.doi.org/10.3390/ijms21218298] [PMID: 33167474]

[20] Buarque F, Gautério G, Coelho M, Lemes A, Ribeiro B. Aqueous two-phase systems based on ionic liquids and deep eutectic solvents as a tool for the recovery of non-protein bioactive compounds—a review. Processes (Basel) 2022; 11(1): 31. [http://dx.doi.org/10.3390/pr11010031]

[21] Undri A. Waste polymeric materials valorization through microwave assisted pyrolysis [conference paper]. Florence: University of Florence; 2014. Available from: https://api.semanticscholar.org/CorpusID:189979303

[22] Ai X, Zhang X, Tian Y, Lu M, Wang W. Research status, key technologies and development trends of pharmaceutical waste salt treatment technology: A review. Waste Manag Res: The J Sus Circular Eco 2025; 43(10): 1525-47. [http://dx.doi.org/10.1177/0734242X251326271]

[23] Kumar N, He J, Rusling JF. Electrochemical transformations catalyzed by cytochrome P450s and peroxidases. Chem Soc Rev 2023; 52(15): 5135-71. [http://dx.doi.org/10.1039/D3CS00461A] [PMID: 37458261]

[24] Singh A, Singh DK, Kharwar RN, White JF, Gond SK. Fungal endophytes as efficient sources of plant-derived bioactive compounds and their prospective applications in natural product drug discovery: Insights, avenues, and challenges. Microorganisms 2021; 9(1): 197. [http://dx.doi.org/10.3390/microorganisms9010197] [PMID: 33477910]

[25] Kakaraparthy R, Palivela N, Reddy Karri L G. Chemotherapeutic Challenge: A Case of Acute Kidney Injury During Breast Cancer Management. Indian J Pharm Pract 2025; 19(1): 116-9. [http://dx.doi.org/10.5530/ijopp.9.1.2]

[26] Oller I, Malato S, Sánchez-Pérez JA. Combination of Advanced Oxidation Processes and biological treatments for wastewater decontamination—A review. Sci Total Environ 2011; 409(20): 4141-66. [http://dx.doi.org/10.1016/j.scitotenv.2010.08.061] [PMID: 20956012]

[27] Tran NH, Reinhard M, Gin KYH. Occurrence and fate of emerging contaminants in municipal wastewater treatment plants from different geographical regions-a review. Water Res 2018; 133: 182-207. [http://dx.doi.org/10.1016/j.watres.2017.12.029] [PMID: 29407700]

[28] Bui TX, Choi H. Adsorptive removal of selected pharmaceuticals by mesoporous silica SBA-15. J Hazard Mater 2009; 168(2-3): 602-8. [http://dx.doi.org/10.1016/j.jhazmat.2009.02.072] [PMID: 19327889]

[29] Qu X, Alvarez PJJ, Li Q. Applications of nanotechnology in water and wastewater treatment. Water Res 2013; 47(12): 3931-46. [http://dx.doi.org/10.1016/j.watres.2012.09.058] [PMID: 23571110]

[30] Shannon MA, Bohn PW, Elimelech M, Georgiadis JG, Mariñas BJ, Mayes AM. Science and technology for water purification in the coming decades. Nature 2008; 452(7185): 301-10. [http://dx.doi.org/10.1038/nature06599] [PMID: 18354474]

[31] Kümmerer K. The presence of pharmaceuticals in the environment due to human use – present knowledge and future challenges. J Environ Manage 2009; 90(8): 2354-66. [http://dx.doi.org/10.1016/j.jenvman.2009.01.023] [PMID: 19261375]

[32] Mountouris A, Voutsas E, Tassios D. Solid waste plasma gasification: Equilibrium model development and exergy analysis. Energy Convers Manage 2006; 47(13-14): 1723-37. [http://dx.doi.org/10.1016/j.enconman.2005.10.015]

[33] Zhang F, Zhao P, Niu M, Maddy J. The survey of key technologies in hydrogen energy storage. Int J Hydrogen Energy 2016; 41(33): 14535-52. [http://dx.doi.org/10.1016/j.ijhydene.2016.05.293]

[34] Wamba SF, Gunasekaran A, Akter S, Ren SJ, Dubey R, Childe SJ. Big data analytics and firm performance: Effects of dynamic capabilities. J Bus Res 2017; 70: 356-65. [http://dx.doi.org/10.1016/j.jbusres.2016.08.009]

[35] Ventura SPM, e Silva FA, Quental MV, Mondal D, Freire MG, Coutinho JAP. Ionic-liquid-mediated extraction and separation processes for bioactive compounds: past, present, and future trends. Chem Rev 2017; 117(10): 6984-7052. [http://dx.doi.org/10.1021/acs.chemrev.6b00550] [PMID: 28151648]

[36] Rizzo L, Malato S, Antakyali D, *et al.* Consolidated *vs* new advanced treatment methods for the removal of contaminants of emerging concern from urban wastewater. Sci Total Environ 2019; 655: 986-1008. [http://dx.doi.org/10.1016/j.scitotenv.2018.11.265] [PMID: 30577146]

[37] Vogna D, Marotta R, Andreozzi R, Napolitano A, d'Ischia M. Kinetic and chemical assessment of the UV/H2O2 treatment of antiepileptic drug carbamazepine. Chemosphere 2004; 54(4): 497-505.

[http://dx.doi.org/10.1016/S0045-6535(03)00757-4] [PMID: 14581052]

[38] Muthuraman G, Ramu AG, McAdam E, Moon IS. Sustainable removal of N_2O by mediated electrocatalytic reduction at ambient temperature electro-scrubbing using electrogenerated Ni(I) electron mediator. J Hazard Mater 2019; 378: 120765.
[http://dx.doi.org/10.1016/j.jhazmat.2019.120765] [PMID: 31226591]

[39] Heberlein J, Murphy AB. Thermal plasma waste treatment. J Phys D Appl Phys 2008; 41(5): 053001.
[http://dx.doi.org/10.1088/0022-3727/41/5/053001]

[40] García-Serna J, Pérez-Barrigón L, Cocero MJ. New trends for design towards sustainability in chemical engineering: Green engineering. Chem Eng J 2007; 133(1-3): 7-30.
[http://dx.doi.org/10.1016/j.cej.2007.02.028]

[41] Zayoud A, Dao Thi H, Kusenberg M, *et al.* Pyrolysis of end-of-life polystyrene in a pilot-scale reactor: Maximizing styrene production. Waste Manag 2022; 139: 85-95.
[http://dx.doi.org/10.1016/j.wasman.2021.12.018] [PMID: 34953380]

[42] Semple KT, Riding MJ, McAllister LE, Sopena-Vazquez F, Bending GD. Impact of black carbon on the bioaccessibility of organic contaminants in soil. J Hazard Mater 2013; 261: 808-16.
[http://dx.doi.org/10.1016/j.jhazmat.2013.03.032] [PMID: 23608746]

CHAPTER 6

The Role of the Pharmaceutical Industry in Sustainable Waste Recycling

Prashant Singh[1,*], **Dilip Kumar Mishra**[2], **Shambaditya Goswami**[3], **Asheesh Kumar Singh**[4] and **Pradeep Singh**[5]

[1] *Department of Pharmaceutics, Buddha Institute of Pharmacy, GIDA, Gorakhpur, Uttar Pradesh, India*

[2] *Faculty of Pharmaceutical Sciences, Mahayogi Gorakhnath University, Gorakhpur, Uttar Pradesh, India*

[3] *Department of Pharmaceutical Chemistry, Divine College of Pharmacy, Ziradei, Siwan, Bihar, India*

[4] *Department of Pharmacognosy, Buddha Institute of Pharmacy, GIDA, Gorakhpur, Uttar Pradesh, India*

[5] *Department of Pharmaceutics, Sultanpur Institute of Pharmacy, Sultanpur, Uttar Pradesh, India*

Abstract: This chapter critically analyses the pharmaceutical sector's evolving role in green waste recycling practice. The pharmaceutical industry is shifting away from conventional waste management methods toward circular economy models that emphasise resource recovery and environmental responsibility. We examine ongoing recycling efforts across various pharmaceutical waste streams, including production residues, expired drugs, packaging materials, and laboratory consumables. Novel technologies that facilitate the recovery of valuable compounds, solvents, and rare materials from pharmaceutical waste receive specific attention here. Regulatory regimes vary considerably across regions, and we assess how industry influence, economic incentives, and implementation challenges shape current practice. Case studies highlight industry success stories, outline best practices, and document measurable environmental gains. Our discussion concludes by proposing a forward-looking framework for the recycling of pharmaceutical waste. This framework considers ecological protection, resource conservation, public health concerns, and economic viability while offering pragmatic suggestions for industry actors, policymakers, and researchers working in this space.

* **Corresponding author Prashant Singh:** Department of Pharmaceutics, Buddha Institute of Pharmacy, GIDA, Gorakhpur, Uttar Pradesh, India; E-mail: prashantsingh30785@gmail.com

Suman Gautam, Jai Narayan Mishra, Preeti Mishra, Preeti Verma & Sudhanshu Mishra (Eds.)

Keywords: Circular economy, Environmental risk mitigation, Environmental stewardship, Extended producer responsibility, Green pharmacy, Life cycle assessment, Medication take-back programs, Resource recovery, Sustainable manufacturing, Zero-waste initiatives.

INTRODUCTION

Fundamentally rooted in drug discovery, development, and therapeutic delivery, the pharmaceutical industry sustains modern healthcare by advancing human and animal health while addressing environmental concerns that affect the planet. Its contributions to life extension and quality-of-life enhancement remain indisputable. Nevertheless, this essential sector simultaneously generates substantial pharmaceutical waste streams, a reality often overshadowed in discourse despite its significance for operational sustainability. These waste matrices encompass manufacturing residues, expired pharmaceuticals and therapeutics, depleted inventory, and protective packaging systems (primarily blister pack configurations) designed to maintain product stability and bioavailability before clinical administration. Inadequate or inappropriate disposal practices pose multifaceted environmental and ecological hazards, with documented impacts on aquatic ecosystems, terrestrial biodiversity, and both animal and human health trajectories (Fig. **1**). Consequently, sustainable recycling technologies and methodologies have emerged as critical imperatives. This chapter examines the pharmaceutical industry's pivotal role in advancing sustainable waste-stream recovery and resource-recirculation strategies [1].

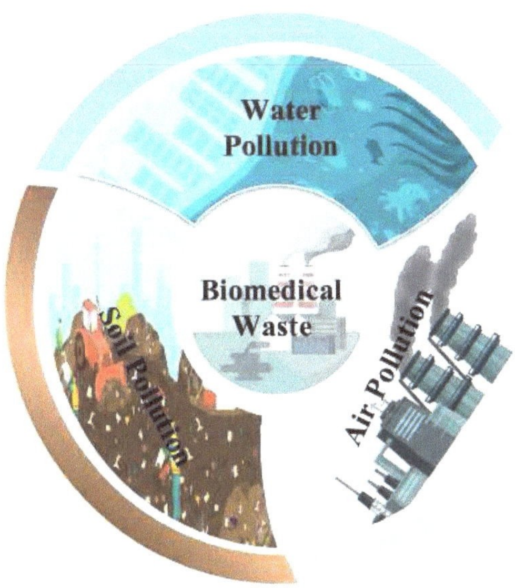

Fig. (1). Types of pollution caused by pharmaceutical waste.

THE SCALE OF THE CHALLENGE: UNDERSTANDING PHARMACEUTICAL WASTE GENERATION

A comprehensive understanding of pharmaceutical waste sources is essential for designing effective recycling strategies. The pharmaceutical product lifecycle, spanning manufacture through disposal, presents multiple points at which waste is generated. Specifically, pharmaceutical waste streams (Fig. **2**) emerge at distinct stages throughout the product lifecycle, from initial production phases to final end-of-life management [2].

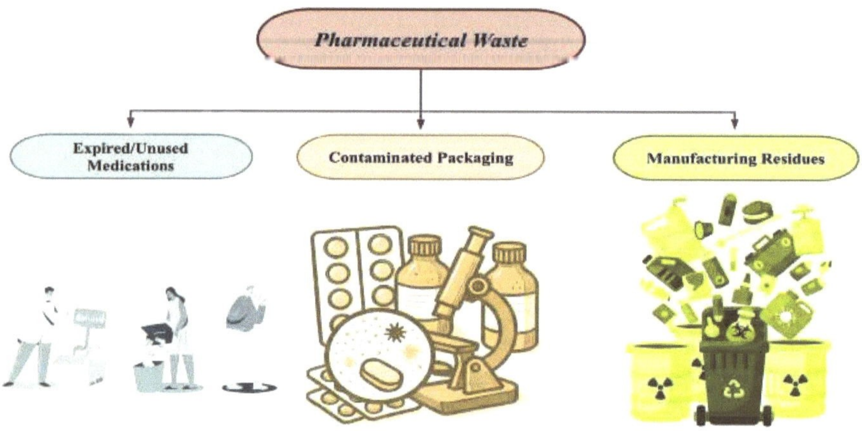

Fig. (2). Types of pharmaceutical waste.

Sources of Pharmaceutical Waste Across the Value Chain

Pharmaceutical products generate substantial waste throughout their entire supply chain, from the synthesis and manufacturing of active pharmaceutical ingredients to distribution networks, clinical administration, and ultimate end-of-life management.

Manufacturing Facilities

Pharmaceutical manufacturing is a multi-stage process that encompasses the synthesis of active pharmaceutical ingredients (APIs), the integration of excipients, drug formulation, and rigorous quality assurance protocols. This complex operational framework generates both inevitable byproducts and intentional disposal outputs, resulting in various streams of pharmaceutical waste. API manufacturing, in particular, produces substantial solvent residues, unreacted process intermediates, and batch failures due to stringent quality control specifications. The heterogeneous nature of pharmaceutical waste necessitates specialised handling and disposal methodologies to prevent environmental contamination and subsequent bioaccumulation through aquatic ecosystems and terrestrial food chains. While essential to therapeutic drug production, contemporary manufacturing processes invariably generate multiple, distinct pharmaceutical waste streams that require systematic characterisation and management [3].

Healthcare Institutions (Hospitals, Clinics, Pharmacies)

Healthcare institutions, including hospitals, clinics, and community pharmacies, represent a substantial nexus of pharmaceutical waste. Daily pharmaceutical inventory management within these settings generates heterogeneous waste streams: expired medications, partially depleted formulations, and medications no longer therapeutically indicated for patient management. Surgical procedures and parenteral therapies generate contaminated sharps, IV administration sets, and syringes contaminated with pharmaceutical residues. Pharmaceutical packaging significantly contributes to the accumulation of medical waste volumes. Cytotoxic and controlled substances necessitate particularly stringent regulatory protocols, given their documented abuse potential and environmental hazard profiles. Healthcare delivery inherently generates continuous waste flows, demanding sophisticated, systematically integrated institutional waste management frameworks [4].

Pharmaceutical research and development activities represent a distinct waste stream of considerable complexity. From initial drug discovery through preclinical evaluation and subsequent clinical investigation, these processes generate substantial chemical and biological byproducts, including experimental reagents, biological specimens, and unsuitable synthetic intermediates, as well as lead compounds that are precluded from commercial advancement. The particular challenge lies in characterising waste of novel or unknown chemical composition, mandating stringent containment protocols due to uncertain environmental and toxicological profiles. Though therapeutically essential, exploratory research inherently produces chemical and biological materials whose environmental consequences remain largely undetermined, underscoring the necessity for rigorous waste control strategies [5].

Consumer-level pharmaceutical disposal constitutes a final yet significant source. Household disposal of unused, expired, or therapeutically surplus medications *via* municipal sewage systems or general refuse streams results in environmental contamination and associated management complications. Active pharmaceutical ingredients readily permeate conventional water treatment processes, compromising aquatic ecosystems and bioaccumulating through food webs. Insufficient public education and inadequate accessible disposal infrastructure perpetuate inappropriate disposal practices, directly contaminating soil and marine environments. Expanded pharmaceutical take-back programs and targeted community engagement on appropriate disposal methods remain critical to mitigating household-derived pharmaceutical pollution [6, 7].

Global Trends and Statistics in Pharmaceutical Waste Generation

Pharmaceutical waste poses a pressing global challenge that demands intensified regulatory and operational attention. Contemporary market assessments highlight the substantial economic implications: valued at approximately USD 38–40 billion in 2023, the global pharmaceutical waste management sector is projected to experience exponential expansion to USD 65–77 billion by 2032–2033, representing a compound annual growth rate (CAGR) of 7.7–7.8%. This market trajectory underscores both the severity and economic consequences of pharmaceutical waste across healthcare systems worldwide. The hazardous fraction comprises the dominant market segment, accounting for roughly 70% of 2023 valuations. This predominance reflects the inherent toxicological properties of numerous pharmaceutical compounds, necessitating the development of sophisticated containment and treatment protocols to safeguard the integrity of environmental and human health [8, 9].

Regional pharmaceutical waste generation and management practices exhibit considerable heterogeneity. North America and Europe currently function as established market leaders, whilst the Asia-Pacific region demonstrates accelerated growth trajectories. Notably, higher-income nations paradoxically generate higher hazardous waste volumes per hospital bed than lower-income economies, a disparity reflecting differences in healthcare infrastructure sophistication, regulatory stringency, and pharmaceutical utilisation patterns. Developed healthcare systems frequently generate greater hazardous waste due to complex treatment modalities and rigorous quality control mechanisms, whereas resource-limited settings often face infrastructural constraints that limit waste segregation sophistication [10].

The coronavirus disease 2019 (COVID-19) pandemic has substantially intensified the complexities of pharmaceutical and medical waste management. The accelerated demand for personal protective equipment, diagnostic reagents, and immunological therapeutics led to a marked escalation in waste generation during the pandemic response phases. This phenomenon highlights the vulnerability of waste management infrastructure to acute health crises and underscores the necessity for adaptive, scalable operational frameworks. Such epidemiological disruptions typically catalyse elevated pharmaceutical consumption and the deployment of single-use medical devices, demonstrating how geopolitical health emergencies directly amplify waste stream burdens [11].

Contemporary epidemiological surveillance and market characterisation are systematically catalogued in companion analyses (Table **1**: global and regional hazard classification frameworks; Table **2**: regional pharmaceutical waste generation stratification; Table **3**: compositional pharmaceutical waste categorisation and handling specifications).

Table 1. Global and regional hazardous waste management market overview.

Region	Market Size (2023, USD Billion)	Projected Market Size (2033, USD Billion)	Fastest Growing Market	Largest Market (2023)	Hazardous Waste Share (2023)
Global	38-40	65-77	Asia Pacific	North America	~70%
North America	~1.7	-	-	North America	-
Europe	-	-	-	Europe	-
Asia Pacific	-	-	Asia Pacific	-	-
High-Income	-	-	-	-	Up to 0.5 kg/bed/day
Low-Income	-	-	-	-	Up to 0.2 kg/bed/day

Table 2. Global pharmaceutical waste generation statistics by region.

Region	Hazardous Waste per Bed per Day (High-Income Countries) [1]	Hazardous Waste per Bed per Day (Low-Income Countries) [2]	Total Pharmaceutical Waste Collected in New Zealand (2019) [3]
High-Income Countries	Up to 0.5 kg	-	-
Low-Income Countries	-	Up to 0.2 kg	-
North America	8.4–10.7 kg (USA)	-	-
Europe	2.7–4.4 kg (France, Spain)	-	-
Asia	0.6–6.10 kg (China, Jordan)	-	-
South America	2.09–3.3 kg (Ecuador, Brazil)	-	-
Africa	0.38–1.8 kg (Sudan, Ethiopia)	-	-
New Zealand (as a country)	-	-	542 tonnes

Table 3. Composition of pharmaceutical waste.

Waste Category	Description	Examples
P-Listed Waste	Acutely hazardous waste from discarded commercial chemical products.	Warfarin (P001), Epinephrine (P042)
U-Listed Waste	Hazardous waste from discarded commercial chemical products.	Cyclophosphamide (U058), Diethylstilbestrol (DES)
Characteristic Hazardous Waste	Waste exhibiting ignitability, corrosivity, reactivity, or toxicity.	Alcohol-based cough syrups (ignitable), Glacial acetic acid (corrosive), Acetyl chloride (reactive), Mercury (toxic)
Non-Hazardous Pharmaceutical Waste	Medications not classified as hazardous but still requiring careful disposal.	Expired or unused medications not meeting hazardous waste criteria.
Cytotoxic and Cytostatic Waste	Waste from cancer treatments containing dangerous medicines.	Chemotherapy drugs and their metabolites
Infectious Waste	Waste contaminated with microorganisms or viruses that can cause infection.	Used syringes and bandages contaminated with bodily fluids
Radioactive Waste	Waste containing radioactive materials.	Waste from radiopharmaceutical production
Chemical Waste	Waste containing expired or unused disinfectants or laboratory reagents.	Solvents, waste with high heavy metal content
General/Other Waste	Non-hazardous waste like packaging, paper, and food scraps.	Empty bottles, non-blood intravenous tubing

PHARMACEUTICAL WASTE'S EFFECTS ON ECOSYSTEMS AND HUMAN HEALTH: THE ENVIRONMENTAL IMPERATIVE

The generation of pharmaceutical waste, which is escalating at an alarming rate, presents multifaceted environmental and public health challenges with profound ecological consequences. Recognition of these impacts spanning ecosystem disruption and human health vulnerability across diverse populations remains fundamental to catalysing evidence-based transitions toward sustainable waste stream recirculation methodologies.

Pollution of Water Sources and Their Environmental Effects

Pharmaceutical contaminants enter aquatic ecosystems through multiple pathways, including human and veterinary drug metabolism and excretion, disposal of unused medications, and inadequate treatment during municipal wastewater processing. Standard wastewater treatment plants often lack sufficient capacity for comprehensive removal of pharmaceutical residues, allowing pharmacologically active metabolites to persist in treated effluent discharged into fluvial and lacustrine environments [12].

The ecological consequences prove multifaceted and extensively documented. Endocrine disruption represents one of the most problematic effects of pharmaceutical compounds that interfere with hypothalamic-pituitary-gonadal axes in aquatic fauna, frequently manifesting as reproductive dysfunction and sex reversal in fish populations, including impaired gamete production and feminisation of males. Beyond reproductive pathology, pharmaceutical exposure modulates fish behaviour, decreasing predator avoidance reflexes and increasing predation vulnerability. Certain pharmaceuticals directly damage aquatic invertebrates and macrophytes, effectively destabilising the trophic base of food webs [13].

Antibiotic persistence in aquatic systems generates particularly concerning selective pressures. Even subtherapeutic antibiotic concentrations establish ecological niches that favour bacterial resistance phenotypes, thereby accelerating the emergence of antimicrobial resistance, now recognised as a critical global health threat. Furthermore, lipophilic pharmaceuticals undergo bioaccumulation, accumulating in organismal tissues at concentrations exceeding environmental levels and progressively increasing through successive trophic levels [14].

The confluence of endocrine disruption, altered behavioural phenotypes, and selection for antimicrobial resistance poses substantial threats to the stability and function of aquatic ecosystems. Pharmaceutical-contaminated aquatic environments thus represent a significant threat to both ecological integrity and downstream human health security [15].

Soil Pollution and Threats to Terrestrial Life

Soil serves as a significant repository for pharmaceuticals through multiple exposure pathways, including the application of biosolids in agricultural systems, the excretion of veterinary drugs in livestock waste, and improper disposal practices. Upon soil incorporation, pharmaceuticals disrupt microbial communities that are essential for biogeochemical cycling processes, critically affecting nutrient mobilisation and ecosystem function. Phytotoxic uptake mechanisms enable the accumulation of pharmaceutical residues in plants, potentially facilitating trophic transfer through herbivory or direct human consumption, thereby compromising the integrity of the food chain [16].

The diclofenac-induced vulture population collapse in South Asian ecosystems exemplifies the catastrophic impacts of pharmaceuticals on terrestrial fauna. Non-steroidal anti-inflammatory drug residues in livestock carcasses caused acute nephrotic syndrome in scavenging vulture populations, precipitating species-specific declines exceeding 95% in certain geographical regions. This ecological disaster highlights the capacity of pharmaceutical compounds to induce profound trophic disruption and the potential for species extinction within terrestrial systems [17].

Soil thus functions as a persistent sink for pharmaceuticals, mediating ecosystem-wide contamination cascades that affect both microbial communities and terrestrial macrofauna. The interconnectedness of biogeochemical compartments means that pharmaceutical pollution readily migrates across aqueous, pedospheric, and biotic domains, generating cascading ecological perturbations that extend across multiple organismal taxa and functional groups [18].

Air Pollution from Improper Waste Disposal Practices

Improper thermal processing of pharmaceutical waste poses a substantial air quality hazard, particularly through uncontrolled open burning of medical waste streams. Incomplete combustion at suboptimal temperatures generates a complex mixture of polychlorinated dibenzo-p-dioxins and dibenzofurans, recognised carcinogenic pollutants with documented associations to multiple adverse health outcomes. Even regulated incineration, when insufficient emission-control infrastructure is in place, can lead to atmospheric release of these persistent organic pollutants. The complexity of pharmaceutical waste's chemical composition, encompassing diverse organic moieties, halogenated compounds, and heteroatom-containing structures, renders thermal processing inherently hazardous without rigorous temperature control and scrubbing technologies. Consequently, inadequately managed thermal waste disposal generates occupational and community exposures to airborne carcinogens, collectively degrading regional air quality and establishing sustained human health risks to proximal populations [18].

The Growing Concern of Pharmaceutical Residues in the Food Chain

Aqueous and pedospheric pharmaceutical contamination precipitates bioavailability to primary producers and lower trophic organisms, establishing persistent dietary exposure pathways. Terrestrial plants directly accumulate pharmaceutical residues from contaminated soil matrices; aquatic organisms sequester contaminants from ambient aqueous and sedimentary reservoirs. Humans occupy apical trophic positions within multiple food webs, receiving continuous and cumulative pharmaceutical exposures through the dietary consumption of botanicals and fauna. Certain lipophilic compounds undergo biomagnification, progressively concentrating at higher trophic levels as trophic transfers accumulate residues. The chronic, low-level pharmaceutical exposures derived from nutritional pathways remain poorly characterised regarding long-term health implications, yet warrant rigorous epidemiological investigation and precautionary management strategies. Human population segments occupy terminal positions within food chains, rendering even minimal organismal pharmaceutical accumulation potentially consequential for population-level health trajectories; the toxicological consequences of protracted subclinical pharmaceutical exposures remain substantially undetermined, necessitating careful biomonitoring and risk characterisation [19].

Beyond Conventional Methods: Why Sustainable Recycling is Essential

Conventional pharmaceutical waste disposal methodologies, notably landfilling and thermal incineration, are inadequate for addressing the chronic, large-scale burden of pharmaceutical waste. This operational insufficiency mandates a paradigmatic reorientation toward circular economy frameworks, emphasising resource recovery and waste-stream valorisation [20].

LIMITATIONS OF TRADITIONAL PHARMACEUTICAL WASTE MANAGEMENT (LANDFILLING, INCINERATION)

Conventional pharmaceutical waste disposal modalities, landfilling and thermal incineration, each present distinct environmental and operational constraints [21].

Landfilling

Designated landfill repositories theoretically contain waste materials whilst preventing immediate environmental dispersal. However, this approach offers negligible consideration for pharmaceutical-specific treatment. Pharmaceutical waste landfill disposal presents substantial leaching hazards, contaminant mobilisation into adjacent soil matrices, and consequent groundwater contamination represents a critical failure mode. Beyond environmental contamination risks, landfilling diverts finite land resources from alternative productive applications. The chemical heterogeneity of pharmaceutical waste, characterized by complex organic structures and potentially hazardous constituents, creates long-term environmental consequences incompatible with landfill containment methods. Groundwater and soil quality degradation emerge as inevitable outcomes rather than anomalies, rendering landfill disposition fundamentally unsustainable [22].

Incineration

Thermal oxidation at elevated temperatures effectively reduces the volume of and inactivates pathogens, while potentially eliminating specific pharmaceutical moieties. Inadequately regulated combustion processes, however, lead to substantial air quality deterioration through the emission of polychlorinated dibenzo-p-dioxin and dibenzofuran. Pharmaceutical waste incineration proves to be energy-intensive, particularly for moisture-containing substrates that require sustained high temperatures to be effectively treated. Incomplete combustion of certain pharmaceutical compounds generates hazardous atmospheric emissions or residual ash-phase contaminants. Sophisticated emission control technologies remain essential to mitigate air pollution risks, a capital and operational expense that substantially limits deployment accessibility. Thus, whilst thermally destructive, incineration necessitates complex technological infrastructure to avoid creating alternative environmental contamination pathways [23].

The Principles of Sustainable Recycling and the Circular Economy

Sustainable pharmaceutical waste recycling represents a fundamental departure from linear disposal paradigms, embodying circular economy principles that emphasise extended material lifecycles and resource valorisation. Rather than conceptualising waste as a terminal byproduct, this framework repositions discarded or underutilised pharmaceutical materials as functional feedstocks. By maximising resource utility duration and recirculating materials and products through successive service iterations, circular approaches substantially mitigate gross environmental burdens whilst reducing dependency on virgin raw material extraction. This operational philosophy directly contrasts conventional "take-make-dispose" models, instead implementing closed-loop architectures in which waste streams become secondary resources rather than environmental liabilities [24].

The Economic and Environmental Benefits of Recycling Pharmaceutical Waste

The economic and environmental dimensions of pharmaceutical waste recycling manifest through complementary mechanisms. Resource recovery initiatives that extract active pharmaceutical ingredients, packaging components, and other recoverable materials from discarded formulations simultaneously reduce environmental contamination while generating revenue streams through the commercialisation of recovered materials. This dual benefit structure creates a genuine financial incentive architecture that supports ecologically responsible industry practices. Beyond remediated ecological quality and natural resource preservation, resource recovery diminishes operational disposal expenditures whilst establishing profitable circular revenue channels. Consequently, sustainable recycling fundamentally reorients pharmaceutical industry economics toward regenerative rather than extractive models [25].

INNOVATIVE TECHNOLOGIES FOR RECYCLING PHARMACEUTICAL WASTE

Emerging technological developments are substantially accelerating the implementation of circular pharmaceutical waste management. Green chemistry methodologies, bioremediation systems, advanced separation techniques, and solvent recovery platforms collectively enhance recovery efficiency, operational safety, and economic viability. These technological innovations facilitate the extraction of valuable compounds while minimising environmental footprints, critically enabling material recirculation at scale (Fig. **3**). Contemporary technological trajectories demonstrate substantial promise for transforming pharmaceutical waste management toward genuinely sustainable operational frameworks [26].

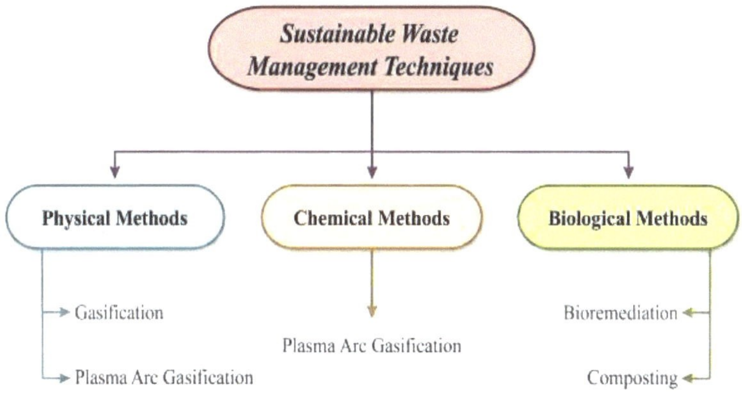

Fig. (3). Advanced treatment methods.

ADVANCED THERMAL TREATMENT METHODS: PYROLYSIS AND GASIFICATION

Advanced thermal treatment methodologies, such as pyrolysis and gasification, represent environmentally sophisticated alternatives to conventional pharmaceutical waste disposal. These high-temperature, oxygen-limited processes decompose complex pharmaceutical compounds into simpler, frequently recoverable materials whilst substantially mitigating hazardous emission profiles. Compared to standard incineration, such technologies facilitate superior emission control, enabling cleaner energy recovery and more sustainable waste management strategies (Fig. **3**) [27].

Pyrolysis

Pyrolytic thermal decomposition, typically conducted within 300–800°C temperature windows, occurs under anoxic or severely oxygen-limited conditions.

This approach proves particularly efficacious for pharmaceutical waste streams. Complex organic pharmaceutical molecules undergo efficient fragmentation, yielding valuable byproducts: biochar (a carbon-enriched solid), syngas (a hydrogen-carbon monoxide mixture), and bio-oil. These products function as alternative energy vectors or industrial feedstock precursors. By converting pharmaceutical hazards into potentially valuable materials within controlled, thermally regulated, oxygen-depleted environments, pyrolysis simultaneously addresses environmental contamination whilst enabling resource recovery pathways [28].

Gasification

Gasification represents an alternative high-temperature thermal process that produces synthesis gas through partial oxidation of pharmaceutical waste under limited oxygen, air, or steam conditions, typically operating at temperatures of 700–1400°C. Unlike complete combustion, partial oxidation converts organic components into combustible mixtures predominantly comprising carbon monoxide, hydrogen, and methane. This syngas serves as a fuel or chemical feedstock, providing cleaner and more energy-efficient alternatives to conventional incineration. Syngas extraction enables the valorisation of pharmaceutical waste energy while substantially reducing environmental contamination and hazardous emissions. Combustible gaseous products support downstream industrial energy generation or electricity production, providing practical energy recovery mechanisms through pharmaceutical waste-derived gaseous feedstocks [29].

CHEMICAL RECYCLING: RECOVERING VALUABLE COMPOUNDS AND MATERIALS

Chemical recycling emphasises molecular-level waste deconstruction, facilitating the recovery of therapeutically and commercially valuable compounds. Solvent extraction methodologies recover active pharmaceutical ingredients and other high-value chemicals from expired formulations or manufacturing waste streams. Specialised chemical processes enable the recycling of blister packs and complex pharmaceutical packaging materials. Chemical recycling establishes high-value feature extraction pathways, thereby reducing terminal disposal requirements and dependencies on virgin resources. Through chemical decomposition, waste materials yield functional building blocks that support the synthesis of novel products, thereby operationalising circular economy principles [30].

BIOLOGICAL TREATMENT APPROACHES: BIOREMEDIATION AND ANAEROBIC DIGESTION

Biological treatment technologies utilise the metabolic capacity of organisms for the sustainable management of pharmaceutical waste [31].

Bioremediation

Microorganism-mediated bioremediation converts complex pharmaceutical contaminants into less harmful molecular species. Bacterial and fungal systems exploit inherent metabolic pathways that degrade pharmaceutically active compounds. Bioremediation offers environmental advantages over purely chemical or thermal approaches for specific categories of pharmaceutical waste. By exploiting natural enzymatic metabolic pathways, microorganisms establish sustainable treatment mechanisms that convert complex organic compounds into simpler, substantially less toxic products [32].

Anaerobic Digestion

Anaerobic microbial decomposition of organic material generates methane-enriched biogas in the absence of oxygen. This technology addresses organic pharmaceutical waste, including wastewater streams from pharmaceutical manufacturing. Anaerobic digestion proves particularly valuable for waste treatment, coupled with renewable energy recovery. The generated biogas serves as a harvestable renewable energy source, supporting both thermal and electrical generation. Concurrent organic pharmaceutical waste management and renewable energy production establish genuinely circular waste treatment frameworks. Oxygen-free organic decomposition yields methane-rich biogas, which is amenable to energy recovery applications [33].

Composting

Composting represents an alternative biological treatment method for non-hazardous pharmaceutical waste components, particularly those derived from paper- or cardboard-based packaging and certain organic pharmaceutical compounds. Controlled microbial decomposition generates nutrient-enriched compost suitable for soil amelioration. Composting offers viable management pathways for non-hazardous organic pharmaceutical waste fractions. Natural biodegradable decomposition converts suitable materials into soil-enriching products [34].

SUSTAINABLE PACKAGING SOLUTIONS: MINIMISING WASTE THROUGH DESIGN

Pharmaceutical product packaging has a substantial influence on cumulative sector waste generation. Sustainable packaging innovations are proving critical for mitigating this impact [35].

Pharmaceutical waste generation reflects a substantial contribution from packaging, particularly multi-layered plastic-intensive materials such as blister packs. While packaging remains therapeutically essential for protecting drugs, maintaining stability, and ensuring efficacy, the complexity of composites creates recycling impediments due to their heterogeneous material composition. Stringent pharmaceutical storage regulations often mandate intricate and expansive packaging designs, inadvertently escalating waste production trajectories. This circumstance urgently necessitates innovative, environmentally viable packaging solutions that strike a balance between planetary sustainability and rigorous product protection requirements [36].

Encouragingly, pharmaceutical manufacturers are increasingly embracing sustainable packaging innovations that reduce their environmental footprints. Emerging approaches include biodegradable materials, mono-material designs, and recyclable or reusable packaging systems reflecting institutional, consumer, and regulatory sustainability pressures throughout pharmaceutical supply chains [37].

Biodegradable polymers represent a significant advance in pharmaceutical packaging, frequently derived from renewable resources such as cellulose, polylactic acid (PLA), and starch. These materials decompose naturally within industrial composting facilities, substantially reducing the long-term environmental burdens of packaging waste compared to the persistence of conventional plastics. Biodegradable polymers offer genuine alternatives to synthetic polymers, substantially reducing packaging waste and environmental impact, and promoting genuinely sustainable waste management approaches [38, 39].

Mono-material packaging solutions constitute another substantial pharmaceutical packaging trend utilising single plastic materials (polyethene or polypropylene). This approach significantly simplifies recycling processes, circumventing the challenges of separating multi-material components inherent in heterogeneous packaging. Mono-material formulations substantially enhance recyclability, minimise contamination in recycling streams, and support genuinely circular packaging frameworks. Streamlined recycling processes facilitate material recovery [40].

Reusable pharmaceutical packaging systems are increasingly gaining market traction, representing environmentally superior alternatives to ubiquitous single-use containers. These systems facilitate repeated medication refills within identical or recyclable containers, substantially reducing demand for disposable packaging. Reuse of approaches promotes extended-lifecycle sustainability throughout pharmaceutical supply chains, diminishing cumulative waste generation and encouraging circular consumption patterns. Exemplary initiatives, such as return-and-reuse programs for insulin pens and inhalers, have demonstrated a substantial reduction in demand for single-use packaging [41].

Pharmaceutical manufacturers increasingly investigate paper-based packaging alternatives. Paperboard applications for blister pack substrates or pill containers provide environmentally friendlier alternatives to traditional plastics. Paper materials possess inherent advantages, including renewable sourcing, straightforward recyclability, and typical biodegradability, which establish genuinely sustainable pharmaceutical packaging options [42].

Case Studies of Sustainable Packaging Adoption

Contemporary pharmaceutical manufacturers actively implement sustainable packaging strategies. Novo Nordisk's Returpen initiative enables international insulin pen return and recycling programs through pharmacy networks. GSK, Chiesi, and Teva established UK and Ireland-based initiatives to collect and recycle used inhalers, despite the complex material composition and propellant complications. Blueprint Medicines collaborated with specialised recycling enterprises managing substantial plastic laboratory waste. Johnson & Johnson initiated comprehensive material recycling and reuse initiatives across operational facilities. Bayer HealthCare developed comprehensive environmental strategies that incorporated data-driven waste management systems throughout its pharmaceutical operations. These case studies demonstrate the practical feasibility of implementing sustainability and the ecological benefits derivable from adopting sustainable pharmaceutical packaging [43].

GREEN CHEMISTRY AND LEAN MANUFACTURING: PREVENTING WASTE AT THE SOURCE

Beyond sustainable packaging and recycling, the pharmaceutical sector innovation emphasises green chemistry and lean manufacturing methodologies for upstream waste prevention [44].

Applying Green Chemistry Principles in Pharmaceutical Production

Green chemistry minimises or eliminates the use and generation of hazardous chemicals throughout the design, manufacture, and application of chemical products. Pharmaceutical applications emphasise safer chemical alternatives and sustainable procedures during drug synthesis and manufacturing. Production process reoptimisation reduces wasteful byproduct generation, whilst selective substitution of conventional chemicals, catalysts, and solvents favours safer, more sustainable alternatives. Green chemistry establishes inherently sustainable manufacturing processes, substantially reducing pharmaceutical waste generation through prioritisation of foundational environmental responsibility [45].

The Role of Lean Manufacturing in Reducing Waste Generation

Lean manufacturing methodology systematically maximises operational value whilst minimising manufacturing waste. Pharmaceutical manufacturers employ the "5S" methodologies — Sort, Set in Order, Shine, Standardise, Sustain — to simplify processes and eliminate upstream waste sources. Lean approaches identify and eliminate inefficiencies and non-value-adding activities, substantially reducing cumulative waste production. Workflow and resource utilisation optimisation minimises manufacturing inefficiencies and waste generation throughout pharmaceutical production cycles [46].

Pharmaceutical manufacturers increasingly implement production-phase waste recovery techniques. Distillation and advanced filtration enable the recovery of liquids and processing aids, facilitating their reintegration within manufacturing cycles. Such approaches reduce hazardous waste generation whilst diminishing virgin raw material dependencies. Integrated resource recovery mechanisms within production infrastructure substantially reduce cumulative waste streams, enhance resource efficiency, and foster genuinely sustainable manufacturing practices [47, 48].

REGULATORY FRAMEWORKS: NAVIGATING COMPLEX COMPLIANCE LANDSCAPES

Pharmaceutical waste management governance involves intricate, multilevel regulatory frameworks that encompass national legislation and international regulatory standards. Core regulatory objectives establish balanced approaches that ensure the safe disposal, recycling, and treatment of pharmaceutical waste, while safeguarding public health and environmental integrity. Effective waste management necessitates region-specific regulatory compliance expertise, as governance structures vary substantially across jurisdictions [49, 50].

United States Regulatory Framework

United States' pharmaceutical waste management operates under a comprehensive regulatory architecture substantially influenced by the Resource Conservation and Recovery Act (RCRA). The Environmental Protection Agency (EPA) establishes federal standards governing the handling, storage, treatment, transport, and disposal of hazardous and non-hazardous waste. The EPA promulgated pharmaceutical-sector-specific regulations, notably "Management Standards for Hazardous Waste Pharmaceuticals" (RCRA Subpart P), designed to facilitate compliance among healthcare providers through clarified, cost-effective guidelines for identifying, classifying, and disposing of pharmaceutical hazards. The Drug Enforcement Administration (DEA) specifically regulates controlled substance disposal, precluding environmental dispersal and diversion. DEA regulations explicitly prohibit the flushing of hazardous pharmaceutical waste from any source. While complex, the United States' regulatory framework establishes substantive pharmaceutical waste management standards, with recent modifications most notably Subpart P reflecting ongoing efforts to simplify compliance for healthcare facilities and promote safer disposal practices [51 - 55].

Regulatory Frameworks in the European Union (EMA and Related Directives)

The European Medicines Agency (EMA) oversees the evaluation and regulation of medicinal products for human and veterinary therapeutic applications throughout the European Union. While the EMA primarily addresses the safety and efficacy of pharmaceuticals, it also provides guidance on environmental risk assessment for human medicinal products. These directives evaluate and mitigate the potential environmental impacts of pharmaceuticals throughout their entire product lifecycle, incorporating waste management considerations. EU general environmental protection and waste management regulations apply to the pharmaceutical sector, establishing comprehensive frameworks that address the ecological effects of pharmaceuticals throughout their lifecycle, from development to disposal. The EU regulatory architecture systematically targets pharmaceutical environmental impacts, minimising environmental releases while promoting sustainable sector-wide practices [56].

The Influence of Regulations on Sustainable Practices

National and international regulations function as critical drivers promoting sustainable pharmaceutical waste management and recycling implementation. Regulatory provisions frequently specify mandatory disposal methodologies, establish emissions thresholds, and actively encourage or mandate environmentally conscious practices. Navigating regulatory compliance presents substantial complexity for pharmaceutical manufacturers and healthcare providers; evolving requirements necessitate continuous regulatory monitoring. Rigorous enforcement mechanisms prove essential for regulatory effectiveness. By establishing legal standards and environmental criteria, regulatory systems drive the pharmaceutical industry's transition toward sustainable waste management. Regulations effectively compel comprehensive waste minimisation, the adoption of recycling, and secure handling procedures for pharmaceutical byproducts. Regulatory frameworks ultimately encourage manufacturers to institutionalise sustainability throughout their operational infrastructure, facilitating the achievement of national and international environmental objectives [57].

CHALLENGES AND OPPORTUNITIES IN TRANSITIONING TO SUSTAINABLE RECYCLING

Pharmaceutical waste management transitions toward genuinely sustainable recycling present both substantive challenges and significant innovation opportunities. Whilst logistical, legal, and technical obstacles necessitate systematic resolution, these transitions simultaneously enable genuine innovation in waste prevention, valuable resource recovery, and environmental harm reduction. Enhanced efficiency and resource valorisation generate both ecological benefits and tangible financial advantages emerging from sustainable operational adoption [58].

Technological Barriers and the Need for Innovation

Significant technological limitations hinder the widespread adoption of sustainable pharmaceutical waste recycling. Complex pharmaceutical waste streams, including multi-layered packaging or medications containing hazardous chemicals, require advanced, specialised treatment techniques that are frequently in developmental phases or have limited accessibility. Fortunately, substantial technological advancements progressively bridge existing gaps. Chemical recycling shows particular promise for breaking down complex polymeric structures. Advanced thermal methodologies, such as pyrolysis and gasification, convert waste into usable energy or valuable byproducts. Emergent artificial intelligence and Internet of Things-enabled waste management systems substantially enhance tracking efficiency, sorting precision, and treatment optimisation. While technological constraints temporarily limit the widespread adoption of sustainable recycling, continuous development progressively establishes increasingly feasible solutions. The compositional uniqueness of pharmaceutical waste frequently necessitates purpose-designed recycling technologies [59].

Economic Considerations: Investment and Return on Sustainable Practices

The adoption of advanced recycling technology encounters substantial initial expenditure obstacles. However, the economic feasibility of sustainable recycling progressively increases as environmental regulations intensify and conventional disposal expenses, particularly landfill fees, escalate. The recovery potential of pharmaceutical waste material substantially offsets initial investment costs, potentially generating a revenue stream. While the establishment of sustainable recycling infrastructure requires considerable initial capital allocation, long-term economic advantages driven by escalating disposal costs and intensifying environmental regulations render sustainability increasingly attractive. Sustainable practices progressively achieve cost competitiveness as economic landscapes evolve, supporting ecologically responsible approaches.

The Importance of Collaboration Among Stakeholders

Widespread recognition of sustainable pharmaceutical waste recycling depends fundamentally on comprehensive collaboration among stakeholders. Requisite participants encompass legislators establishing supportive regulatory frameworks, pharmaceutical manufacturers championing sustainable operational paradigms, healthcare providers guiding appropriate patient disposal practices, specialised waste management enterprises providing innovative solutions, and consumers actively participating in take-back initiatives. Public awareness campaigns prove absolutely vital, educating populations about the health and environmental hazards of pharmaceutical waste while encouraging participation in take-back programmes. The successful implementation of sustainable pharmaceutical waste recycling depends fundamentally on coordinated stakeholder engagement that spans the entire pharmaceutical value chain. Manufacturers, healthcare providers, policymakers, and consumers must work together actively to resolve complex issues and achieve widespread acceptance of practical solutions.

Engaging Consumers in Responsible Disposal Practices

Fundamental objectives necessitate raising public awareness about the health and environmental hazards associated with pharmaceutical disposal. Consumer education must translate into direct action, encouraging active participation in take-back programs and adherence to professional disposal guidelines. Consumer engagement proves essential for minimising environmental pharmaceutical waste infiltration. Informed consumers demonstrate a substantially greater likelihood of making responsible disposal choices, directly contributing to the development of sustainably robust waste management systems. Consumer participation constitutes an utterly crucial framework implementation component.

CASE STUDIES: SUCCESS STORIES IN PHARMACEUTICAL WASTE RECYCLING

Examining the successful implementation of comprehensive sustainable waste recycling initiatives by pharmaceutical enterprises inspires broader adoption of this practice and provides valuable analytical insights. Prominent manufacturers, including Novo Nordisk, GSK, Chiesi, Teva, Blueprint Medicines, Johnson & Johnson, and Bayer HealthCare, employ diverse strategies, such as take-back programmes, specialised product recycling, and comprehensive environmental management systems. Particular tactical examination and favourable outcome analysis provide instructive lessons that inspire the adoption of expanded, sustainable pharmaceutical waste recycling. Real-world examples demonstrate the viability of sustainable waste management techniques and their practical feasibility of implementation.

CONCLUSION: EMBRACING A SUSTAINABLE FUTURE FOR THE PHARMACEUTICAL INDUSTRY

Pharmaceutical waste management constitutes an increasingly pressing global challenge that demands a comprehensive and expedited response. Conventional disposal methodologies such as landfilling and incineration persist despite their inherent environmental and potential health risks. This circumstance underscores the urgency for paradigmatic reorientation toward sustainable practices. This analysis has delineated the pathways of pharmaceutical waste genesis, documented the ecosystem and human health consequences, and highlighted the limitations of conventional disposal techniques. Critically, it has highlighted promising alternatives, including advanced thermal treatments, chemical recycling, biological approaches, circular economy frameworks, and sustainable recycling methodologies, which represent viable pathways forward.

Encouraging industry developments include strengthened environmental protection and operational integration. Emphasising material innovation and prioritising enhanced reusability and recycling establishes genuinely effective waste reduction mechanisms. Lean manufacturing and green chemistry principles offer substantial potential for preventing waste at the source. Nevertheless, sustainable practice transitions necessitate navigating complex legal environments, particularly within the United States and European regulatory landscapes that substantially influence environmental management.

Despite demonstrated progress and emerging innovative approaches, substantial challenges persist, particularly regarding the requisite advanced technologies and the considerable capital requirements for recycling infrastructure. However, sustainable recycling benefits, including the potential for valuable resource recovery, long-term financial savings, and enhanced environmental stewardship, remain genuinely compelling, warranting a sustained commitment. Meaningful systemic change requires robust multi-stakeholder collaboration: policymakers, medical professionals, pharmaceutical enterprises, waste management specialists, and individual consumers. Public awareness and responsible consumer disposal practices are vital for the effectiveness of the solution.

The success of sustainable pharmaceutical waste management depends fundamentally on sustained research and development investment, the establishment of comprehensive value chain partnerships, and genuinely supportive regulatory environments. By actively championing sustainable practices, the pharmaceutical industry occupies a uniquely influential position, safeguarding environmental and planetary health across intergenerational timeframes. Providing emerging practitioners with a rigorous understanding of these challenges and opportunities equips future leaders to advance the pharmaceutical industry's sustainable transformation.

REFERENCES

[1] Janik-Karpinska E, Brancaleoni R, Niemcewicz M, *et al.* Healthcare waste is a serious problem for global health. Healthcare (Basel) 2023; 11(2): 242. [http://dx.doi.org/10.3390/healthcare11020242] [PMID: 36673610]

[2] Deshmukh G, Umap S, Bhapkar T, *et al.* Pharmaceutical Waste is a Global Challenge to the Ecosystem. Chron Aquat Sci 2024; 1(10): 53-64.

[3] Mitkidis K, Mitkidis P. "Homemade": the vicious circle of household pharmaceutical waste. Eur J Risk Regul 2020; 11(3): 693-7. [http://dx.doi.org/10.1017/err.2020.57]

[4] Paut Kusturica M, Jevtic M, Ristovski JT. Minimizing the environmental impact of unused pharmaceuticals: Review focused on prevention. Front Environ Sci 2022; 10: 1077974. [http://dx.doi.org/10.3389/fenvs.2022.1077974]

[5] Rogowska J, Zimmermann A. Household pharmaceutical waste disposal as a global problem: a review. Int J Environ Res Public Health 2022; 19(23): 15798. [http://dx.doi.org/10.3390/ijerph192315798] [PMID: 36497873]

[6] Çetin E, Esenlikçi Yıldız İA, Öz Yaşar Ç, Yulistyorini A. Life Cycle Assessment of Medical Waste Management: Case Study for Istanbul. Appl Sci (Basel) 2025; 15(8): 4439. [http://dx.doi.org/10.3390/app15084439]

[7] Han J, He S, Lichtfouse E. Waves of pharmaceutical waste. Environ Chem Lett 2023; 21(3): 1251-5. [http://dx.doi.org/10.1007/s10311-022-01491-0] [PMID: 35975196]

[8] Wise J. Covid-19: Pandemic waste threatens human and environmental health, says WHO. BMJ 2022; 376: o266. [http://dx.doi.org/10.1136/bmj.o266] [PMID: 35105547]

[9] Ye J, Song Y, Liu Y, Zhong Y. Assessment of medical waste generation, associated environmental impact, and management issues after the outbreak of COVID-19: A case study of the Hubei Province in China. PLoS One 2022; 17(1): e0259207. [http://dx.doi.org/10.1371/journal.pone.0259207] [PMID: 35073321]

[10] Luhar I, Luhar S, Abdullah M. Challenges and impacts of COVID-19 pandemic on global waste

management systems: a review. J Compos Sci 2022; 6(9): 271.
[http://dx.doi.org/10.3390/jcs6090271]

[11] Daoud AO, Elattar H, Abdelatif G, Morsy KM, Peters RW, Mostafa MK. Implications of the COVID-19 pandemic on the management of municipal solid waste and medical waste: a comparative review of selected countries. Biomass (Basel) 2024; 4(2): 555-73.
[http://dx.doi.org/10.3390/biomass4020030]

[12] Jayasinghe PA, Jalilzadeh H, Hettiaratchi P. The impact of COVID-19 on waste infrastructure: lessons learned and opportunities for a sustainable future. Int J Environ Res Public Health 2023; 20(5): 4310.
[http://dx.doi.org/10.3390/ijerph20054310] [PMID: 36901318]

[13] Peng Y, Wu P, Schartup AT, Zhang Y. Plastic waste release caused by COVID-19 and its fate in the global ocean. Proc Natl Acad Sci USA 2021; 118(47): e2111530118.
[http://dx.doi.org/10.1073/pnas.2111530118] [PMID: 34751160]

[14] Ejeromedoghene O, Nwosisi MC, Tesi GO, Noraghon EI, Akinyeye RO. Impact of pharmaceutical waste generation and handling on environmental health in developing countries: COVID–19 pandemic in perspective! J Appl Sci Environ Manag 2021; 25(3): 385-96.
[http://dx.doi.org/10.4314/jasem.v25i3.12]

[15] Ashiwaju BI, Uzougbo CG, Orikpete OF. Environmental impact of pharmaceuticals: a comprehensive review. Matrix Science Pharma 2023; 7(3): 85-94.
[http://dx.doi.org/10.4103/mtsp.mtsp_15_23]

[16] Barrett JR. The Yin and Yang of exposure: chemical combinations may explain feminization of wild fish. Environ Health Perspect 2009; 117(5): A211.
[PMID: 19478990]

[17] Gross-Sorokin MY, Roast SD, Brighty GC. Assessment of feminization of male fish in English rivers by the Environment Agency of England and Wales. Environ Health Perspect 2006; 114(Suppl 1) (Suppl. 1): 147-51.
[PMID: 16818261]

[18] Christiansen LB, Winther-Nielsen M, Helweg C. Feminisation of fish The effect of estrogenic compounds and their fate in sewage treatment plants and nature. Environmental Project 2002; p. 729.

[19] Kidd KA, Blanchfield PJ, Mills KH, *et al.* Collapse of a fish population after exposure to a synthetic estrogen. Proc Natl Acad Sci USA 2007; 104(21): 8897-901.
[http://dx.doi.org/10.1073/pnas.0609568104] [PMID: 17517636]

[20] Tyler CR, Jobling S. Roach, sex, and gender-bending chemicals: The feminization of wild fish in English rivers. Bioscience 2008; 58(11): 1051-9.
[http://dx.doi.org/10.1641/B581108]

[21] Solar I I, Donaldson E M, Charles J. The effect of three estrogens on the direct feminisation of Chinook salmon (Oncorhynchus tshawytscha). West Vancouver: Department of Fisheries and Oceans; 1994. 20 p. Canadian Technical Report of Fisheries and Aquatic Sciences No. 1955. Available from: https://publications.gc.ca/collections/collection_2014/mpo-dfo/Fs97-6-1955-eng.pdf

[22] Wojnarowski K, Podobiński P, Cholewińska P, Smoliński J, Dorobisz K. Impact of estrogens present in environment on health and welfare of animals. Animals (Basel) 2021; 11(7): 2152.
[http://dx.doi.org/10.3390/ani11072152] [PMID: 34359280]

[23] Khan AHA, Barros R. Pharmaceuticals in water: risks to aquatic life and remediation strategies. Hydrobiology 2023; 2(2): 395-409.
[http://dx.doi.org/10.3390/hydrobiology2020026]

[24] Polianciuc SI, Gurzău AE, Kiss B, Ştefan MG, Loghin F. Antibiotics in the environment: causes and consequences. Med Pharm Rep 2020; 93(3): 231-40.
[http://dx.doi.org/10.15386/mpr-1742] [PMID: 32832887]

[25] Larsson DGJ, Flach CF. Antibiotic resistance in the environment. Nat Rev Microbiol 2022; 20(5):

257-69.
[http://dx.doi.org/10.1038/s41579-021-00649-x] [PMID: 34737424]

[26] Resources N. Interactions of Soil Chemical Contaminants, Soil Health, and Human Health.Exploring Linkages Between Soil Health and Human Health. US: National Academies Press 2024; p. 6. Available from: https://www.ncbi.nlm.nih.gov/books/NBK609355/

[27] Zhang C, Barron LP, Stürzenbaum SR. Pollution of Soil by Pharmaceuticals: Implications for Metazoan and Environmental Health. Annu Rev Pharmacol Toxicol 2024; 65(1): 547-565.
[PMID: 39227350]

[28] Pérez-Lucas G, Navarro S. How Pharmaceutical Residues Occur, Behave, and Affect the Soil Environment. J Xenobiot 2024; 14(4): 1343-77.
[http://dx.doi.org/10.3390/jox14040076] [PMID: 39449417]

[29] Earl K, Sleight H, Ashfield N, Boxall ABA. Are pharmaceutical residues in crops a threat to human health? J Toxicol Environ Health A 2024; 87(19): 773-91.
[http://dx.doi.org/10.1080/15287394.2024.2371418] [PMID: 38959023]

[30] Boxall ABA. The environmental side effects of medication. EMBO Rep 2004; 5(12): 1110-6.
[http://dx.doi.org/10.1038/sj.embor.7400307] [PMID: 15577922]

[31] Arnold KE, Brown AR, Ankley GT, Sumpter JP. Medicating the environment: assessing risks of pharmaceuticals to wildlife and ecosystems. Philos Trans R Soc Lond B Biol Sci 2014; 369(1656): 20130569.
[http://dx.doi.org/10.1098/rstb.2013.0569] [PMID: 25405959]

[32] Bindra P. Declining vulture population can cause a health crisis. Mongabay-India. [internet]. 2018 Feb 6. Available from: https://india.mongabay.com/2018/02/declining-vulture/

[33] Oaks JL, Gilbert M, Virani MZ, *et al.* Diclofenac residues as the cause of vulture population decline in Pakistan. Nature 2004; 427(6975): 630-3.
[http://dx.doi.org/10.1038/nature02317] [PMID: 14745453]

[34] Prakash V, Bishwakarma MC, Chaudhary A, *et al.* The population decline of Gyps vultures in India and Nepal has slowed since veterinary use of diclofenac was banned. PLoS One 2012; 7(11): e49118.
[http://dx.doi.org/10.1371/journal.pone.0049118] [PMID: 23145090]

[35] Shultz S, Baral HS, Charman S, *et al.* Diclofenac poisoning is widespread in declining vulture populations across the Indian subcontinent. Proc Biol Sci 2004; 271(Suppl 6) (Suppl. 6): S458-60.
[PMID: 15801603]

[36] Eapen JV, Thomas S, Antony S, George P, Antony J. A review of the effects of pharmaceutical pollutants on humans and aquatic ecosystem. Explor Drug Sci 2024; 2(5): 484-507.
[http://dx.doi.org/10.37349/eds.2024.00058]

[37] Zenker A, Cicero MR, Prestinaci F, Bottoni P, Carere M. Bioaccumulation and biomagnification potential of pharmaceuticals with a focus to the aquatic environment. J Environ Manage 2014; 133: 378-87.
[http://dx.doi.org/10.1016/j.jenvman.2013.12.017] [PMID: 24419205]

[38] Richmond EK, Rosi EJ, Walters DM, *et al.* A diverse suite of pharmaceuticals contaminates stream and riparian food webs. Nat Commun 2018; 9(1): 4491.
[http://dx.doi.org/10.1038/s41467-018-06822-w] [PMID: 30401828]

[39] Xie Z, Lu G, Yan Z, Liu J, Wang P, Wang Y. Bioaccumulation and trophic transfer of pharmaceuticals in food webs from a large freshwater lake. Environ Pollut 2017; 222: 356-66.
[http://dx.doi.org/10.1016/j.envpol.2016.12.026] [PMID: 28034558]

[40] Sokołowski A, Mordec M, Caban M, *et al.* Bioaccumulation of pharmaceuticals and stimulants in macrobenthic food web in the European Arctic as determined using stable isotope approach. Sci Total Environ 2024; 909: 168557.
[http://dx.doi.org/10.1016/j.scitotenv.2023.168557] [PMID: 37979847]

[41] Bataduwaarachchi V, Weeraratne C. Global medication waste management practices: challenges and opportunities in developing countries. Int J Basic Clin Pharmacol 2016; 5(6): 2290-4. [http://dx.doi.org/10.18203/2319-2003.ijbcp20164081]

[42] Su G, Ong HC, Ibrahim S, Fattah IMR, Mofijur M, Chong CT. Valorisation of medical waste through pyrolysis for a cleaner environment: Progress and challenges. Environ Pollut 2021; 279: 116934. [http://dx.doi.org/10.1016/j.envpol.2021.116934] [PMID: 33744627]

[43] Mgharbel M, Halawy L, Milane A, Zeaiter J, Saad W. Pyrolysis of pharmaceuticals as a novel means of disposal and material recovery from waste for a circular economy. J Anal Appl Pyrolysis 2023; 172: 106014. [http://dx.doi.org/10.1016/j.jaap.2023.106014]

[44] Abad-Grillo T, McNaughton-Smith G. Chemical Upcycling of Expired Pharmaceuticals as a Source of Value-Added Chemicals for Organic Synthesis and Medicinal Chemistry. Molecules 2024; 29(20): 4811. [http://dx.doi.org/10.3390/molecules29204811] [PMID: 39459183]

[45] Amirahmadi H, FarshiFasih H, Saviz S, Nobakhti MH. Experimental and modeling study of medical waste based on plasma gasification. Waste Manag 2024; 186: 198-204. [http://dx.doi.org/10.1016/j.wasman.2024.06.017] [PMID: 38909443]

[46] Tamošiūnas A, Milieška M, Gimžauskaitė D, *et al.* Plasma Gasification of Medical Plastic Waste to Syngas in a Greenhouse Gas (CO2). Environ Sustain (Singap) 2025; 17(5): 2040.

[47] Kumar D, Malviya R, Singh DP. Innovative Techniques for Pharmaceutical Waste Management: Enhancing Drug Recovery and Environmental Sustainability. Curr Green Chem 2025; 12(2): 138-45. [http://dx.doi.org/10.2174/0122133461322762240926072018]

[48] Aboagye EA, Chea JD, Yenkie KM. Systems level roadmap for solvent recovery and reuse in industries. iScience 2021; 24(10): 103114. [http://dx.doi.org/10.1016/j.isci.2021.103114] [PMID: 34622166]

[49] Srinivasan K, Hariharapura RC, Mallikarjuna SV. Pharmaceutical waste management through microbial bioremediation. Environ Monit Assess 2025; 197(4): 488. [http://dx.doi.org/10.1007/s10661-025-13912-y] [PMID: 40163141]

[50] Randhawa GK, Kullar JS. Bioremediation of pharmaceuticals, pesticides, and petrochemicals with gomeya/cow dung. ISRN Pharmacol 2011; 2011: 1-7. [http://dx.doi.org/10.5402/2011/362459] [PMID: 22084712]

[51] Bali A. Bioremediation of pharmaceutical wastes.Handbook of research on inventive bioremediation techniques. IGI Global 2017; pp. 364-93. [http://dx.doi.org/10.4018/978-1-5225-2325-3.ch016]

[52] Shah A, Shah M. Characterisation and bioremediation of wastewater: A review exploring bioremediation as a sustainable technique for pharmaceutical wastewater. Groundw Sustain Dev 2020; 11: 100383. [http://dx.doi.org/10.1016/j.gsd.2020.100383]

[53] Azizan NAZ, Yuzir A, Abdullah N. Pharmaceutical compounds in anaerobic digestion: A review on the removals and effect to the process performance. J Environ Chem Eng 2021; 9(5): 105926. [http://dx.doi.org/10.1016/j.jece.2021.105926]

[54] Asplund K. Removal of pharmaceutical compounds by anaerobic digestion of sewage sludge [Master's thesis]. Vasa: Novia University of Applied Sciences; 2022. Available from: https://www.theseus.fi/bitstream/handle/10024/755160/ Asplund_Katrin.pdf?sequence=2

[55] Zupančič GD, Žgajnar Gotvajn A. Anaerobic treatment of pharmaceutical waste fermentation broth. Chem Biochem Eng Q 2009; 23(4): 485-92.

[56] Kazimierowicz J, Dębowski M, Zieliński M. Effect of pharmaceutical sludge pre-treatment with

Fenton/Fenton-like reagents on toxicity and anaerobic digestion efficiency. Int J Environ Res Public Health 2022; 20(1): 271.
[http://dx.doi.org/10.3390/ijerph20010271] [PMID: 36612592]

[57] Enright AM, McHugh S, Collins G, O'Flaherty V. Low-temperature anaerobic biological treatment of solvent-containing pharmaceutical wastewater. Water Res 2005; 39(19): 4587-96.
[http://dx.doi.org/10.1016/j.watres.2005.08.037] [PMID: 16242171]

[58] Popović K, Živanović S, Jevtić I. Biopolymer packaging materials in the pharmaceutical industry. AIDASCO Reviews 2024; 2(1): 46-56.
[http://dx.doi.org/10.59783/aire.2024.43]

[59] Desai M, Njoku A, Nimo-Sefah L. Comparing environmental policies to reduce pharmaceutical pollution and address disparities. Int J Environ Res Public Health 2022; 19(14): 8292.
[http://dx.doi.org/10.3390/ijerph19148292] [PMID: 35886145]

CHAPTER 7

Role of Advanced Technologies in Transforming Pharmaceutical Waste Management

Aarti Tiwari[1], **Ajay Kumar Shukla**[1,*], **Rahul Kumar Maurya**[2], **Rama Sankar Dubey**[3], **Shivali Singla**[4] and **Joohee Pradhan**[5]

[1] *Institute of Pharmacy, Dr Rammanohar Lohia Avadh University, Ayodhya, Uttar Pradesh, India*

[2] *National Ayurveda Research Institute for Panchakarma, Cheruthuruthy, Thrissur, Kerala, India*

[3] *Department of Pharmacy, Madan Mohan Malaviya University of Technology, Gorakhpur, Uttar Pradesh, India*

[4] *Department of Anesthesiology & Critical Care Medicine, University of New Mexico School of Medicine, Albuquerque, New Mexico, USA*

[5] *Department of Pharmaceutical Sciences, Mohanlal Sukhadia University, Udaipur, Rajasthan, India*

Abstract: Managing pharmaceutical waste is a significant challenge to environmental integrity and public health, necessitating innovative ways to mitigate its adverse effects. The advancement of innovative technology has fundamentally transformed the management, recycling, and disposal of pharmaceutical waste, offering efficient and sustainable alternatives. Emerging technologies such as bioremediation, nanotechnology, green chemistry, artificial intelligence (AI), and machine learning (ML) are transforming the management of pharmaceutical waste. Nanotechnology offers innovative materials for effective waste filtration and degradation, while artificial intelligence (AI) and machine learning (ML) facilitate predictive modelling and optimisation of waste management systems. Green chemistry minimises hazardous waste generation by promoting the development of biodegradable excipients and eco-friendly pharmaceutical formulations. Moreover, pharmaceutical contaminants can be ecologically detoxified by bioremediation techniques utilising microorganisms and enzymes. The integration of blockchain and the Internet of Things (IoT) enhances waste disposal systems by improving transparency, traceability, and regulatory compliance. This chapter examines the advancements, challenges, and prospects of technology-driven pharmaceutical waste management, emphasising the importance of global collaboration and innovative legislation to ensure environmental sustainability and public health safety.

[*] **Corresponding author Ajay Kumar Shukla:** Institute of Pharmacy, Dr Rammanohar Lohia Avadh University, Ayodhya, Uttar Pradesh, India; E-mail: ashukla1007@gmail.com

Suman Gautam, Jai Narayan Mishra, Preeti Mishra, Preeti Verma & Sudhanshu Mishra (Eds.)

Keywords: Advanced technologies, Artificial intelligence, Bioremediation, Green chemistry, Machine learning, Nanotechnology, Pharmaceutical waste management.

INTRODUCTION

The management of pharmaceutical waste is an increasing concern due to the escalating global consumption of medications and the associated threats to human health and the environment. Inappropriate disposal of expired, unused, or contaminated medications can result in water contamination, antimicrobial resistance, and ecological disruption. Advanced technologies are crucial for transforming conventional waste management systems into more efficient, safer, and more sustainable processes to tackle these difficulties. Pharmaceutical products can be intelligently tracked throughout their lifecycle thanks to digital technologies like Radio Frequency Identification (RFID) and the Internet of Things (IoT). These systems make it easier to monitor trash generation, disposal, storage, and segregation in real time. These technologies are used by hospitals and the pharmaceutical industry to make sure that hazardous and non-hazardous wastes are handled correctly and in compliance with regulations. Despite its effectiveness, manual waste sorting is losing efficiency as garbage quantities rise and human resources become scarcer. Resource recovery and recyclability are improved by source segregation, especially into wet and dry streams. Wet waste, which is often turned into compost or biogas, can be used as a source of energy and as a substitute for artificial fertilisers. It is possible to recycle or reuse metallic waste. Source segregation guarantees better material quality for recycling, lowering transportation expenses and occupational hazards even in the face of industrial segregators. Alternative techniques, including pre-shredding or sensor-based sorting, are being researched to deal with excessive garbage. For high waste quantities, sensor-based sorting presents a viable option. The installation of smart dustbins offers a practical and affordable way to separate waste in homes and public areas. These bins move waste to the proper containers for direct processing by using sensors to differentiate between wet and dry waste according to moisture content. Smart dustbins simplify garbage management by automating the sorting process, encouraging recycling, and lowering the need for manual sorting. By guaranteeing premium materials for recycling and reducing the amount of waste dumped in landfills or incinerators, this strategy improves resource recovery and environmental sustainability. It also maximises the use of available resources and lessens reliance on physical effort, which helps create a waste management system that is more sustainable and effective (Fig. **1**) [1, 2].

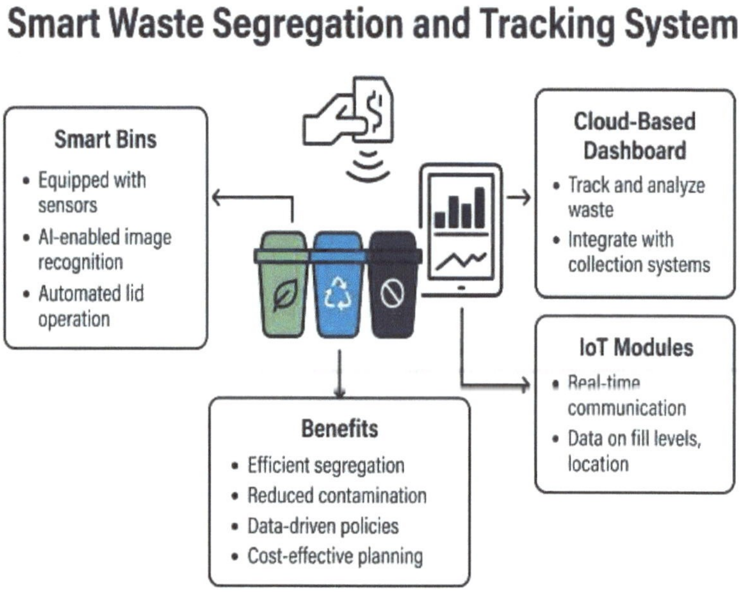

Fig. (1). Smart waste segregation and tracking systems.

ADVANCED OXIDATION PROCESSES (AOPS)

AOPs are being used more and more to break down complex pharmaceutical chemicals in wastewater, such as ozonation, photocatalysis, and Fenton reactions. These techniques produce extremely reactive hydroxyl radicals, which decompose persistent organic contaminants into innocuous byproducts such as carbon dioxide and water. AOPs are particularly good at treating hospital and pharmaceutical industrial effluents.

Due to urbanisation, industrialisation, and the overuse of chemicals, water pollution has emerged as one of the world's most urgent environmental issues. The removal of heavy metals, dyes, pharmaceuticals, persistent organic pollutants (POPs), and other new contaminants is frequently beyond the scope of conventional water and wastewater treatment methods. Advanced Oxidation Processes (AOPs) have become strong and promising technologies for the degradation and mineralisation of a variety of hazardous pollutants in aqueous systems in order to overcome these restrictions.

The *in situ* production of extremely reactive species, mainly hydroxyl radicals (•OH), which can non-selectively attack and degrade complex organic compounds into innocuous byproducts like water, carbon dioxide, and inorganic ions, is what defines AOPs [2].

Principles of Advanced Oxidation Processes

AOPs' primary mechanism is the generation of hydroxyl radicals (•OH), one of the strongest oxidising agents known to exist in aqueous environments, with an oxidation potential of 2.8 V. Depending on the type of AOP used, these radicals are produced using a variety of physical and chemical processes.

General Oxidation Reaction in AOPs

Organic Pollutant+ OH→CO2+H2O+Inorganic Acids

Explanation:

In this reaction:

•OH represents the hydroxyl radical, a powerful oxidizing agent.

It attacks the organic pollutant, breaking it down into:

Carbon dioxide (CO_2)

Water (H_2O)

Other inorganic compounds or acids, depending on the structure of the original pollutant (*e.g.*, HCl, HNO_3, H_2SO_4).

Classification of AOPs

AOPs can be broadly classified based on the method of •OH radical generation:

Photochemical AOPs

UV/H_2O_2: Ultraviolet light decomposes hydrogen peroxide to produce •OH radicals.

UV/TiO_2 (Photocatalysis): Semiconductor catalysts like titanium dioxide absorb UV light and generate electron-hole pairs, leading to the formation of •OH.

Photo-Fenton: Combines UV light with Fenton's reagent (Fe^{2+}/H_2O_2) for enhanced radical generation.

Ozone-Based AOPs

O_3/H_2O_2: Synergistic action of ozone and hydrogen peroxide increases •OH production.

O_3/UV: Ozone decomposition under UV light leads to radical generation.

O_3/Fe^{2+} (Peroxone-Fenton): Combines the oxidizing potential of ozone with Fenton's chemistry.

Electrochemical AOPs

Electro-Fenton: Electrochemical generation of H_2O_2*in situ* using electrodes, which then reacts with Fe^{2+}.

Anodic oxidation: Direct oxidation of pollutants at the anode surface, often using boron-doped diamond (BDD) electrodes [3].

Fenton and Photo-Fenton Processes

The traditional **Fenton reaction** uses Fe^{2+} and H_2O_2 to generate •OH in acidic media.

Photo-Fenton enhances the process under light irradiation, regenerating Fe^{2+} and improving efficiency.

Heterogeneous Catalytic AOPs

Use of solid catalysts (*e.g.*, Fe_3O_4, MnO_2, CuO) to activate oxidants such as H_2O_2, persulfates, or ozone for radical generation [4, 5].

Mechanisms of Degradation

The key mechanism in AOPs is the abstraction of hydrogen atoms or addition reactions involving hydroxyl radicals:

Hydrogen abstraction: •OH attacks C-H bonds, forming water and carbon radicals.

Electron transfer: •OH abstracts an electron, leading to ionized intermediate compounds.

Radical recombination: Secondary radicals combine or undergo further reactions to yield final products.

Applications of AOPs

AOPs have found widespread applications in the degradation of various contaminants:

Industrial Wastewater Treatment

Removal of dyes, phenols, pesticides, and surfactants from textile, tannery, and pharmaceutical effluents.

Drinking Water Purification

Elimination of taste and odor-causing compounds, natural organic matter, and endocrine-disrupting chemicals.

Groundwater Remediation

Effective for chlorinated solvents, polycyclic aromatic hydrocarbons (PAHs), and heavy metals.

Emerging Contaminants

Degradation of pharmaceuticals, personal care products, and microplastics.

Advantages of AOPs

- High efficiency in degrading non-biodegradable and toxic pollutants.
- Complete mineralization potential (conversion to CO_2 and H_2O).
- No sludge production compared to biological treatment methods.
- Effective for a wide range of contaminants.

Limitations and Challenges

- Despite their benefits, AOPs have some limitations:
- High operational costs due to the use of energy and reagents.
- Sensitivity to pH, temperature, and the presence of radical scavengers.
- Need for post-treatment (*e.g.*, for removal of residual iron in Fenton's process).
- Complex reaction kinetics and by-product formation in some cases [6].

Recent Advances and Future Prospects

Recent research has focused on enhancing AOP efficiency and reducing costs:

Nanomaterials: Use of nano-sized catalysts with higher surface area and reactivity.

Hybrid systems: Combining AOPs with biological or membrane processes for synergistic effects.

Solar-driven AOPs: Utilizing solar energy to reduce energy input and improve sustainability.

Persulfate-based AOPs: Sulfate radicals ($SO_4•^-$) offer longer lifetimes and different reactivity profiles compared to •OH.

AI and modeling: Application of machine learning to optimize operational parameters and predict degradation pathways.

A dynamic and adaptable collection of technologies, advanced oxidation processes can help solve the rising problem of water pollution from both new and persistent contaminants. Future sustainable water treatment solutions are projected to heavily rely on AOPs due to ongoing advancements in materials, process integration, and cost-efficiency. For wider industrial applications, scaling up and guaranteeing cost-effective execution are still crucial issues that need to be resolved [5 - 9].

BIOTECHNOLOGICAL SOLUTIONS

Pharmaceutical waste presents a considerable environmental concern because of its enduring and hazardous characteristics. The pervasive and frequently unselective application of medications has resulted in the accumulation of residues in both aquatic and terrestrial ecosystems. These leftovers can disturb the natural equilibrium and perhaps infiltrate the human food chain, posing significant public health risks. Conventional pharmaceutical waste disposal options, including cremation and chemical treatment, frequently prove inadequate due to elevated costs, insufficient degradation, and the production of secondary pollutants. In light of these constraints, biotechnology methods have arisen as sustainable, environmentally benign, and highly efficient options for the breakdown and detoxification of pharmaceutical pollutants [10].

Microbial Degradation of Pharmaceutical Waste

Natural Microbial Biodegradation

Bacteria, fungi, and actinomycetes are essential microorganisms in the spontaneous decomposition of organic substances. Specific microbial species have exhibited the capacity to break down medicinal substances, employing them as a carbon or energy source. Species such as *Pseudomonas, Bacillus, Rhodococcus*, and *Phanerochaete* have been documented to degrade antibiotics, analgesics, and anti-inflammatory medications. These bacteria generate several enzymes that can cleave intricate drug compounds into simpler, less detrimental metabolites.

Genetically Engineered Microbes

Recent advancements in genetic engineering have resulted in the creation of microbial strains with improved skills for pharmaceutical breakdown. Scientists have developed "designer microbes" by integrating specific genes that encode drug-degrading enzymes into microbial genomes, enabling these organisms to effectively target and decompose particular pharmaceutical molecules. Genetically modified *E. coli* strains have been engineered to produce laccase and peroxidase enzymes, which efficiently degrade various pharmaceutical contaminants, including endocrine-disrupting chemicals and synthetic hormones [11].

Microbial Consortia

The utilisation of microbial consortia communities of diverse microbial species functioning synergistically has demonstrated greater efficacy in the degradation of complex pharmacological combinations compared to reliance on individual microbial strains. These consortia integrate the enzymatic functions of many species, facilitating sequential and complementary degradation processes. This method enhances the efficacy and thoroughness of pharmaceutical waste degradation while minimising the risk of intermediate hazardous metabolite accumulation.

ENZYMATIC DEGRADATION TECHNIQUES

Enzymes are biological catalysts that promote the decomposition of complex compounds. The utilisation of pure or immobilised enzymes in the treatment of pharmaceutical waste presents numerous benefits, including selectivity, fast action, and functionality under mild conditions [12].

Laccases and Peroxidases

Laccases (multi-copper oxidases) and peroxidases are extensively researched enzymes for the biodegradation of pharmaceuticals. They are capable of oxidising a diverse array of phenolic and non-phenolic substances, encompassing antibiotics, hormones, and analgesics. These enzymes facilitate the conversion of poisonous molecules into less damaging or inert substances, frequently *via* radical-mediated processes.

Amidohydrolases and Esterases

These enzymes efficiently degrade amide and ester linkages found in many pharmaceutical compounds, including non-steroidal anti-inflammatory medications (NSAIDs) and antibiotics. Their action leads to the destruction of the active drug moiety, making the molecule physiologically inert and more susceptible to additional microbial degradation.

Immobilized Enzyme Systems

Employing immobilised enzymes on solid substrates improves the stability and reusability of biocatalysts, rendering the method more economical for large-scale applications. Immobilised enzyme reactors can be incorporated into wastewater treatment facilities for the continuous breakdown of pharmaceutical contaminants.

Applications and Case Studies

Numerous pilot-scale and full-scale implementations of microbial and enzymatic degrading technologies have been executed globally. A treatment facility in Germany utilised laccase-based enzymatic reactors to process hospital wastewater, effectively diminishing the levels of prevalent drugs, including diclofenac and carbamazepine. Microbial consortia extracted from pharmaceutical sector effluents have been utilised to create bioreactors proficient at decomposing ciprofloxacin and paracetamol in industrial wastewater.

Studies in the United States have shown the efficacy of genetically modified Pseudomonas putida strains in decomposing environmental oestrogens present in sewage sludge [13 - 16].

NANOTECHNOLOGY IN WASTE REMEDIATION

The rapid expansion of industrialisation and urbanisation has markedly exacerbated environmental pollution, including air, water, and soil degradation. Conventional waste remediation systems frequently encounter constraints regarding cost, efficiency, and sustainability. In this setting, nanotechnology has emerged as a transformative instrument providing novel options for environmental remediation. Owing to their distinctive physicochemical characteristics, nanoparticles can engage with contaminants at the molecular level, hence facilitating more effective and precise remediation methods.

Principles of Nanotechnology in Waste Management

Nanotechnology is the manipulation of matter at the nanometre scale (1–100 nm), where materials display unique traits like a high surface area-to-volume ratio, enhanced reactivity, and adjustable optical and magnetic characteristics. These characteristics allow nanoparticles to adsorb, degrade, or alter dangerous pollutants in diverse environmental matrices [17].

The key principles of nanotechnology applied in waste remediation include:

Surface modification to enhance pollutant affinity.

Catalytic activity for the degradation of complex pollutants.

Redox reactions for the transformation of toxic compounds.

Magnetic properties for easy recovery and reuse [18, 19].

Types of Nanomaterials Used in Waste Remediation

Zero-Valent Metal Nanoparticles (nZVMs)

Nanoscale zero-valent iron (nZVI) and other zero-valent metals are widely employed for the remediation of groundwater and soil. nZVI particles can effectively reduce various contaminants, such as chlorinated solvents, heavy metals, and pesticides, *via* redox processes [20].

Example: nZVI has been successfully used for the dechlorination of trichloroethylene (TCE), converting it into less toxic compounds.

Metal Oxide Nanoparticles

Nanoparticles, including titanium dioxide, zinc oxide, and iron oxide, have superior photocatalytic and adsorptive characteristics. These are employed in the breakdown of organic contaminants and the adsorption of heavy metals.

Example: TiO_2 nanoparticles under UV light can effectively degrade dyes, phenols, and pharmaceuticals in wastewater.

Carbon-Based Nanomaterials

Carbon nanotubes (CNTs), graphene oxide, and fullerenes exhibit substantial surface areas and superior adsorption capabilities. These materials are optimal for the extraction of heavy metals, organic pollutants, and microbes from water.

Example: Functionalized CNTs have shown high affinity for adsorbing lead, arsenic, and mercury from contaminated water.

Nanocomposites

Hybrid nanomaterials that integrate two or more functional nanostructures improve remediation efficacy. Magnetic nanocomposites can be readily extracted from the environment after treatment utilising external magnetic fields [21].

Example: Magnetic graphene oxide composites have been used for dye removal and can be reused after magnetic separation.

Mechanisms of Nano Remediation

Nanomaterials can remediate environmental pollutants through several mechanisms, including:

Adsorption: Binding of contaminants to the surface of nanoparticles.

Catalysis: Acceleration of chemical reactions to degrade pollutants.

Photocatalysis: Light-activated degradation of pollutants using semiconducting nanoparticles.

Redox Reactions: Electron transfer to transform contaminants into less harmful substances.

Membrane Filtration: Nanofiber membranes for physical separation of pollutants [22, 23].

Applications in Environmental Sectors

Water and Wastewater Treatment

Nanotechnology plays a vital role in purifying industrial effluents, municipal wastewater, and drinking water. Applications include:

Removal of heavy metals such as lead, cadmium, and chromium.

Degradation of dyes, pesticides, and pharmaceuticals.

Pathogen disinfection using antimicrobial nanoparticles like silver and copper.

Soil Remediation

Nanoparticles can penetrate soil matrices and inactivate pollutants *in situ*. They are particularly effective for:

Degradation of petroleum hydrocarbons

Immobilization of heavy metals and radionuclides.

Air Pollution Control

Nanocatalysts and nanofilters are employed to:

- Capture volatile organic compounds (VOCs)
- Reduce NOx, SOx emissions.
- Adsorb greenhouse gases like CO_2.

Advantages of Nanotechnology in Waste Remediation

- High efficiency and selectivity.
- Rapid reaction kinetics due to high surface area.
- Minimal secondary waste generation.
- Potential for *in situ* treatment.
- Reusability of magnetic nanomaterials.

Challenges and Limitations

- Despite promising potential, nanoremediation faces certain challenges:
- Environmental toxicity and long-term fate of nanoparticles.
- High production cost of some nanomaterials.
- Lack of regulation and standardization.
- Need for large-scale field validation [24, 25].

ARTIFICIAL INTELLIGENCE (AI) AND DATA ANALYTICS

The incorporation of Artificial Intelligence (AI) and Data Analytics into waste management systems has become a vital strategy for tackling the escalating issues posed by urbanisation, industrialisation, and environmental sustainability. These modern technologies are transforming conventional waste management processes by providing data-driven, predictive, and automated solutions that improve efficiency, save costs, and ensure adherence to environmental requirements [26].

Role of AI in Waste Management

Natural language processing (NLP), computer vision, deep learning, and machine learning (ML) are some of the technologies that make up artificial intelligence. Systems can now mimic human intelligence and decision-making skills because of these technologies. AI is widely used in waste management to automate procedures, forecast outcomes, and optimise operations.

Predicting Waste Generation Patterns

Predicting the amount and kinds of trash produced in commercial, industrial, and urban settings is becoming more and more common with AI algorithms. Artificial intelligence (AI) systems may accurately predict future trash generation trends by evaluating past waste data in conjunction with real-time inputs, including population growth, consumer behaviour, seasonal fluctuations, and economic indicators. Authorities and trash management firms may more effectively plan collection, transportation, and disposal operations thanks to these insights [27].

Optimizing Collection and Disposal Routes

Route optimisation is one of the major advantages of AI in trash management. To identify the most effective routes for waste collection vehicles, machine learning algorithms can examine traffic patterns, bin fill levels, meteorological conditions, and operational limitations. This minimises carbon emissions and traffic congestion in addition to fuel usage and operating expenses [28 - 30].

Enhancing Recycling Efficiency

Artificial intelligence-driven sorting devices are being implemented in recycling facilities to autonomously categorise waste materials. Employing computer vision and robotics, these systems can accurately and swiftly identify and categorise recyclable materials, including plastics, metals, glass, and paper, from heterogeneous waste streams. This automation optimises the purity of recovered materials, diminishes manual labour, and increases overall recycling rates.

Data Analytics in Waste Management

Data analytics entails the methodical examination of extensive datasets to derive significant insights and facilitate decision-making. Data analytics is essential in waste management for assessing system performance, detecting inefficiencies, and formulating enhancement strategies [31 - 37].

Risk Identification and Mitigation

Sophisticated data analytics techniques can identify anomalies, irregularities, and potential problems in waste management processes. For instance, abrupt alterations in trash composition or anomalous sensor readings at landfill sites may be identified for more scrutiny. Prompt identification of such issues facilitates prompt response and mitigates the danger of environmental pollution or equipment malfunction.

Improving Waste Handling Practices

Data analytics can reveal patterns and trends that identify areas for enhancement by examining data gathered from many sources, like GPS trackers, smart bins, and sensor networks. Subsequent recommendations may be formulated for enhanced trash segregation, refined collection schedules, or optimised staff allocation. These enhancements result in increased operational efficiency and improved resource utilisation [38].

Ensuring Regulatory Compliance

Data analytics offers a consistent way to monitor compliance given stricter environmental rules. It keeps correct records of waste volumes, disposal strategies, emissions, and treatment results. Automated reporting systems and real-time dashboards help companies to remain compliant with local and global waste management guidelines, therefore preventing fines and improving their environmental reputation [39 - 44].

AI in Waste Treatment Plant Design and Monitoring

AI technologies are also being leveraged in the design and operation of waste treatment plants. Simulation models based on AI can evaluate various design scenarios and predict their performance under different conditions. This helps in selecting the most cost-effective and sustainable plant configuration.

During operations, AI-enabled monitoring systems continuously assess parameters such as temperature, pressure, chemical composition, and processing time. These systems can detect inefficiencies, predict equipment failures, and suggest real-time adjustments to optimize performance and reduce downtime [45 - 48]. The adoption of AI and data analytics in waste management is poised to grow further with advancements in sensor technologies, cloud computing, and the Internet of Things (IoT). Future systems are expected to be more autonomous, intelligent, and integrated, providing end-to-end waste management solutions with minimal human intervention. However, challenges remain, including data privacy concerns, the need for standardized data formats, integration with legacy systems, and the requirement for skilled personnel. Addressing these challenges will be crucial to fully realizing the potential of AI and data analytics in waste management.

Artificial Intelligence and Data Analytics are redefining the landscape of waste management. By enabling smart, data-driven decision-making, these technologies contribute significantly to environmental sustainability, operational efficiency, and regulatory compliance. As technology continues to evolve, their role in creating cleaner, smarter, and more resilient waste management systems will become increasingly indispensable [49, 50].

GREEN CHEMISTRY APPROACHES

Green chemistry, also known as sustainable chemistry, represents a proactive strategy toward designing products and processes that reduce or eliminate the use and generation of hazardous substances. This approach aligns well with the growing global concern for environmental sustainability, particularly in the pharmaceutical industry, where large-scale manufacturing often leads to the generation of toxic by-products and considerable energy consumption [51].

Introduction to Green Chemistry

The concept of green chemistry was introduced by Paul Anastas and John Warner in the 1990s and has since evolved into a foundational principle guiding sustainable scientific practices. In the pharmaceutical domain, green chemistry not only addresses ecological concerns but also enhances the safety, cost-efficiency, and performance of chemical processes. The primary aim is to minimize the environmental impact throughout a drug's lifecycle from synthesis and formulation to disposal without compromising therapeutic efficacy [52 - 54].

Principles of Green Chemistry

There are twelve core principles of green chemistry, many of which are particularly relevant to pharmaceutical development:

Prevention of Waste: Emphasis is placed on designing processes that do not generate waste, rather than managing it after formation.

Atom Economy: Maximizing the incorporation of all materials used in the process into the final product.

Less Hazardous Chemical Syntheses: Use of safer reagents and reaction conditions to reduce toxicity.

Designing Safer Chemicals: Molecules are designed to perform their function while minimizing toxicity.

Safer Solvents and Auxiliaries: Avoiding the use of harmful solvents and auxiliaries where possible.

Energy Efficiency: Conducting reactions at ambient temperature and pressure to conserve energy.

Use of Renewable Feedstocks: Utilizing raw materials that are renewable rather than depleting.

Reduce Derivatives: Minimizing the use of blocking or protecting groups in chemical synthesis.

Catalysis: Employing catalytic reactions rather than stoichiometric ones to enhance efficiency.

Design for Degradation: Designing products that break down into harmless substances after use.

Real-time Analysis for Pollution Prevention: Monitoring processes in real time to prevent emissions.

Inherently Safer Chemistry for Accident Prevention: Choosing materials and processes that minimize the potential for chemical accidents [51 - 53].

Green Chemistry in Drug Design and Development

Pharmaceutical manufacturing traditionally involves the use of organic solvents, heavy metals, and toxic reagents. Green chemistry seeks to replace or reduce these elements through innovative alternatives:

Solvent-Free Syntheses: Reactions carried out without the use of solvents significantly decrease environmental pollution and lower production costs. Mechanochemical synthesis, microwave-assisted reactions, and ultrasonic methods are among the techniques employed to avoid harmful solvents.

Biodegradable Excipients: Incorporating excipients derived from natural sources such as starch, cellulose, chitosan, or gums like tamarind and fenugreek ensures that the inactive components of drug formulations degrade safely after disposal.

These excipients are renewable, non-toxic, and eco-friendly [54].

Renewable Raw Materials: Utilizing plant-based compounds and biomaterials not only aligns with sustainability goals but also opens new avenues in drug discovery, particularly in phytopharmaceuticals and herbal medicines.

Green Catalysis: The use of enzyme catalysis and metal-free organic catalysts (organocatalysts) reduces reliance on heavy metals, thus minimizing toxic waste and improving reaction specificity [55].

Applications of Green Chemistry in Pharmaceutical Technology

Green chemistry principles have found wide-ranging applications across the pharmaceutical development spectrum [56]:

Process Optimization: Pharmaceutical industries are adopting greener synthetic pathways that reduce the number of steps, simplify purification, and use milder reaction conditions.

Nanoformulation Techniques: Green synthesis of nanoparticles using plant extracts as reducing and stabilizing agents avoids toxic chemicals and supports eco-friendly biomedical applications.

Drug Delivery Systems: The use of natural polymers in the development of sustained release formulations, transdermal patches, and nanocarriers exemplifies the successful integration of green chemistry in dosage form design [51, 57, 58].

Waste Management Reduction: By minimizing hazardous inputs and maximizing process efficiency, green chemistry helps reduce the volume and toxicity of waste, thereby decreasing the burden on downstream waste treatment systems [59, 60].

Regulatory and Economic Implications

Global regulatory authorities, including the U.S. Food and Drug Administration (FDA) and the European Medicines Agency (EMA), are increasingly supporting green initiatives. Guidelines and incentives are being developed to encourage the adoption of sustainable practices. Economically, green chemistry reduces production costs through efficient resource utilization, reduced waste handling expenses, and lower energy consumption. Moreover, it enhances a company's public image and compliance with environmental standards.

Nevertheless, continued research and collaboration between academia and industry are expected to overcome these challenges. Innovations in synthetic biology, green engineering, and AI-driven process design will likely play crucial roles in advancing sustainable pharmaceutical manufacturing.

Green chemistry offers a transformative approach to pharmaceutical development, focusing on sustainability without compromising efficacy. By incorporating solvent-free synthesis, biodegradable materials, and renewable resources, the industry can significantly reduce its environmental footprint. The integration of green principles from the initial stages of drug development not only benefits the planet but also enhances safety, cost-effectiveness, and regulatory compliance. As the field evolves, green chemistry is poised to become a standard practice rather than an optional strategy in pharmaceutical science [61].

PLASMA GASIFICATION AND PYROLYSIS

The growing accumulation of pharmaceutical waste, including expired, unused, or returned medications, poses a significant threat to environmental and public health. Traditional disposal methods such as landfilling or incineration are increasingly being scrutinized due to their potential to release toxic compounds into the environment. In this context, advanced thermal treatment methods like plasma gasification and pyrolysis have emerged as sustainable and efficient technologies for the safe disposal and conversion of pharmaceutical waste into useful forms of energy [62, 63].

Pyrolysis: Decomposition in the Absence of Oxygen

Pyrolysis is another thermal treatment process that decomposes organic materials at elevated temperatures (typically 400°C to 800°C) in an oxygen-free environment. Unlike incineration, which involves combustion, pyrolysis transforms pharmaceutical waste into valuable by-products such as syngas, bio-oil, and biochar.

Syngas: Similar to plasma gasification, pyrolysis also produces syngas, which can be used to generate heat or electricity.

Bio-oil: A liquid product that can be refined and used as a renewable energy source.

Biochar: A carbon-rich solid that can be utilized as a soil amendment, in filtration systems, or even for carbon sequestration.

Applications and Advantages in Pharmaceutical Waste Management

Plasma gasification and pyrolysis are particularly suited for the treatment of large volumes of expired or returned pharmaceutical products, including those containing hazardous active pharmaceutical ingredients (APIs). These methods offer several distinct advantages are:

High Destruction Efficiency: Both methods achieve near-complete decomposition of complex organic molecules, including persistent pharmaceutical compounds.

Energy Recovery: The processes not only eliminate waste but also recover energy in the form of syngas, bio-oil, or electricity.

Minimal Emissions: Compared to conventional incineration, these processes generate significantly lower quantities of harmful emissions such as dioxins and furans.

Versatility: Effective for a wide range of pharmaceutical formulations, including tablets, capsules, liquids, and injectables [64, 65].

Challenges and Considerations

Despite their benefits, plasma gasification and pyrolysis technologies face several challenges that must be addressed for widespread adoption:

High Capital Costs: The initial setup cost for plasma and pyrolysis facilities can be substantial.

Operational Complexity: Requires skilled operators and regular maintenance.

Feedstock Preparation: Pre-treatment of pharmaceutical waste is often necessary to remove moisture and non-organic contaminants.

Future Prospects

With increasing regulatory pressure and environmental awareness, plasma gasification and pyrolysis are expected to gain traction in pharmaceutical waste management. Ongoing research and technological advancements aim to reduce costs, improve energy efficiency, and scale these solutions for broader implementation.

Plasma gasification and pyrolysis represent transformative technologies in the realm of pharmaceutical waste management. By converting hazardous waste into valuable energy resources, these processes not only address environmental concerns but also contribute to circular economy goals. Their integration into pharmaceutical waste disposal strategies holds promise for a more sustainable and health-conscious future.

BLOCKCHAIN FOR SECURE WASTE DISPOSAL

The management and disposal of pharmaceutical waste have become increasingly critical due to rising environmental concerns, regulatory requirements, and public health issues. Improper disposal of pharmaceutical byproducts and expired or unused medications can lead to serious ecological and human health hazards, including contamination of soil and water, antibiotic resistance, and toxic exposure. Traditional waste disposal systems often lack transparency and traceability, making it difficult to identify the source of malpractice or non-compliance.

Blockchain technology, with its decentralized, tamper-resistant ledger system, offers an innovative solution to these challenges. By providing secure, immutable records of waste generation, transportation, treatment, and disposal, blockchain ensures transparency, traceability, and accountability at every stage of the waste management process.

Application of Blockchain in Pharmaceutical Waste Management

Transparent Waste Tracking

One of the significant advantages of using blockchain in pharmaceutical waste disposal is the ability to track waste throughout its lifecycle. Each stage of waste handling, from generation to final disposal, is recorded as a digital transaction on the blockchain. This allows stakeholders to monitor the waste movement from origin to endpoint, ensuring that it is handled in accordance with environmental and legal standards [66].

Immutable and Tamper-Proof Records

Blockchain's cryptographic structure ensures that once a transaction is recorded, it cannot be modified or deleted without consensus from the entire network. This immutability guarantees that waste disposal records are trustworthy and verifiable, minimizing the risk of data manipulation or fraud. It also facilitates audits by regulatory agencies, as all activities are recorded in a secure and unchangeable format [67].

Enhanced Compliance and Regulation

Compliance with waste management laws and environmental regulations is crucial in the pharmaceutical industry. Blockchain facilitates this by providing auditable and transparent records of waste handling practices. Regulators can access real-time data to verify compliance, reducing the need for on-site inspections and lengthy paperwork. Furthermore, automatic alerts and smart contracts can be integrated to notify authorities of any non-compliant behaviour or deviations from standard protocols [68].

Prevention of Illegal Dumping and Diversion

Illegal dumping of pharmaceutical waste poses severe risks to the environment and public health. Blockchain can help prevent this by making every transaction in the waste disposal chain visible and traceable. Unauthorized deviations from the planned route or unrecorded waste handoffs can be flagged immediately, enabling prompt intervention. This level of accountability discourages illicit practices and promotes ethical waste handling.

Smart Contracts in Waste Disposal Systems

Smart contracts are self-executing contracts with predefined conditions coded into them. In pharmaceutical waste management, smart contracts can automate various processes, such as:

- Triggering payments upon successful waste delivery and treatment.
- Sending alerts for overdue disposal activities.
- Enforcing contractual obligations between waste generators and disposal firms.

These contracts reduce human error, eliminate administrative overhead, and ensure timely compliance with regulatory obligations [69 - 71].

Integration with IoT and AI

Blockchain can be further strengthened by integrating with Internet of Things (IoT) devices and Artificial Intelligence (AI):

IoT Devices: Sensors placed in waste containers can monitor temperature, fill levels, and movement. These devices can send real-time data to the blockchain, ensuring that the waste is stored and transported under optimal conditions.

AI Algorithms: AI can analyze blockchain data to predict waste generation trends, identify inefficiencies, and optimize waste handling operations.

Together, these technologies create a robust and intelligent waste management ecosystem.

Case Studies and Implementation Examples

Several pilot programs and research initiatives have demonstrated the viability of blockchain in waste management:

MediLedger Project (USA): Originally designed for pharmaceutical supply chain transparency, its framework has been extended to include waste traceability.

Plastic Bank (Global): Though not specific to pharmaceuticals, this initiative uses blockchain to reward individuals for collecting plastic waste, showcasing the potential for similar incentive-based pharmaceutical waste programs.

These case studies highlight how blockchain can be adapted to diverse waste streams and regulatory environments.

Challenges and Limitations

While promising, the implementation of blockchain in waste disposal faces several challenges:

Scalability Issues: Managing large volumes of transactions in real-time can be computationally intensive.

Initial Costs: Infrastructure setup and training require significant investment.

Interoperability: Integration with existing systems and regulatory frameworks may be complex.

Data Privacy: Ensuring confidential data protection while maintaining transparency is a delicate balance.

Addressing these challenges requires cross-sector collaboration, government support, and continued technological innovation [72 - 75].

Future Prospects

With increasing focus on sustainability and digital transformation, the use of blockchain in waste management is expected to grow. Future developments may include:

Nationwide blockchain waste management networks.

Blockchain-based carbon credit tracking for eco-friendly disposal.

Decentralized applications (DApps) for waste tracking and community engagement.

Blockchain has the potential to revolutionize waste management by fostering trust, transparency, and environmental responsibility.

Blockchain technology presents a transformative approach to pharmaceutical waste disposal, addressing the longstanding challenges of transparency, traceability, and accountability. By providing a secure and verifiable ledger of waste-related activities, blockchain enhances regulatory compliance, deters illegal practices, and promotes environmentally responsible disposal. As the technology continues to mature, its integration with IoT, AI, and smart contracts will further optimize waste management systems, paving the way for a cleaner, safer, and more sustainable future.

CONCLUSION

The integration of advanced technologies into pharmaceutical waste management has revolutionized the way waste is monitored, treated, and disposed of. By adopting smart systems, biotechnological solutions, nanotechnology, and AI-driven tools, the pharmaceutical sector can significantly reduce its environmental impact while ensuring public health safety. Continued innovation and investment in these technologies are essential for building a sustainable and responsible pharmaceutical ecosystem.

REFERENCES

[1] Pulparambil S, Al-Busaidi A, Al-Hatimy Y, Al-Farsi A. Internet of things-based smart medical waste management system. Telematics and Informatics Reports 2024; 15: 100161. [http://dx.doi.org/10.1016/j.teler.2024.100161]

[2] Gogate PR, Pandit AB. A review of imperative technologies for wastewater treatment I: oxidation technologies at ambient conditions. Adv Environ Res 2004; 8(3-4): 501-51. [http://dx.doi.org/10.1016/S1093-0191(03)00032-7]

[3] Esplugas S, Bila DM, Krause LGT, Dezotti M. Ozonation and advanced oxidation technologies to remove endocrine disrupting chemicals (EDCs) and pharmaceuticals and personal care products (PPCPs) in water effluents. J Hazard Mater 2007; 149(3): 631-42. [http://dx.doi.org/10.1016/j.jhazmat.2007.07.073] [PMID: 17826898]

[4] Wang J, Wang S. Removal of pharmaceuticals and personal care products (PPCPs) from wastewater: A review. J Environ Manage 2016; 182: 620-40. [http://dx.doi.org/10.1016/j.jenvman.2016.07.049] [PMID: 27552641]

[5] Poyatos JM, Muñio MM, Almecija MC, Torres JC, Hontoria E, Osorio F. Advanced Oxidation

Processes for Wastewater Treatment: State of the Art. Water Air Soil Pollut 2010; 205(1-4): 187-204. [http://dx.doi.org/10.1007/s11270-009-0065-1]

[6] Oturan MA, Aaron JJ. Advanced Oxidation Processes in Water/Wastewater Treatment: Principles and Applications. A Review. Crit Rev Environ Sci Technol 2014; 44(23): 2577-641. [http://dx.doi.org/10.1080/10643389.2013.829765]

[7] Ibhadon A, Fitzpatrick P. Heterogeneous Photocatalysis: Recent Advances and Applications. Catalysts 2013; 3(1): 189-218. [http://dx.doi.org/10.3390/catal3010189]

[8] Klavarioti M, Mantzavinos D, Kassinos D. Removal of residual pharmaceuticals from aqueous systems by advanced oxidation processes. Environ Int 2009; 35(2): 402-17. [http://dx.doi.org/10.1016/j.envint.2008.07.009] [PMID: 18760478]

[9] Rizzo L, Manaia C, Merlin C, *et al.* Urban wastewater treatment plants as hotspots for antibiotic resistant bacteria and genes spread into the environment: A review. Sci Total Environ 2013; 447: 345-60. [http://dx.doi.org/10.1016/j.scitotenv.2013.01.032] [PMID: 23396083]

[10] Kümmerer K. The presence of pharmaceuticals in the environment due to human use – present knowledge and future challenges. J Environ Manage 2009; 90(8): 2354-66. [http://dx.doi.org/10.1016/j.jenvman.2009.01.023] [PMID: 19261375]

[11] Chang F, Simcik MF, Capel PD. Occurrence and fate of the herbicide glyphosate and its degradate aminomethylphosphonic acid in the atmosphere. Environ Toxicol Chem 2011; 30(3): 548-55. [http://dx.doi.org/10.1002/*etc.*431] [PMID: 21128261]

[12] Lin H, Lin S, Awasthi MK, Wang Y, Xu P. Exploring the bacterial community and fermentation characteristics during silage fermentation of abandoned fresh tea leaves. Chemosphere 2021; 283: 131234. [http://dx.doi.org/10.1016/j.chemosphere.2021.131234] [PMID: 34153916]

[13] Ali H, Khan E. What are heavy metals? Long-standing controversy over the scientific use of the term 'heavy metals' – proposal of a comprehensive definition. Toxicol Environ Chem 2018; 100(1): 6-19. [http://dx.doi.org/10.1080/02772248.2017.1413652]

[14] Singh Arora D, Kumar Sharma R. Ligninolytic fungal laccases and their biotechnological applications. Appl Biochem Biotechnol 2010; 160(6): 1760-88. [http://dx.doi.org/10.1007/s12010-009-8676-y] [PMID: 19513857]

[15] Gavrilescu M, Demnerová K, Aamand J, Agathos S, Fava F. Emerging pollutants in the environment: present and future challenges in biomonitoring, ecological risks and bioremediation. N Biotechnol 2015; 32(1): 147-56. [http://dx.doi.org/10.1016/j.nbt.2014.01.001] [PMID: 24462777]

[16] Deegan AM, Shaik B, Nolan K, *et al.* Treatment options for wastewater effluents from pharmaceutical companies. Int J Environ Sci Technol 2011; 8(3): 649-66. [http://dx.doi.org/10.1007/BF03326250]

[17] Duraisamy P, Sekar J, Arunkumar AD, Ramalingam PV. Kinetics of Phenol Biodegradation by Heavy Metal Tolerant Rhizobacteria *Glutamicibacter nicotianae* MSSRFPD35 From Distillery Effluent Contaminated Soils. Front Microbiol 2020; 11(Jul): 1573. [http://dx.doi.org/10.3389/fmicb.2020.01573] [PMID: 32760369]

[18] Rickerby DG, Morrison M. Nanotechnology and the environment: A European perspective. Sci Technol Adv Mater 2007; 8(1-2): 19-24. [http://dx.doi.org/10.1016/j.stam.2006.10.002]

[19] Zhang W xian. Nanoscale Iron Particles for Environmental Remediation: An Overview. J Nanopart Res 2003; 5(3–4): 323-32.

[20] Khin MM, Nair AS, Babu VJ, Murugan R, Ramakrishna S. A review on nanomaterials for

environmental remediation. Energy Environ Sci 2012; 5(8): 8075. [http://dx.doi.org/10.1039/c2ee21818f]

[21] Crane RA, Scott TB. Nanoscale zero-valent iron: Future prospects for an emerging water treatment technology. J Hazard Mater 2012; 211-212: 112-25. [http://dx.doi.org/10.1016/j.jhazmat.2011.11.073] [PMID: 22305041]

[22] Liu R, Zhao D. Reducing leachability and bioaccessibility of lead in soils using a new class of stabilized iron phosphate nanoparticles. Water Res 2007; 41(12): 2491-502. [http://dx.doi.org/10.1016/j.watres.2007.03.026] [PMID: 17482234]

[23] Theron J, Walker JA, Cloete TE. Nanotechnology and water treatment: applications and emerging opportunities. Crit Rev Microbiol 2008; 34(1): 43-69. [http://dx.doi.org/10.1080/10408410701710442] [PMID: 18259980]

[24] Mauter MS, Elimelech M. Environmental applications of carbon-based nanomaterials. Environ Sci Technol 2008; 42(16): 5843-59. [http://dx.doi.org/10.1021/es8006904] [PMID: 18767635]

[25] Qu X, Alvarez PJJ, Li Q. Applications of nanotechnology in water and wastewater treatment. Water Res 2013; 47(12): 3931-46. [http://dx.doi.org/10.1016/j.watres.2012.09.058] [PMID: 23571110]

[26] Sarmadi M, Rahimi S, Evensen D, Kazemi Moghaddam V. Interaction between meteorological parameters and COVID-19: an ecological study on 406 authorities of the UK. Environ Sci Pollut Res Int 2021; 28(47): 67082-97. [http://dx.doi.org/10.1007/s11356-021-15279-2] [PMID: 34244943]

[27] Kumar A, Samadder SR. A review on technological options of waste to energy for effective management of municipal solid waste. Waste Manag 2017; 69: 407-22. [http://dx.doi.org/10.1016/j.wasman.2017.08.046] [PMID: 28886975]

[28] Sharma R. Leveraging AI and IoT for Sustainable Waste Management. In: Whig P, Silva N, Elngar A A, Aneja N, Sharma P, Eds. Sustainable Development through Machine Learning, AI and IoT ICSD 2023. Cham: Springer 2023; pp. 145-58. [http://dx.doi.org/10.1007/978-3-031-47055-4_12]

[29] Lee E, Seo Y D, Oh S R, *et al.* Device description in HYDRA middleware. IEEE Access 2021; 9: 56233-44.

[30] Munawir M, Nasional B S, Susanta G. Penentuan alternatif lokasi Tempat Pembuangan Akhir (TPA) sampah di kabupaten sidoarjo. Energies 2022; 15(19): 7214-30.

[31] Kasar P, Sharma DK, Ahmaruzzaman M. Thermal and catalytic decomposition of waste plastics and its co-processing with petroleum residue through pyrolysis process. J Clean Prod 2020; 265: 121639. [http://dx.doi.org/10.1016/j.jclepro.2020.121639]

[32] Aghamiri AR, Lahijani P. Catalytic conversion of biomass and plastic waste to alternative aviation fuels: A review. Biomass Bioenergy 2024; 183: 107120. [http://dx.doi.org/10.1016/j.biombioe.2024.107120]

[33] Nanda S, Berruti F. Thermochemical conversion of plastic waste to fuels: a review. Environ Chem Lett 2021; 19(1): 123-48. [http://dx.doi.org/10.1007/s10311-020-01094-7]

[34] Wan Mahari WA, Chong CT, Cheng CK, *et al.* Production of value-added liquid fuel *via* microwave co-pyrolysis of used frying oil and plastic waste. Energy 2018; 162: 309-17. [http://dx.doi.org/10.1016/j.energy.2018.08.002]

[35] An L, Kou Z, Li R, Zhao Z. Research Progress in Fuel Oil Production by Catalytic Pyrolysis Technologies of Waste Plastics. Catalysts 2024; 14(3): 212. [http://dx.doi.org/10.3390/catal14030212]

[36] Tamizhdurai P, Mangesh VL, Santhosh S, *et al.* Sustainable synthesis: High-efficiency ZrO2/KIT-6 catalyst to hydroprocess waste plastics into fuels. Process Saf Environ Prot 2024; 182: 960-74. [http://dx.doi.org/10.1016/j.psep.2023.12.030]

[37] Madrid B, Wortman S, Hayes D G, *et al.* End-of-life management options for agricultural mulch films in the United States—a review Front Sustain Food Syst 2022; 6: 921496.

[38] Azmi NN, Mohd Shahrum MA, Ahmad Redzuan AN, Mahmud J. Compressive failure behaviour of glass epoxy and graphite epoxy composite laminates due to the effects of different cut-out sizes and variations in fibre orientation. Mater Today Proc 2022; 48: 1936-40. [http://dx.doi.org/10.1016/j.matpr.2021.10.065]

[39] Ugwuanyi C, Okoro O, Adeel M S, Adegbite S. A comprehensive review of waste-to-energy technologies and their potential in African countries. Sustainability 2022; 14(20): 13578.

[40] Althubiti SA, Kumar Sen S, Altaf Ahmed M, *et al.* Automated biomass recycling management system using modified grey wolf optimization with deep learning model. Sustain Energy Technol Assess 2023; 55: 102936. [http://dx.doi.org/10.1016/j.seta.2022.102936]

[41] Mookkaiah SS, Thangavelu G, Hebbar R, Haldar N, Singh H. Design and development of smart Internet of Things–based solid waste management system using computer vision. Environ Sci Pollut Res Int 2022; 29(43): 64871-85. [http://dx.doi.org/10.1007/s11356-022-20428-2] [PMID: 35476273]

[42] Nasir I, Aziz Al-Talib GA. Waste Classification Using Artificial Intelligence Techniques:Literature Review. Tech Rom J Appl Sci Technol 2023; 5: pp. 49-59.

[43] Arashpour M. AI explainability framework for environmental management research. J Environ Manage 2023; 342: 118149. [http://dx.doi.org/10.1016/j.jenvman.2023.118149] [PMID: 37187074]

[44] Abdallah M, Abu Talib M, Feroz S, Nasir Q, Abdalla H, Mahfood B. Artificial intelligence applications in solid waste management: A systematic research review. Waste Manag 2020; 109: 231-246.

[45] Jiang P, Zhang L, You S, *et al.* Blockchain technology applications in waste management: Overview, challenges and opportunities. J Clean Prod 2023; 421: 138466. [http://dx.doi.org/10.1016/j.jclepro.2023.138466]

[46] Yang Z, Xue F, Lu W. Handling missing data for construction waste management: machine learning based on aggregated waste generation behaviors. Resour Conserv Recycl. 2021; 175: p. 105809.

[47] Rodrigo N, Omrany H, Chang R, Zuo J. Leveraging digital technologies for circular economy in construction industry: a way forward. 2024; 13 (1): 85–116.

[48] Chang X, Huang Y, Li M, Bo X, Kumar S. Efficient Detection of Environmental Violators: A Big Data Approach. Prod Oper Manag 2021; 30(5): 1246-70. [http://dx.doi.org/10.1111/poms.13272]

[49] Vafeiadis T, Nizamis A, Pavlopoulos V, *et al.* Data Analytics Platform for the Optimization of Waste Management Procedures. In: 15th International Conference on Distributed Computing in Sensor Systems (DCOSS), Santorini, Greece, 2019, pp. 333-338. [http://dx.doi.org/10.1109/DCOSS.2019.00074]

[50] Kedia P. Big data analytics for efficient waste management. Int J Res Eng Technol 2016; 5: 208-211.

[51] Sharma S, Das J, Braje WM, Dash AK, Handa S. A Glimpse into Green Chemistry Practices in the Pharmaceutical Industry. ChemSusChem 2020; 13(11): 2859-2875.

[52] Pramanik R, Hazra S Role of green chemistry in pharmaceutical industry: a review. 2021; 23(10): 114-124.

[53] Cue BW, Zhang J. Green process chemistry in the pharmaceutical industry. Green Chem Lett Rev 2009; 2(4): 193-211.
[http://dx.doi.org/10.1080/17518250903258150]

[54] Mishra M, Sharma M, Dubey R, Kumari P, Ranjan V, Pandey J. Green synthesis interventions of pharmaceutical industries for sustainable development. Curr Res Green Sust Chem 2021; 4: 100174.
[http://dx.doi.org/10.1016/j.crgsc.2021.100174]

[55] Roschangar F, Sheldon RA, Senanayake CH. Overcoming barriers to green chemistry in the pharmaceutical industry – the Green Aspiration Level™ concept. Green Chem 2015; 17(2): 752-68.
[http://dx.doi.org/10.1039/C4GC01563K]

[56] Ciriminna R, Pagliaro M. Green Chemistry in the Fine Chemicals and Pharmaceutical Industries. Org Process Res Dev 2013; 17(12): 1479-84.
[http://dx.doi.org/10.1021/op400258a]

[57] Kar S, Sanderson H, Roy K, Benfenati E, Leszczynski J. Green Chemistry in the Synthesis of Pharmaceuticals. Chem Rev 2022; 122(3): 3637-710.
[http://dx.doi.org/10.1021/acs.chemrev.1c00631] [PMID: 34910451]

[58] Fetter B, Zilahy G. Challenges of the green supply chain management in the pharmaceutical industry. St Petersburg University Journal of Economic Studies 2022; 38(2): 235-58.
[http://dx.doi.org/10.21638/spbu05.2022.204]

[59] Dunn PJ, Wells AS, Williams MT. Green Chemistry in the Pharmaceutical Industry. Weinheim: Wiley-VCH; 2010. Pp. 384.
[http://dx.doi.org/10.1002/9783527629688]

[60] Santi M, Sancineto L, Nascimento V, *et al.* Flow biocatalysis: A challenging alternative for the synthesis of APIs and natural compounds. Int J Mol Sci 2021; 22(3): 990.
[http://dx.doi.org/10.3390/ijms22030990] [PMID: 33498198]

[61] Byrne FP, Jin S, Paggiola G, *et al.* Tools and techniques for solvent selection: green solvent selection guides. 2016; 4(1): 7.

[62] Tang L, Huang H, Hao H, Zhao K. Development of plasma pyrolysis/gasification systems for energy efficient and environmentally sound waste disposal. J Electrost 2013; 71(5): 839-47.
[http://dx.doi.org/10.1016/j.elstat.2013.06.007]

[63] Cai X, Cai H, Shang C, Du C. Two-Stage Pyrolysis/Gasification and Plasma Conversion Technology for the Utilization of Solid Waste. IEEE Trans Plasma Sci 2021; 49(1): 191-213.
[http://dx.doi.org/10.1109/TPS.2020.3044534]

[64] Sikarwar V S, Mašláni A, Hlína M, *et al.* Thermal plasma assisted pyrolysis and gasification of RDF by utilizing sequestered CO2 as gasifying agent. Journal of CO2 Utilization 2022; 66: 102275.

[65] Hrabovsky M, Jeremias M, van Oost G. Plasma Gasification and Pyrolysis. 1st ed.. Boca Raton: CRC Press 2022; p. 246.
[http://dx.doi.org/10.1201/9781003096887]

[66] Bamakan SMH, Malekinejad P, Ziaeian M. Towards blockchain-based hospital waste management systems; applications and future trends. J Clean Prod 2022; 349: 131440.
[http://dx.doi.org/10.1016/j.jclepro.2022.131440]

[67] Rajendiran K, Sridhar A, Cassinadane A V. Data Consistency, Transparency, and Privacy in Healthcare Systems Using Blockchain Technology. In: Sood K, Dhanaraj R K, Balusamy B, Kadry S, Eds. Blockchain Technology in Corporate Governance. Hoboken: John Wiley & Sons 2022; pp. 125-41.
[http://dx.doi.org/10.1002/9781119865247.ch6]

[68] Coffee J C, Lowenstein L, Rose-Ackerman S. Knights, Raiders, and Targets: The Impact of the Hostile Takeover. The Journal of Finance 1990; 45(1): 311-3.

[69] Sen Gupta Y, Mukherjee S, Dutta R, Bhattacharya S. A blockchain-based approach using smart contracts to develop a smart waste management system. Int J Environ Sci Technol 2022; 19(8): 7833-56.
[http://dx.doi.org/10.1007/s13762-021-03507-8]

[70] Ahmad RW, Salah K, Jayaraman R, Yaqoob I, Omar M. Blockchain for Waste Management in Smart Cities: A Survey. IEEE Access 2021; 9: 131520-41.
[http://dx.doi.org/10.1109/ACCESS.2021.3113380]

[71] Bułkowska K, Zielińska M, Bułkowski M. Implementation of Blockchain Technology in Waste Management. Energies 2023; 16(23): 7742.
[http://dx.doi.org/10.3390/en16237742]

[72] Gong Y, Wang Y, Frei R, Wang B, Zhao C. Blockchain application in circular marine plastic debris management. Ind Mark Manage 2022; 102: 164-76.
[http://dx.doi.org/10.1016/j.indmarman.2022.01.010]

[73] Moulika M, Muhammad S, Sreerag R. Transportation and disposal of medical waste using block chain technology. International Journal of Innovative Research in Information Security 2024; 10(2): 14-24.

[74] Gopalakrishnan P, Ramaguru R. Blockchain Based Waste Management. International Journal of Engineering and Advanced Technology 2019; 8(5): 548-52.

[75] Paturi M, Puvvada S, Ponnuru B S, Simhadri M S, Egala B, Pradhan A K. Smart Solid Waste Management System using Blockchain and IoT for Smart Cities. Proceedings - 2021 IEEE International Symposium on Smart Electronic Systems (iSES). 440-3.

CHAPTER 8

Pharmaceutical Waste Management in Healthcare Facilities: Challenges and Solutions

Rufaida Wasim[1], **Tarique Mahmood**[1,*], **Saba Parveen**[2] and **Sumaiya Azmi**[3]

[1] *Department of Pharmacology, Faculty of Pharmacy, Integral University, Lucknow, Uttar Pradesh, India*

[2] *Department of Pharmaceutical Science & Technology, Madan Mohan Malaviya University of Technology, Gorakhpur, Uttar Pradesh, India*

[3] *Department of Periodontics, Career Post Graduate Institute of Dental Sciences and Hospital, Lucknow, Uttar Pradesh India*

Abstract: Pharmaceutical waste comprises several waste streams that reflect the variety and complexity of substances used in pharmaceuticals. Several activities within a healthcare institution may generate pharmaceutical waste, including intravenous (IV) preparation, general compounding, spills or breakages, partially used vials and syringes, abandoned or unused preparations, patients' prescriptions, and expired pharmaceuticals. Except for chemotherapy medications, which are regularly moved to a regulated medical waste incinerator, pharmaceutical waste at hospitals is typically disposed of in landfills. Legislation about hazardous waste was not well understood when these processes were developed. Additionally, certain medications have hazardous properties that make them challenging to manage without the required procedures and tools. The lack of precise standards for identifying pharmaceutical waste is one of the biggest challenges, leading to disparate disposal methods across medical institutions. Often, healthcare workers receive inadequate training in waste segregation, leading to the mixing of hazardous and non-hazardous waste. Waste management's operational and financial costs are another difficulty, particularly for smaller organizations with little funding. Healthcare organizations should develop comprehensive waste management strategies that address these issues by implementing ecologically safe disposal methods, proper waste segregation, and staff training. Working together with competent waste management companies may ensure that pharmaceutical waste is handled appropriately and in compliance with regional regulations.

Keywords: Hazardous, Health care, Pharmaceutical waste, Waste management.

* **Corresponding author Tarique Mahmood:** Department of Pharmacology, Faculty of Pharmacy, Integral University, Lucknow, Uttar Pradesh, India; E-mail: tmahmood@iul.ac.in

Suman Gautam, Jai Narayan Mishra, Preeti Mishra, Preeti Verma & Sudhanshu Mishra (Eds.)

INTRODUCTION

Pharmaceutical waste management involves the appropriate handling, storage, treatment, and disposal of pharmaceutical products and drugs that are no longer required, are considered dangerous, or have expired. To minimize adverse impacts on human health, pharmaceutical waste management in hospital settings must be done effectively. As healthcare processes get more complicated and the amount of pharmaceutical waste increases, it becomes difficult to dispose of these materials safely [1]. Hospitals, pharmacies, and long-term care facilities are among the healthcare facilities that produce various kinds of pharmaceutical waste, including hazardous chemicals, controlled substances, and unused or expired medication. Keeping a clean and safe hospital environment requires that pharmaceutical waste be disposed of properly. Since the development of contemporary medical therapies, patients are routinely prescribed and given medications. Waste gets produced if these medications are unused, broken, or expired. Hospitals accumulate unnecessary pharmaceuticals owing to the need for specialized drugs, and these drugs need to be disposed of safely. Pharmaceutical waste must be managed properly for the environment and public health to be protected, as well as for healthcare institutions to operate safely [1]. Serious repercussions may result from improper disposal of pharmaceutical waste. Air, soil, and water sources may get contaminated when narcotics are handled or disposed of improperly. When discharged into the environment, many pharmaceutical compounds may have long-lasting effects on aquatic life, ecosystems, and perhaps human populations, making environmental issues serious. Inadequate disposal may also result in the misuse of controlled medications, such as opioids, which can be used for drug addiction and abuse [2]. Therefore, healthcare facilities must manage pharmaceutical waste according to the best standards to reduce these dangers.

Regulatory frameworks are essential to the management of pharmaceutical waste. To guarantee the safe disposal of pharmaceutical waste, a number of national and international organizations provide policies and procedures. Hazardous pharmaceutical waste is regulated by the Environmental Protection Agency (EPA) in the United States following the Resource Conservation and Recovery Act (RCRA). Regarding the disposal of outdated medications, the Food and Drug Administration (FDA) also establishes regulations [3]. Under the Secure and Responsible Drug Disposal Act, the Drug Enforcement Administration (DEA) is also in charge of managing the disposal of restricted narcotics [4]. In both industrialized and developing nations, the World Health Organization (WHO) offers guidelines for managing pharmaceutical waste, particularly concerning waste reduction and ecologically friendly disposal methods.

Many healthcare institutions still struggle to manage pharmaceutical waste in an efficient manner in spite of these rules. Inadequate infrastructure, a lack of employee training, and the high expenses of putting in place acceptable disposal procedures are some of these difficulties. Furthermore, there is often a misunderstanding about the classification of pharmaceutical waste, especially concerning what qualifies as prohibited or hazardous compounds. In order to guarantee that the right procedures are followed, this emphasizes the need for thorough waste management systems and ongoing training for healthcare personnel [5]. Healthcare providers must implement strong pharmaceutical waste management plans that put public health, environmental preservation, and legal compliance first in light of these difficulties. Clear waste segregation guidelines, safe pharmaceutical storage, and the use of authorized disposal techniques like incineration or reverse distribution schemes are all a part of this. The objective is to reduce the hazards related to pharmaceutical waste while maintaining the safe and effective functioning of medical facilities [5].

TYPES OF PHARMACEUTICAL WASTE

There are many categories into which pharmaceutical waste at healthcare institutions may be divided, each with specific disposal needs and legal constraints. Non-hazardous pharmaceutical waste, hazardous pharmaceutical waste, regulated substances, infectious pharmaceutical waste, and unused or expired medications are the main categories of pharmaceutical waste [6]. To ensure that pharmaceutical waste is handled and disposed of appropriately, minimizing hazards to the environment, human health, and safety, it is crucial to comprehend the different categories of pharmaceutical waste. Fig. (**1**) shows different types of pharmaceutical waste.

Pharmaceutical Non-Hazardous Waste

Medications and pharmaceutical items that do not fit the definition of hazardous waste under laws like the Resource Conservation and Recovery Act (RCRA) in the United States or comparable frameworks in other nations are referred to as non-hazardous pharmaceutical waste. When disposed of properly, these medications do not present a serious risk to the environment or public health. Examples of non-hazardous pharmaceutical waste include: Over-the-counter drugs: Typical drugs include antacids, allergy treatments, and painkillers. Supplements and vitamins: Goods with non-toxic, non-hazardous components. Topical creams and ointments: Non-toxic drugs used topically to treat mild skin irritations.

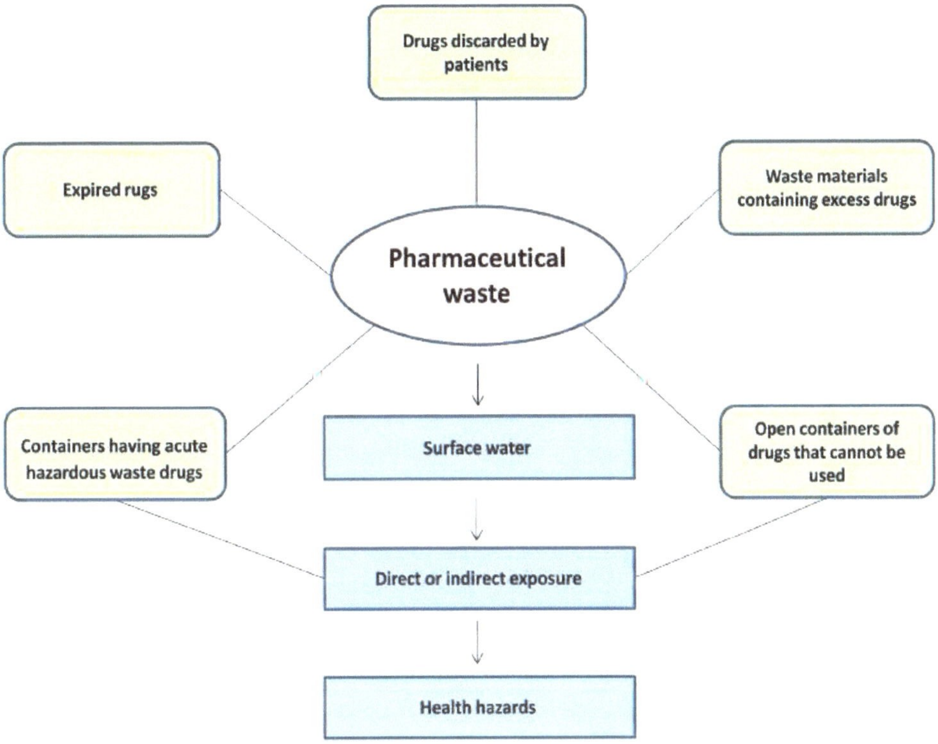

Fig. (1). Types of pharmaceutical waste.

Hazardous Pharmaceutical Waste

Drugs that are deemed poisonous, reactive, or potentially harmful to the environment or human health are referred to as hazardous pharmaceutical waste. To reduce the hazards, these medications must be handled and disposed of carefully. Because of its potential to cause damage, hazardous pharmaceutical waste is subject to stricter regulations than non-hazardous waste [6].

The following are some examples of hazardous pharmaceutical waste:

• Cytotoxic substances: Drugs that are used in chemotherapy treatments may be dangerous even in small doses. They need to be disposed of *via* certain methods, such as high-temperature incineration [6].
• Some antibiotics: Because they may be harmful, some antibiotics, particularly those given in large dosages or for resistant illnesses, are regarded as dangerous.
• Hormonal therapies: If not disposed of appropriately, medications used for hormone replacement therapy (HRT), contraception, and other hormone-related treatments may have a major negative impact on the environment.

• Mercury-containing drugs: Because of their toxicity and environmental endurance, older drugs that include mercury, including diuretics or antiseptics, are considered dangerous.
Hazardous pharmaceutical waste must be disposed of carefully to reduce the danger of contamination and exposure to harmful substances. These materials are often burned at facilities specifically constructed for the secure disposal of hazardous waste. Before being disposed of, they could sometimes be neutralized using chemical deactivation techniques [7].

Controlled Substances

Governmental organizations like the U.S. Drug Enforcement Administration (DEA) closely monitor drugs classified as controlled substances because of their high potential for misuse or addiction. To avoid abuse, these drugs need to be stored and disposed of with extra care. According to their propensity for misuse, they are divided into several schedules; Schedule V medications are less restricted, while Schedule I substances are subject to strict regulations.

Controlled drugs include, for example:

• Opioids: In addition to being very addictive, painkillers like morphine and oxycodone may be extremely harmful if used regularly at large doses [8].
• Benzodiazepines: Medications used to treat anxiety and sleep problems, such as diazepam and alprazolam, may cause dependence and misuse [8].
• Stimulants: Drugs used to treat attention deficit hyperactivity disorder (ADHD), such as methylphenidate and amphetamines, have a significant potential for abuse.
• Barbiturates and sedatives: Medications used for anesthesia or sedation are also prone to abuse.

Certain legal and regulatory criteria regulate the disposal of prohibited chemicals. For instance, the DEA in the United States requires healthcare institutions to dispose of banned medications according to stringent guidelines, which may involve incineration *via* certified facilities or the use of reverse distribution methods [8]. To guarantee compliance and avoid diversion, healthcare professionals must keep detailed records of the disposal procedure.

Infectious Pharmaceutical Waste

Medications and pharmaceuticals used to treat infectious illnesses or that have come into contact with potentially infectious substances, such as blood or bodily fluids, are considered infectious pharmaceutical waste. Medications intended to treat patients with communicable illnesses are also included in this category. Pharmaceutical waste that is contagious includes:

• Antibiotics: Frequently used to treat infections, these drugs may be categorized as infectious pharmaceutical waste if they come into contact with bodily fluids [9].
• Chemotherapeutic agents: If chemotherapy medications come into contact with the patient's bodily fluids, they may sometimes be regarded as infectious waste [9].
• IV fluids and administration sets: Products that have come into contact with body fluids or contaminated patients, such as saline bags or intravenous tubing.
Because infectious pharmaceutical waste might contain harmful microbes, it must be handled carefully. Usually, it is handled following procedures established by healthcare facilities for the disposal of biohazardous waste. Before being disposed of, the waste is sterilized (autoclaving, for example) or burned to remove any infectious pathogens [9]. To safeguard employees and patients, healthcare institutions must follow local, state, or federal laws pertaining to the processing and disposal of infectious pharmaceutical waste.

Unused or Expired Drugs

Medications that have reached their expiry dates or are no longer needed are referred to as expired pharmaceuticals. Patient returns, leftover medication from treatment plans, or other factors may make these medications. If used by mistake, abused, or disposed of inappropriately, unused or expired medications may be dangerous. Among the medications that are unused or expired are:

• Prescription drugs for transient illnesses: prescription drugs for acute diseases that the patient did not take until the end [10].
• Expired OTC pharmaceuticals: These include painkillers, cough treatments, and allergy medications that have passed their expiry date.
• Medications that patients return: In some instances, patients may return unwanted drugs, particularly prohibited pharmaceuticals, which need to be disposed of appropriately to prevent consumption [10].

REGULATORY FRAMEWORK GOVERNING PHARMACEUTICAL WASTE

Pharmaceutical waste is handled and disposed of according to strict regulations, protecting the environment and the general public from the harmful effects of medications. These laws at the international, national, and local levels address certain guidelines for the appropriate management and treatment of pharmaceutical waste. Healthcare facilities must follow the rules and guidelines set forth by significant regulatory bodies such as the World Health Organization (WHO), the Environmental Protection Agency (EPA), the United Nations Environment Programme (UNEP), and the Occupational Safety and Health Administration (OSHA) [11]. The management of prohibited drugs—prescriptions with a high risk of abuse—raises additional regulatory concerns. Below, we look closely at the regulatory framework that governs pharmaceutical waste, including national, international, and specialized regulatory bodies.

International Regulations

World Health Organization (WHO): In low- and middle-income nations where waste management infrastructure may be less established, the World Health Organization (WHO) is especially important in setting international standards for pharmaceutical waste management. The WHO's recommendations are centered on encouraging ecologically friendly disposal methods and reducing the dangers related to pharmaceutical waste. These recommendations place a strong emphasis on lowering the amount of pharmaceutical waste produced by implementing measures, including appropriate stock management and procurement procedures [11]. The WHO's recommendations for pharmaceutical waste include the following:

- Waste Minimization: To lower the harmful effects of waste, healthcare institutions are urged to refrain from excessive pharmaceutical stockpiling. Regular audits and inventory management may help guarantee that medications are utilized within their expiration dates.
- Appropriate Segregation and Disposal: Ensuring that pharmaceutical waste is divided into categories that are hazardous and non-hazardous so that suitable disposal techniques may be used. For certain types of pharmaceutical waste, WHO recommends ecologically friendly practices, including incineration or the use of specialist landfills. The World Health Organization places a strong emphasis on the proper handling and storage of hazardous and toxic medications, particularly those used in hormonal and chemotherapy treatments, which call for particular disposal procedures to prevent environmental contamination [11].

United Nations Environment Programme (UNEP)

The United Nations Environment Programme (UNEP) addresses pharmaceutical waste as part of its broader initiatives on chemical waste and sustainable development. UNEP's Guidance on the Environmentally Sound Management of Chemicals provides recommendations for managing pharmaceuticals in a way that minimizes harm to the environment. UNEP's guidelines align with the principles of the basel convention on the control of transboundary movements of hazardous wastes and their disposal, which includes pharmaceuticals as part of the waste streams that require special handling due to their toxic, persistent, and bioaccumulative properties [11].

UNEP Emphasizes

Pharmaceutical Waste as Chemical Waste: Recognizing pharmaceuticals as a type of chemical waste that requires specific disposal methods to avoid environmental contamination, especially in water bodies where pharmaceutical residues are frequently detected [11].

International Cooperation: UNEP promotes international cooperation to help developing nations adopt effective pharmaceutical waste management practices and comply with international treaties [11].

National Regulations

UNEP's guidance on the environmentally sound management of chemicals provides recommendations for managing pharmaceuticals to minimize damage to the environment. Pharmaceuticals constitute one of the waste streams that need particular management due to their hazardous, persistent, and bioaccumulative properties; UNEP's standards are basedon the Basel Convention on the control of transboundary movements of hazardous wastes and their disposal [11]. The UNEP emphasizes:

- Chemical Waste from Pharmaceuticals: It is well recognized that medications are a specific kind of chemical waste that must be disposed of in accordance with certain regulations to avoid contaminating the environment, especially in water bodies where pharmaceutical residues are often discovered [11].
- International Cooperation: UNEP promotes international cooperation to help developing nations follow international agreements and put effective pharmaceutical waste management plans into place [11]. The Environmental Protection Agency (EPA), the Drug Enforcement Administration (DEA), and the Food and Drug Administration (FDA) are among the federal authorities that regulate pharmaceutical waste in the United States. Certain facets of pharmaceutical waste management are governed by each agency.
- EPA, or the Environmental Protection Agency: The EPA divides pharmaceutical waste into hazardous and non-hazardous categories under the Resource

Conservation and Recovery Act (RCRA), and there are stringent rules on how to dispose of hazardous pharmaceutical waste. Pharmaceutical waste may be classified as hazardous according to toxicity, reactivity, or ignitability, according to the EPA's hazardous waste rules [11]. Hazardous Pharmaceuticals: Certain antibiotics, chemotherapeutic drugs, and other toxic pharmaceuticals are categorized as hazardous waste and need to be handled appropriately. In order to reduce the dangers to the environment and public health, the EPA requires that these medications be burned or disposed of in some other way [11]. Non-Hazardous Pharmaceuticals: Despite not being dangerous, these drugs must be disposed of properly to avoid contamination and abuse. For non-hazardous pharmaceutical waste, techniques including cremation, landfilling, and reverse distribution schemes are typical [12].

• Food and Drug Administration (FDA): The FDA is in charge of disposing of pharmaceutical items that have been recalled, expired, or unused. Secure disposal techniques, such as drug take-back programs and incineration for prohibited drugs, are advised by the agency's recommendations to avoid abuse [12].
• Drug Enforcement Administration (DEA): The Controlled Substances Act (CSA) is the DEA's regulatory tool for restricted drugs. Pharmaceutical medications having a significant potential for misuse are among the prohibited substances for which the DEA has devised comprehensive disposal protocols [12]. With a focus on permitted collection locations and reverse distribution networks, the Secure and Responsible Drug Disposal Act of 2010 permits the safe collection and disposal of banned narcotics.

• The European Union (EU) has clear rules and regulations for pharmaceutical waste. By classifying pharmaceutical waste into several categories according to the substance's properties and possible risks, the European Union (EU) highlights the need to reduce pharmaceutical waste and guarantee its appropriate disposal.
• The 2008/98/EC Waste Directive: General waste management concepts are outlined in this regulation, such as the waste hierarchy, which places an emphasis on recycling and waste avoidance above disposal. With an emphasis on reusing and recycling wherever feasible, it promotes reducing the production of pharmaceutical waste [12].
• EU legislation 1272/2008 on the Classification, Labeling, and Packaging of Substances and Mixtures (CLP Regulation): This legislation establishes the standards for classifying dangerous compounds, including medications, according to their toxicity, effects on the environment, and other characteristics. Specialized disposal methods, such as high-temperature burning, are necessary for drugs that are categorized as hazardous [12].

Role of Environmental Protection Agencies (EPA, OSHA)

Environmental Protection Agency (EPA): The primary agency in charge of overseeing pharmaceutical waste disposal in the US is the EPA. Pharmaceutical waste management is based on the Resource Conservation and Recovery Act (RCRA) of the EPA, which defines hazardous waste and establishes guidelines for its secure disposal. In order to guarantee the safe handling of hazardous pharmaceutical waste and the proper disposal of non-hazardous waste, the EPA enforces standards for pharmaceutical firms as well as healthcare institutions [13]. In order to ensure that controlled substances are disposed of in a way that avoids diversion or abuse, the EPA collaborates with the FDA and DEA to regulate them.

Occupational Safety and Health Administration (OSHA): The safety of healthcare personnel managing pharmaceutical waste is the responsibility of the Occupational Safety and Health Administration (OSHA). In order to safeguard employees from exposure to harmful chemicals, OSHA offers standards for the proper treatment of hazardous pharmaceutical waste. In order to reduce exposure hazards, healthcare personnel who handle medications like chemotherapeutic agents or regulated chemicals need to be well educated in safe handling procedures, which include using personal protective equipment (PPE) and engineering controls [13].

Special Considerations for Controlled Substances: Pharmaceuticals with a high potential for abuse, including addiction or misuse, are classified as controlled drugs. Because of their potential for harm, they are subject to stricter regulations than other kinds of pharmaceutical waste. The main federal organization in charge of regulating the disposal of prohibited narcotics in the US is the Drug Enforcement Administration (DEA) [13]. Important factors for restricted drugs are as follows:

• Reverse Distribution systems: These systems, which return unwanted controlled medications to the manufacturer for secure disposal, are often employed by healthcare institutions [13].
• Secure Collection and Disposal: To avoid diversion, controlled drugs must be gathered and disposed of safely. This entails following stringent documentation guidelines and using approved collecting locations.
• Incineration: Since it guarantees the total annihilation of the narcotics and eliminates any chance of diversion, incineration is often the recommended method of disposal for prohibited substances [13].

WASTE SEGREGATION IN HEALTHCARE FACILITIES

In healthcare institutions, waste segregation is an essential feature of waste management, especially when it comes to pharmaceutical waste management. Pharmaceutical waste is disposed of in a way that is efficient, safe for the environment, and compatible with the law when it is properly segregated [9]. Segregation is the process of classifying and arranging waste into discrete categories according to its characteristics, hazards, and needs for disposal. By doing this, contamination is reduced, environmental risks are avoided, and economic waste management techniques are encouraged. Pharmaceutical waste segregation lowers the risk of hazardous material exposure for healthcare workers and helps avoid cross-contamination of waste kinds in healthcare environments [14]. The significance of waste segregation, the best methods for classifying various pharmaceutical waste categories, regulatory requirements, and the labeling and marking of pharmaceutical waste containers are all covered in this section (Table **1**). Table **1** shows waste segregation facilities using colour coding.

Table 1. Waste segregation in healthcare facilities, covering common categories, their descriptions, and colour coding.

Waste Category	Description	Colour Coding	Reference
Normal waste	Non-hazardous waste like paper, plastics, and packaging.	Black	[13]
Infectious Waste	Waste contaminated with blood, body fluids, and cultures.	Yellow	[13]
Hazardous Waste	Chemicals, pharmaceuticals, cytotoxic drugs, and pesticides.	Purple (for cytotoxic), Red for hazardous	[14]
Pharmaceutical Waste	Expired or unused medications, vaccines.	Blue	[14]
Chemical Waste	Laboratory chemicals, solvents, and reagents.	White	[14]

Importance of Segregation

Healthcare institutions must effectively separate their waste for a variety of reasons.

1. Health and Safety: Adequate segregation lowers the possibility of coming into contact with dangerous materials, especially those included in hazardous pharmaceutical waste. Healthcare professionals who handle pharmaceuticals, including opioids, cytotoxic drugs, and prohibited substances, should pay particular attention to this. Workers may unintentionally come into contact with infectious or dangerous chemicals if strict segregation is not followed, which might result in environmental pollution, infection, or poisoning [14].

2. Environmental Protection: Significant harm to the environment may result from improper disposal of pharmaceutical waste, particularly toxic medications. When pharmaceuticals find their way into water systems, they may damage aquatic life, upset ecosystems, and endanger human health over time by contaminating drinking water. Segregation guarantees that harmful pharmaceutical waste is disposed of in ways that avoid contamination, including landfills or high-temperature burning.

3. Regulation Compliance: To guarantee adherence to several regional, national, and worldwide requirements, pharmaceutical waste must be segregated. The proper handling, storage, and disposal of pharmaceutical waste are governed by regulations set out by regulatory agencies such as the World Health Organization (WHO), Drug Enforcement Administration (DEA), and Environmental Protection Agency (EPA). There may be legal repercussions for breaking these rules, such as fines or punishments [14].

4. Cost-Efficiency: By separating waste at the point of development, costly treatment techniques are not required, allowing for more effective disposal. For instance, incineration is required for hazardous pharmaceutical waste, which is more expensive than recycling or landfilling. Healthcare institutions may save disposal expenses by separating hazardous and non-hazardous waste [15].

5. Diversion and Misuse Reduction: The danger of abuse or diversion is decreased when controlled pharmaceuticals and expired prescriptions are properly segregated. Opioids and other controlled medications are particularly prone to misuse, and inappropriate disposal may result in theft or unapproved usage. These medications are disposed of safely and without diversion when they are segregated [15].

Legal Requirements for Waste Segregation

Numerous national and international rules that enforce waste segregation rules regulate the handling of pharmaceutical waste in healthcare institutions.

1. U.S. Regulations: Resource Conservation and Recovery Act (RCRA): RCRA is a law that the EPA uses to manage pharmaceutical waste that is deemed hazardous because of its toxic, corrosive, or reactive qualities [16]. The DEA oversees the regulation of banned chemicals, including their disposal, under the Banned Chemicals Act (CSA). To avoid diversion or abuse, healthcare institutions must adhere to stringent regulations for the storage and disposal of regulated drugs [16]. o State rules: Many U.S. states have extra rules governing pharmaceutical waste management in addition to federal legislation. These restrictions include stricter guidelines for the disposal of prohibited and hazardous drugs.

2. European Union Regulation: Directive 2008/98/EC on Waste: This directive mandates that healthcare institutions adopt waste management procedures that include waste segregation, paying particular attention to pharmaceutical and hazardous waste [16]. Pharmaceutical waste is categorized by the European Waste Catalogue (EWC), which also mandates that waste be separated according to its toxicity and other attributes. In order to guarantee appropriate disposal and stay out of trouble, healthcare institutions must adhere to the EWC requirements.

3. International standards: World Health Organization (WHO): Waste segregation is crucial for pharmaceutical waste management, according to WHO standards, in order to avoid human exposure and environmental pollution. According to best practices, the WHO advises healthcare institutions in both developed and developing nations to have waste segregation systems in place [16].

4 Basel Convention: This agreement governs the transboundary transportation of medicines and other hazardous waste. It highlights how important it is to properly separate waste and dispose of pharmaceutical waste in an ecologically responsible manner, particularly in developing countries [16].

Labeling and Marking of Pharmaceutical Waste Containers

Pharmaceutical waste containers must be marked and labelled clearly and accurately for waste segregation to be successful. When waste is properly labelled, healthcare professionals and waste disposal staff can rapidly determine the kind of waste and dispose of it according to the right protocols.

1. Labelling Necessities: The kind of pharmaceutical waste that is included in each container must be identified by labelling it as "Cytotoxic Waste," "Controlled Substances," or "Non-Hazardous Pharmaceutical Waste." The skull and crossbones for poisonous compounds or the corrosive sign for chemicals that might harm skin or eyes are examples of suitable hazard symbols that should be shown on hazardous pharmaceutical waste containers [17].

2. Date of Disposal: According to some regulations, especially in the US, containers holding pharmaceutical waste must include a label indicating the date the waste was first put in the container. Tracking waste creation and making sure it is disposed of properly within the allotted time limits are crucial [17].

3. Marking Containers for Controlled Substances: "Controlled Substance Waste" must be written on containers containing controlled substances, and they must be secured. This labelling guarantees that staff members are aware of how crucial it is to handle these drugs in accordance with stringent guidelines.

4. Colour-coding Systems: Healthcare institutions need to label waste containers and also use a colour-coding system. As an example, red denotes hazardous waste, such as chemotherapy medications [17]. Drugs that are not dangerous are shown in yellow. "Controlled Substance Waste" is clearly labelled and blue for prohibited drugs.

Storage and Handling of Pharmaceutical Waste with Management

A key component of pharmaceutical waste management in healthcare institutions is the appropriate processing and storage of pharmaceutical waste. Health risks, environmental damages, and non-compliance with regulations are reduced when pharmaceutical waste is managed effectively. To maintain safety, legal compliance, and environmental preservation, healthcare institutions must handle and store pharmaceutical waste according to strict guidelines and best practices. The main elements of handling and storing pharmaceutical waste are explained in detail in the section that follows. These include safe storage spaces, safety regulations, the risks of incorrect handling and cross-contamination, and particular storage procedures for hazardous waste and controlled substances [17].

Secure Storage Areas and Facilities

Establishing safe storage spaces in healthcare facilities is one of the most crucial aspects of managing pharmaceutical waste. To avoid unintentional exposure or environmental contamination, these spaces must be built to securely store pharmaceutical waste, especially hazardous and controlled substances [18].

1. Designated Storage Areas: To avoid any mixing with common waste, safe storage spaces should be set aside exclusively for pharmaceutical waste. Only authorised workers should be able to enter these clearly designated zones. To prevent exposure or contamination, the storage spaces should be placed apart from areas used for medical care, food preparation, or other crucial tasks. To further lower the chance of improper handling or cross-contamination, controlled drugs and hazardous pharmaceutical waste should be kept in different locations [18].

2. Physical Security Features: Lockable Doors: To stop unwanted access to pharmaceutical waste, especially controlled drugs, the storage spaces must have lockable doors.

3. Video Systems: To guard against theft or diversion, many healthcare institutions must install video cameras in storage locations that hold controlled drugs.

4. Access Control: The locations used to store pharmaceutical waste should only be accessible by authorised personnel. To monitor who accesses these places and when, a system for recording access and conducting routine audits should be put in place [18]

5. Sufficient Ventilation and Temperature Control: Ventilation: Appropriate ventilation systems have to be installed in the storage spaces, particularly those that hold hazardous pharmaceutical waste. This is essential to avoid the accumulation of toxic gases or vapours that might endanger the environment and healthcare personnel.

6. Temperature Control: Some pharmaceutical wastes may need to be stored in a freezer or refrigerator, especially certain biologics, vaccines, or sensitive drugs. Temperature-controlled spaces, such as freezers or refrigerators, with monitoring systems to guarantee that temperatures stay within predetermined bounds, are essential components of pharmaceutical waste management systems [18].

7. Spill Containment: o Proper materials and equipment for spill containment must be present in storage locations. Trays or spill pallets are included to capture container spills. In order to avoid contamination, waste containers should also be routinely inspected for leaks or other damage, and any compromised containers should be replaced immediately [18].

Safety Standards and Guidelines

Risk of Mismanagement and Cross-Contamination

A number of issues, including health hazards, environmental pollution, legal penalties, and increased costs, may result from improper handling of pharmaceutical waste. It is important to mitigate such risks by implementing appropriate handling and storage procedures.

1. Health Risks: Patients and healthcare personnel may be exposed to hazardous or contagious substances if pharmaceutical waste is not properly managed. For example, there is a chance of unintentional exposure by skin contact, inhalation, or ingestion if medications like opioids or chemotherapeutic chemicals are not handled properly. Long-term illnesses, skin burns, respiratory problems, and reproductive toxicity are just a few of the negative health outcomes that may result from this [19]. Furthermore, if infectious pharmaceutical waste—such as drugs used to treat hepatitis or HIV—is not appropriately confined and disposed of, there is a serious danger of disease transmission to both the environment and workers.

2. Environmental Contamination: The environment may be contaminated as a result of incorrect pharmaceutical waste storage or disposal. When medications are thrown down drains or flushed down toilets, they may get into wastewater systems, which can then reach water bodies and endanger aquatic life. According to studies, pharmaceutical waste in water systems may endanger human health, damage fish, and disturb ecosystems [19]. Cross-contamination happens when several pharmaceutical waste types—including non-hazardous medications, restricted substances, and hazardous drugs—are incorrectly disposed of or kept together. Pharmaceutical waste, especially controlled substances, is susceptible to theft or diversion if not kept properly. This may result in inefficient disposal techniques, increased toxicity, and environmental impact. Because of their significant potential for misuse, controlled medications like benzodiazepines and opioids should be kept in secure, closely watched locations to avoid unwanted access. The continuing opioid crisis and other drug misuse might be exacerbated by the illegal distribution of these drugs due to a lack of security [19].

3. Financial and Legal Risks: Healthcare institutions that improperly handle pharmaceutical waste run the danger of being sued and paying hefty penalties. Organisations that violate waste management standards face severe fines from regulatory agencies, including the EPA, DEA, and OSHA. Additionally, improper handling of pharmaceutical waste may result in loss of accreditation or licensure as well as harm to one's image [19].

PHARMACEUTICAL WASTE DISPOSAL METHODS

One essential part of waste management in healthcare institutions is the disposal of pharmaceutical waste. Using safe and efficient disposal techniques is crucial since pharmaceutical waste has the potential to negatively impact both human health and the environment. Regulations are in place to guarantee that pharmaceutical waste is disposed of in an ecologically conscious way. Incineration, landfilling, chemical deactivation, reverse distribution, take-back programs, and the disposal of prohibited substances and expired medications are some of the main techniques for disposing of pharmaceutical waste that are covered in this section.

Burning

Most people agree that incineration is one of the best and most ecologically friendly ways to dispose of pharmaceutical waste, especially when it comes to hazardous pharmaceuticals. Pharmaceutical waste is burned at high temperatures, which completely destroys the waste materials [20].

Landfilling

Pharmaceutical waste is disposed of in landfills, which are subterranean repositories. Although this approach is less often utilised for controlled pharmaceutical or hazardous pharmaceutical waste, it could work for non-hazardous pharmaceutical waste that is neither ecologically dangerous nor chemically active.

Deactivation of Chemicals:

Chemical deactivation is the process of utilising chemicals to neutralise or make pharmaceutical waste non-toxic. Certain kinds of pharmaceutical waste, such as cytotoxic medicines, which need specific management because of their poisonous nature, are often handled using this manner [20].

Programs for Reverse Distribution and Take-Back:

Programs for reverse distribution and take-back enable patients, medical professionals, and pharmacists to return unwanted or expired medications for appropriate disposal. These initiatives are often planned by government organisations, private organisations, or pharmaceutical corporations.

1. Reverse Distribution: This method entails returning medications that are excess, unused, or expired to the distributor, where they are either securely disposed of or sent back to the manufacturer. Pharmacies may get into agreements with waste management companies or distributors to streamline this procedure. This approach is most often used for non-controlled or non-hazardous substances, such as certain prescription pharmaceuticals and over-the-counter treatments.

2. Take-back Programs: Take-back programs are community- or government-sponsored campaigns that enable people to return unwanted medications to specified collection locations, which are often pharmacies, clinics, or police stations. These initiatives are especially successful in preventing narcotics from falling into the wrong hands. To promote proper disposal, the US Drug Enforcement Administration (DEA) hosts recurring National Prescription Drug Take-Back activities [20].

CHALLENGES IN PHARMACEUTICAL WASTE MANAGEMENT

Healthcare institutions must handle pharmaceutical waste, but there are a number of obstacles that might prevent efficient waste disposal. These difficulties are brought on by budgetary limitations, complicated regulations, environmental issues, and problems with public awareness. The management procedure is further complicated by waste stream contamination and inappropriate handling of regulated drugs.

1. Financial Consequences: The high expense of the appropriate disposal of pharmaceutical waste is one of the main issues facing healthcare institutions. Pharmaceutical waste management requires a large financial outlay for specialised handling, segregation systems, safe storage, and disposal techniques, all of which may be costly [21]. The financial strain also consists of:

• Training costs: It costs more to make sure employees are properly educated to manage pharmaceutical waste.

• Compliance costs: In order to adhere to changing rules, facilities must invest in audits, reporting, and system upgrades.

Particularly in smaller, resource-constrained contexts, healthcare organisations often have to make the tough trade-off between meeting safety and environmental regulations and remaining within their means [22].

2. Issues with Compliance and Regulatory Complexity: There are several national and international legislations pertaining to pharmaceutical waste. These rules may differ widely, which causes misunderstandings and makes it difficult for healthcare facilities to maintain compliance. Penalties, legal action, and professional harm to the organisation may follow noncompliance [22].

3. Education and Public Awareness: Reducing inappropriate medicine disposal and avoiding environmental contamination requires raising public understanding of pharmaceutical disposal practices. However, a lot of individuals still don't know how to properly get rid of unneeded or expired prescriptions, which leads to inappropriate disposal practices, including flushing them down the toilet or throwing them in the garbage [22].

4. Ecological and Environmental Issues: Pharmaceuticals may cause major ecological and environmental problems, especially if they are not disposed of appropriately. Numerous pharmaceutical substances are difficult to decompose and remain in the environment for extended periods of time, which may contaminate soil, water sources, and wildlife [23].

5. Controlled Substance Disposal: Because of the significant danger of abuse and diversion, disposing of controlled drugs poses a special issue. Drug disposal in healthcare settings is a delicate topic since substances, including opioids, benzodiazepines, and stimulants, are especially prone to being diverted for illegal purposes [23].

6. Contamination of Waste Streams: Waste stream contamination, which happens when pharmaceutical waste is improperly separated from other forms of trash, is one of the main problems in pharmaceutical waste management. Cross-contamination and the disposal of dangerous medications in regular waste streams may arise from this, posing serious threats to human health and the environment [24].

CONCLUSION

The rising number of pharmaceutical products and the serious consequences of inappropriate disposal have made pharmaceutical waste management in healthcare a more crucial and complicated problem. The management of pharmaceutical waste must be safe, effective, and environmentally friendly as the healthcare industry develops in order to preserve both the environment and human health. For the management, disposal, storage, and segregation of different kinds of pharmaceutical waste, such as controlled drugs, hazardous compounds, and expired pharmaceuticals, strong systems are needed. Pharmaceutical waste management is fraught with difficulties that include logistical, financial, legal, and environmental issues. Financial limitations often prevent the implementation of sophisticated waste management systems, and healthcare practitioners must be continuously informed about changing regulations due to regulatory difficulties. Environmental issues, such as the impact of inappropriate disposal on ecosystems and water supplies, emphasise how important it is to use green and sustainable disposal methods. Technological developments are opening the door to safer and more effective pharmaceutical waste management. Examples of these developments include enhanced burning techniques, chemical deactivation technologies, and automated waste sorting. However, a large investment and collaboration between manufacturers, regulatory bodies, and healthcare institutions are necessary for the deployment of these technologies. Pharmaceutical businesses are also being urged to assume more responsibility for their goods at every stage of their life cycle, including disposal, by increasing laws and promoting extended producer responsibility (EPR). Since many customers are not aware of the correct ways to dispose of leftover pharmaceuticals, public awareness is still a crucial topic that requires more attention. Governments, healthcare organisations, pharmaceutical producers, and waste management firms must work together to solve the global problem of pharmaceutical waste. Improving disposal procedures and reducing the environmental effect of pharmaceutical waste need international collaboration, take-back initiatives, and educational efforts.

In conclusion, even though substantial progress has been achieved in enhancing pharmaceutical waste management procedures, more work is required to handle the issue's increasing complexity. To create a sustainable, safe, and environmentally friendly future for pharmaceutical waste management, technological innovation, regulatory change, and coordinated effort from all stakeholders in the healthcare and pharmaceutical industries are essential. Adopting these strategies will enable healthcare systems to safeguard the environment and promote public health, leaving a safer and cleaner earth for future generations.

REFERENCES

[1] Fent K, Weston AA, Caminada D. Ecotoxicology of human pharmaceuticals. Aquat Toxicol 2006; 76(2): 122-59. [http://dx.doi.org/10.1016/j.aquatox.2005.09.009] [PMID: 16257063]

[2] Schwartz A. The opioid epidemic: pharmaceutical waste and the public health response. J Environ Health 2019; 81(3): 1-5.

[3] Banjar H, Alrowithi R, Alhadrami S, Magrabi E, Munshi R, Alrige M. An intelligent system for proper management and disposal of unused and expired medications. Int J Environ Res Public Health 2022; 19(5): 2875. [http://dx.doi.org/10.3390/ijerph19052875] [PMID: 35270568]

[4] U.S. Drug Enforcement Administration (DEA). Secure and Responsible Drug Disposal Act of 2010. 2010. Available from: https://www.dea.gov

[5] World Health Organization (WHO). Guidelines on the safe disposal of pharmaceuticals. 2017. Available from: https://www.who.int

[6] Easty AC, Coakley N, Cheng R, *et al.* Safe handling of cytotoxics: guideline recommendations. Curr Oncol 2015; 22(1): 27-37. [http://dx.doi.org/10.3747/co.21.2151] [PMID: 25684994]

[7] U.S. Environmental Protection Agency (EPA). Pharmaceutical Waste 2021. https://www.epa.gov

[8] Hutchison R W Jr. Storage, security, and disposal J Opioid Manag 2019 Sep 01; 15(5): 353-4.

[9] Janik-Karpinska E, Brancaleoni R, Niemcewicz M, *et al.* Healthcare waste—a serious problem for global health. Healthcare (Basel) 2023; 11(2): 242. [http://dx.doi.org/10.3390/healthcare11020242] [PMID: 36673610]

[10] Brechtelsbauer E, Shah S. Update on pharmaceutical waste disposal regulations: Strategies for success. Am J Health Syst Pharm 2020; 77(7): 574-82. [http://dx.doi.org/10.1093/ajhp/zxz360] [PMID: 32050015]

[11] United Nations Environment Programme (UNEP). Guidance on the Environmentally Sound Management of Chemicals. 2019. Available from: https://www.unep.org

[12] European Union (EU). Directive 2008/98/EC on waste. Off J. Eur Union 2008. Available from: http://data.europa.eu/eli/dir/2008/98/oj

[13] Occupational Safety and Health Administration (OSHA). Hazardous Waste Operations and Emergency Response (HAZWOPER). 2020.

[14] Ritchie MA, McAdams C, Fritz N. Exposure risk in the handling and administration of chemotherapy agents: a review and synthesis of the literature. Online J Knowl Synth Nurs 2000; E7(1): 51-60. [http://dx.doi.org/10.1111/j.1524-475X.2000.00051.x] [PMID: 12489036]

[15] Haffajee RL, Abrams MR. Settling the score: maximizing the public health impact of opioid litigation. Ohio St LJ 2019; 80: 701.

[16] Kümmerer K. Pharmaceuticals in the environment: sources, fate, effects and risks. Berlin: Springer 2001. [http://dx.doi.org/10.1007/978-3-662-04634-0]

[17] National Prescription Drug Take-Back Day 2020. https://www.dea.gov/takebackday

[18] Shirazi K M. Green and Sustainable Pharmaceutics: Innovations in Eco Friendly Drug Development Drugs & Clinic 2025 May 29; 40(2): 5-16.

[19] Brechtelsbauer E, Shah S. Update on pharmaceutical waste disposal regulations: strategies for success Am J Health-Syst Pharm 2020 Apr 01; 77(7): 574-82.

[20] Chauhan G, Sevda S. Solid Waste Management. Boca Raton: CRC Press 2023. [http://dx.doi.org/10.1201/9781003189602]

[21] Noudeng V, Pheakdey DV, Minh TTN, Xuan TD. Municipal solid waste management in Laos: comparative analysis of environmental impact, practices, and technologies with ASEAN regions and Japan. Environments 2024; 11(8): 170. [http://dx.doi.org/10.3390/environments11080170]

[22] PharmaCycle. Medications Return Program in Canada [Internet]. Canada: PharmaCycle; 2020.

[23] Porteous A. Energy from waste incineration—a state of the art emissions review with an emphasis on public acceptability Appl Energy 2001 Oct 01; 70(2): 157-67.

[24] Rogowska J, Zimmermann A. Household pharmaceutical waste disposal as a global problem—a review. Int J Environ Res Public Health 2022; 19(23): 15798. [http://dx.doi.org/10.3390/ijerph192315798] [PMID: 36497873]

CHAPTER 9

Sustainable and Eco-Friendly Packaging: A Pathway to Better Recycling

Mukul Yadav[1], **Akhalesh Kumar**[1], **Aastha Sharma**[1,*], **Anjali Chouhan**[1] and **Ravi Shekhar**[1]

[1] *Department of Pharmacy, Institute of Pharmacy & Paramedical Sciences, Dr. Bhimrao Ambedkar University, Agra, Uttar Pradesh, India*

Abstract: As global environmental challenges intensify, sustainable, eco-friendly packaging emerges as a pivotal solution to mitigate ecological degradation and promote circular economies. This chapter examines the complex intersection of material innovation, waste management, and recycling efficiency within the context of sustainable packaging systems. It examines advanced materials, including biodegradable polymers, plant-based alternatives, and recyclable composites, alongside their role in reducing dependence on single-use plastics. Furthermore, it critically analyzes the integration of circular design principles, emphasizing material longevity, reusability, and recyclability while assessing the limitations and opportunities within current recycling infrastructures. By investigating the systemic changes required in packaging design, production, and post-consumer processing, this chapter argues that eco-friendly packaging, when coupled with robust recycling frameworks, can catalyze a more sustainable, closed-loop economy. Ultimately, it underscores the transformative potential of sustainable packaging as a key driver for both environmental and economic resilience in the face of escalating resource scarcity and pollution.

Keywords: Biodegradable, Bioplastic, Biopolymer, Eco-friendly packaging, Ecological degradation, Plastic, Pollution, Recycle, Sustainable packaging, Waste management.

INTRODUCTION

The technology, science, and art of packaging are used to successfully present, preserve, and protect goods for consumers [1]. The materials (Pharmaceutical packaging) are the assemblage of varying components that surround a pharmaceutical product from the time of manufacture until it is used. It offers identification presentation, protection, information, as well as convenience at a fair price from the duration of manufacture until it is utilized. The type of pharma-

* **Corresponding author: Aastha Sharma**, Department of Pharmacy, Institute of Pharmacy & Paramedical Sciences, Dr. Bhimrao Ambedkar University, Agra, Uttar Pradesh, India; E-mail: 1998.aasthasharmaex@gmail.com

Suman Gautam, Jai Narayan Mishra, Preeti Mishra, Preeti Verma & Sudhanshu Mishra (Eds.)

ceutical packaging used depends on the substance and its intended application. Ultimately, research on the stability, storage, sterilization, and testing of specific materials must be conducted to evaluate each packing material. The packaging supports and plays a critical role in maintaining the eminence of therapeutic goods [2].

Sustainable packaging refers to the design, materials, and processes used to create packaging that minimizes environmental impact during its life cycle. The goal is to reduce the ecological footprint of packaging from production to disposal, thereby preserving natural resources and reducing waste. Sustainable packaging supports the principles of reduce, reuse, and recycle while striving to minimize carbon emissions, water usage, and other environmental harms.

Eco-friendly packaging is a subset of sustainable packaging, specifically focused on materials and practices that are not harmful to the environment. Eco-friendly packaging can include recyclable, biodegradable, compostable, or reusable materials. It aims to minimize consumption of non-renewable resources, reduce waste, and lower the pollution associated with packaging production and disposal.

KEY PRINCIPLES [3]

- **Life Cycle Thinking**: Sustainable packaging is designed with its complete life cycle in mind, from fresh material sourcing to end-of-life disposal. The goal is to minimize negative environmental impacts at every stage.
- **Resource Efficiency**: Efficient use of materials, energy, and water in production. Sustainable packaging seeks to reduce waste through efficient design, manufacturing, and transportation processes.
- **Design for Reuse/Recycle**: Packaging should be designed to facilitate reuse or recycling. This includes using single materials, minimizing additives, and making it easier for consumers to dispose of it correctly.

FUNCTIONS OF PACKAGING

- **Barrier Protection** - It serves as a defense against unfavorable external factors that could alter the product's characteristics, such as moisture, light, oxygen, and temperature. Blister packing (pharmaceutical-grade barrier films along with eco-friendly halogenated adhesives that protect the pharmaceutical product from the time of production until the time of free films) can offer this kind of protection.
- **Biological Protection** – It is intended for the defense against biological toxins.
- **Physical Protection** – It is intended for the protection of the pharmaceutical dosage forms against bodily damage.
- **Identification** – It is meant for the proof of identity of the products.

- **Security** - Certain characteristics of pharmaceutical packaging guard against counterfeiting. Additionally, it keeps young children from using the formulation's contents.
- **Convenience** – Packaging needs to be adequate to increase consumer interaction with the products and advance their handling, distribution, sale, and use.

TRADITIONAL MATERIALS USED FOR PACKAGING

Plastic

Because plastics are useful and versatile materials, they can be used for carrying and storing complex instruments, medications, and other medical apparatus. In the health care industry, plastic containers are commonplace. These consist of overwrap, thermoformed blister packs, in addition to trays, vials, bags, pouches, and caps. Synthetic materials, which are frequently oil-based and nonbiodegradable polymers, make up the majority of plastic packaging employed in daily life. Pharmaceutical packaging uses conventional plastics made from non-renewable petroleum-based oils, such as polypropylene, polyethylene, polytetrafluoroethylene, and polyvinyl chloride [4].

These synthetic polymers are most frequently used in pharmaceutical packaging applications due to their exceptional strength, chemical resistance, and lightweight nature [5]. However, sorption, leaching, permeability, chemical responsiveness, and alteration of the properties of the products or plastics are the drawbacks of using plastic materials for pharmaceutical packaging [6]. It takes several decades for these plastics to break down, and as they do, harmful compounds are released. The need to find appropriate alternatives, such as bioplastics with comparable physico-chemical properties to petroleum-based plastics, is increasingly recognized in light of the detrimental effects of conventional plastics.

Tin Plate

The low-carbon steel used to make the tinplate has thin tin coatings applied to both sides. Aerosol containers and packaging closures are commonly made with it. It can be recycled frequently into novel packaging products without losing quality, and it is less expensive than aluminium. It is durable and formable, has a longer shelf life for the dosage form, is appropriate for printing and graphics, provides better barrier protection, is retortable, and, above all, is environmentally friendly [7].

Aluminium

It is primarily used in the manufacturing of aluminium foil laminates and seamless containers. It is an environmentally friendly material for pharmaceutical packaging because it can be recycled into various products [8]. New aluminium packs made solely of recycled materials are possible because the metal is not undermined during the recycling process. Pure aluminium metal can be moved into thin sheets, annealed to create aluminium foils for a diversity of pharmaceutical applications. The main benefit of the films is that they improve the dosage forms' barrier protection against air, moisture, oils, and odors [9].

Steel

Initially, new steel was made from up to 40% recycled steel scrap. Steel comes in a variety of forms, including alloy steel, stainless steel, tool steel, and carbon steel. Magnets can be used to easily and reasonably separate them from mixed waste, which is environmentally beneficial. Primary and secondary steel containers are used to package aerosols and other pharmaceutical products. Bottle caps, as well as closures, also use it as a tamper-proof packaging material. Compared to reprocessing aluminium, recycling steel is inexpensive.

ENVIRONMENTAL IMPLICATIONS OF TRADITIONAL PACKAGING MATERIALS USED

The use of traditional supplies in pharmaceutical packaging has major negative environmental effects. Plastic contributes to the global waste problem by ending up in landfills and along the ocean because it does not decompose. Although metals can be reused, extracting and processing them requires significant energy. Glass production and disposal also involve substantial energy use and emissions. An extensive network of environmental issues is revealed by the lifecycle analysis of these materials, spanning from the mining of raw materials to production, transportation, use, and disposal. Convenience and protection have frequently taken precedence over sustainability in packaging designs, which results in wasteful and excessive material use [10].

A potential remedy for the environmental issues raised by conventional pharmaceutical packaging is biodegradable packaging. New manufacturing techniques and materials are being created to satisfy the demands of a sector that is changing quickly. This section examines these developments, looking at different materials, procedures, and the difficulties they inevitably encounter [11].

BIODEGRADABLE PACKAGING TECHNOLOGIES

Materials

Polylactic Acid

One of the leading materials for biodegradable packaging is PLA (Fig. **1**). A major departure from petroleum-based plastics, renewable sources like sugarcane, corn flour, and cassava are used to make PLA. PLA's composability is what makes it so appealing. PLA can break down in a few months in an industrial composting setting without producing any hazardous byproducts [12]. It is appropriate for a diversity of packaging applications, including blister packs and bottles, due to its transparent appearance and sufficient barrier qualities. However, certain conditions are necessary for PLA to degrade, and temperature, humidity, and the presence of microorganisms can all affect how well PLA performs. When developing PLA-based packaging for pharmaceutical products, these factors must be carefully considered in order to guarantee stability and integrity throughout the product's shelf life [13, 14].

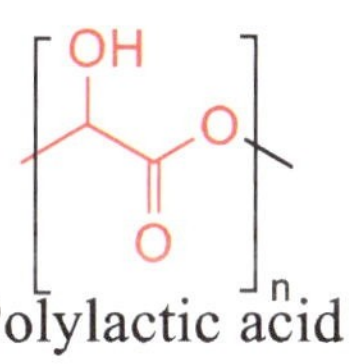

Fig. (1). Chemical structure of polylactic acid.

Polyhydroxyalkanoates

Another intriguing option is provided by PHA, a family of bio-polyesters made by microbial fermentation. PHA, in contrast to PLA, can break down in a variety of settings, such as freshwater, soil, and marine ecosystems [15, 16].

By modifying the microbial fuel and fermentation process, PHA's mechanical qualities can be customized, opening up a variety of uses. PHA's adaptability creates new possibilities for environmentally friendly pharmaceutical packaging, ranging from flexible films to firm containers. A major obstacle to PHA's widespread adoption has been its high production cost, which is caused by the intricacy of microbial cultivation and purification. The goals of ongoing research are to increase PHA's market availability, lower costs, and optimize production [17].

Other Biopolymers

Many more biopolymers are being investigated besides PLA and PHA. The biodegradability and renewable origins of proteins, chitosan, cellulose derivatives, and starch-based plastics are drawing attention. These substances, which are frequently combined with other biopolymers or additives, offer special qualities appropriate for particular uses. The goal of this field's current research is to fully realize its potential while resolving issues with cost, processability, and performance [18, 19].

Chemicals with pharmacological and medical implications for the body that can be either natural or synthetic are known as pharmaceutical products [20]. These products are classified according to their chemical characteristics, therapeutic effects, and mode of administration [21]. According to the author, they also include stimulants, antimalarials, antipyretics, antibiotics, analgesics, statins and tranquilizers. The central nervous, digestive, cardiovascular, endocrine, respiratory and immune systems and organs are among the other potential targets they may target [22]. Pharmaceutical packaging is therefore crucial to guaranteeing that the product achieves necessary objectives.

Production, transportation, storage, sales, delivery, and use are all possible times for this. Pharmaceutical products are protected from contamination, spoiling, and adverse environmental conditions like light, moisture, and oxygen by packaging materials, which also provide details regarding the product and dosage [23].

The majority of pharmaceutical products come in glass, paper, and plastic packaging. The three types of packaging systems are the three categories into which pharmaceutical packaging is separated. The packaging on the exterior of the primary container is the secondary system, whereas the primary system comes into direct contact with the medication. (Fig. **2**) depicts various sustainable options contributing to environmental betterment [24].

ECO-FRIENDLY MATERIAL FOR PHARMACEUTICAL PACKAGING/ CLASSIFICATION

Biodegradable packaging has demonstrated significant promise in addressing the environmental problems associated with conventional pharmaceutical packaging. To meet the demands of a rapidly changing industry, new resources and production methods are being created.

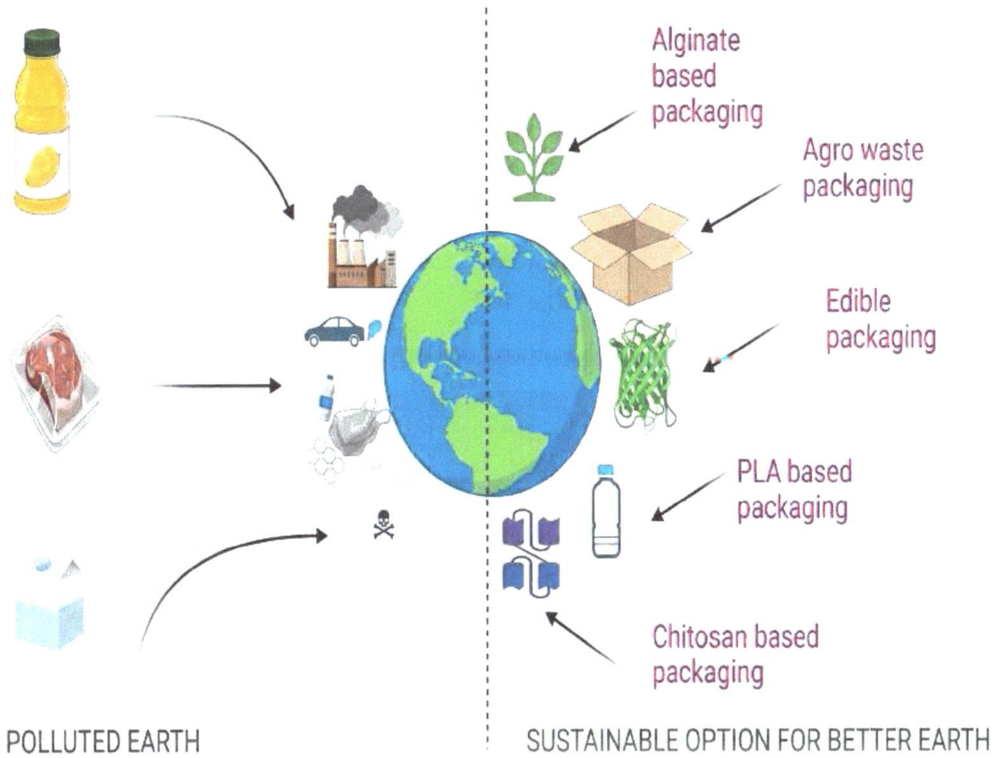

Fig. (2). Various sustainable options contributing to environmental betterment.

There are various ways to categorize environmentally friendly pharmaceutical packaging materials as follows:

a. Based on their intended use
b. Based on chemical composition
c. Presence of different macromolecules.

BASED ON THEIR USES

Packaging can be divided into various classes based on its intended use, including single-use, edible, and multiple-use packaging. Edible packaging aims to provide biologically derived materials for packaging a variety of products. Among the biomaterials that can be utilized for edible packaging are carbohydrates and marine-derived polysaccharides like chitosan, carrageenan, and alginate [25].

The use of reusable packaging has persisted for a very long time. It is an excellent method to maintain the product's functionality while simultaneously obtaining potentially important material and safeguarding the environment. However, a move from reusable to single-use packaging has been observed in recent decades in all countries without strict laws mandating reuse. The shift towards smaller-sized packets discourages reusable solutions even more. This development has resulted in increased material consumption, a rapidly growing amount of trash, and environmental effects related to the use of materials during production. Reaction initiatives to reduce the impact and quantity of material consumption have primarily focused on recycling and lightweighting. However, reusable packaging is a more cost-effective option [26]. Various types of packaging with their examples have been shown in (Table 1).

Table 1. Packaging and its types, including their uses (2).

Types of Packaging	Properties	Examples
Edible packaging	Biodegradable	Wheat bran, starch, *etc.*
Chemical or material recycling packaging	Recycled	Paper, metal, plastics, *etc.*
Multiple-use packaging	Refilled	Glass bottles for injection, syringes, *etc.*
Packaging meant for burning.	Recycled	Cardboard, paper, *etc.*
Single-use packaging	Biodegradable	Biodegradable plastics, paper, *etc.*

BASED ON VARIOUS MACROMOLECULES

Polysaccharides are abundant in many species, such as bacteria, algae, plants, and mammals. Polysaccharides, which are composed of glycosidic bonds with relatively large molecular weights joining the molecules, make up the vast majority of carbohydrates found in nature [27]. These complex carbohydrates are made up of monosaccharides and have either linear or highly branched structures. The diverse structure of this biopolymer enables polysaccharides to carry out a range of functions and be utilized in a wide range of products [28].

One step in addressing the topic of the overproduction and usage of non-biodegradable materials is the development of environmentally friendly packaging composed of biodegradable polymer composites. This enables materials to be disposed of naturally without posing a threat to the environment. It is possible to create such material using polysaccharides derived from plants. The advantages of polysaccharides include their low carbon footprint, biodegradability, and ability to be recovered in nature. Subsequent degradation byproducts are also environmentally safe [29].

Starch

Starch (Fig. **3**) is a common raw material and a polysaccharide that is safe for the environment. There are numerous and varied sources of starch, including cereals and legumes. Rice, corn, wheat, and potatoes are the most widely available sources of starch. Starch is used to make stiff or flexible packaging, bags, and sacks. Since starch packaging materials are naturally brittle, a variety of biodegradable plasticizers, such as urea, polyether, glycerol, and low molecular weight polyhydroxy compounds, are incorporated when an excessive amount of starch is used. Plasticizers stop microbiological growth by decreasing water activity. Based on the types of polymers, there are four types of starch:. thermoplastic starch products, starch polyvinyl alcohol blends, starch polybutylene succinate (PBSA) polyester blends.

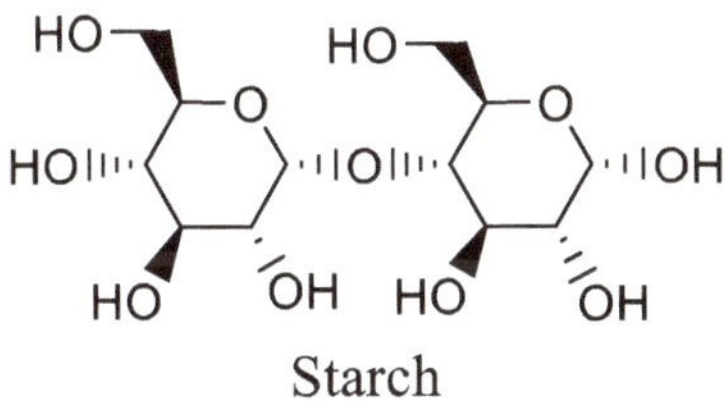

Fig. (3). Chemical structure of starch.

Joshi *et al.* offer a simple process for making biodegradable and biocompatible lightweight structural scaffolds that can be used in place of conventional packaging materials made of plastic. By altering the proportions of polyvinyl alcohol combined with cassava starch, the resulting aerogels' mechanical properties, porosity, and structural integrity can be managed. Because of their remarkable biodegradability, low density, good mechanical modulus, and outstanding thermal stability, starch-based aerogels hold promise as beneficial substitutes for traditional polyolefin thermoplastics and polymer-foam-based packaging materials [30].

By describing the structural, physicochemical, thermal, and morphological characteristics of Cubio (Tropaeolum tuberosum), a native Andean tuber, Daza *et al.* investigated the potential uses of the tuber in the creation of biodegradable packaging material. The films with cubic starch as the primary component demonstrated continuous, porosity-free surfaces, outstanding thermal stability, and remarkable transparency [31].

Cellulose

A linear polymer found in large quantities in nature is cellulose. Bioplastics made from cellulose or its derivatives are highly sought after for use in biomedical and pharmaceutical packaging. Commercial products made from cellulose derivatives include hydroxy cellulose, carboxyl methylcellulose, methylcellulose, cellulose acetate, ethylcellulose, and hydroxypropyl cellulose. Because of its highly promising stiffness and complete biodegradability, cellulose acetate is often employed as a form of packaging in pharmaceutical as well as laboratory settings. In a study, blended polylactic acid and cellulose acetate showed greater toughness and Young's modulus than raw polylactic acid [32, 33].

Natural fibres with nanometric dimensions are used to make a material known as nanocellulose. Cellulose, the key constituent that gives plant cell walls their structure, is their main source. Amorphous nanocellulose (NCA), nanofibril cellulose (NFC), and nanocrystalline cellulose (NCC) are among the various types of nanocellulose. Despite their small size, nanocellulose fibres exhibit remarkable strength, making them suitable for use as backing in composite materials [34]. In the packaging trade, nanocellulose is used to reinforce packaging films, extend the shelf life of packed goods, and improve the liquid and gas barrier. Furthermore, coatings using nanocellulose exhibit improved abrasion resistance, antimicrobial activity, and moisture protection [35].

De Moura *et al.* claim that cellulose-based materials are inexpensive, nontoxic, barrier-like, edible, and biodegradable, among other advantages. The ecological advantages of turning these priceless biomaterials into value-added products for a range of uses, including packaging, would be leveraged by industrial advancement [36].

Xylan

The cell walls of numerous plant and algae species contain this type of carbohydrate. It is possible to create environmentally friendly pharmaceutical packaging materials with this biodegradable xylan. For this reason, the xylophane is employed as an environmentally friendly packaging material. The implementation of xylan-based film in pharmaceutical packaging necessitates addressing its poor mechanical and film-forming qualities. Rao *et al.* employed chitosan, graphene oxide, and carboxymethyl xylan to produce a superior oxygen resistance composite film with the necessary mechanical qualities. These composite films demonstrated superior antibacterial and oxygen barrier qualities. Consequently, the packaging industry may benefit from these composite films [37].

Chitin

Insects, yeast, and other invertebrates are the main sources of chitin. Chitin (Fig. **4**) is extensively utilised as a material for packaging in the pharmaceutical industry due to its antibacterial qualities. Chitin is perfect for use as an edible packaging material because it readily absorbs heavy metal ion contaminants. Another derivative of chitin that is used in pharmaceutical packaging is chitosan. Usually, chitosan cellulose is used to create biodegradable laminations. Chitin is a nitrogenous, white, inelastic polymer. Chitosan is a proton-conducting polymer that is safe for the environment and can be used in cosmetics, batteries, paper finishing, wrapping films, and wastewater purification. In films modified with chitosan, polyethylene glycol is used to lessen the transfer of water vapour. Chitosan can be used in a number of biomedical applications due to its biocompatibility [38].

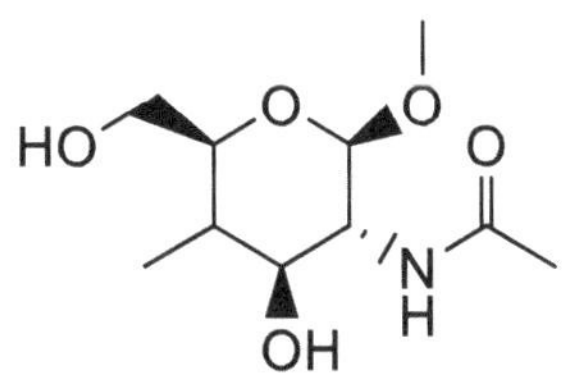

Chitin

Fig. (4). Chemical structure of chitin.

Khan *et al.* fabricated S-chitin-containing chitosan/gelatin active packaging films. Excellent UV-barrier, antibacterial, and antioxidant qualities were demonstrated by S-chitin. The composite films completely inhibited the expansion of E. Coli and L. monocytogenes and demonstrated exceptional antioxidant and antibacterial activity. There is a lot of promise for active packaging with the multifunctional chitosan/gelatin films that integrate chitin [39].

Proteins

Proteins are composed of repeating amino acid units. Protein-based products, derived from renewable and biodegradable agricultural or agro-packaging materials, are used in edible packaging. Protein's side chains can be structurally changed to produce packaging materials. A packaging film that decomposes naturally is produced by cross-linking natural proteins with synthetic monomer units. Animals and plants are the two main sources of protein. Zein, gluten, and soy are examples of plant-based proteins; collagen, keratin, whey, and casein are examples of animal-based proteins (Table **2**) [40] provides examples of the proteins that are commonly utilized to create pharmaceutical packaging materials based on their place of origin. Pharmacies can use biodegradable polymers to improve the shelf life of their products. Due to their combined functional features, multicomponent coatings and films are becoming more and more popular these days. Drug packaging regulations must be followed by green packaging materials.

Table 2. Different plant and animal-originated proteins with their descriptions.

Plant-origin Protein	Description	Animal-origin Protein	Description
Whey	Whey is a byproduct of cheese. For pharmaceutical packaging, it is utilized to make coating and packaging materials.	Collagen	Collagen is employed to make packaging materials that have desired characteristics.
Soy	It is used in the production of biodegradable films and polymers and as a covering for pharmaceutical items.	Keratin	Bioplastics are often made from keratin.
Gluten	It is easy to use and reasonably priced when making films for packaging that is edible.	Gelatin	Vitamins are microencapsulated, and microspheres are prepared using gelatin. It is also used in the preparation of tablet manufacturing and shell encapsulation.
Zein	It is employed for the production of biodegradable packaging materials as well as in the coating of pharmaceutical products.	Casein	Casein is employed for labelling because of its strong adhesive characteristics.

BASED ON CHEMICAL CONSTITUENTS

Bio Plastics

Twenty percent of the total weight of the packaging is made of plastic. Since plastic coating, along with packaging materials, is known to be the main environmental offender, technological advancements are currently in the growth phase in an effort to find more creative ways to reduce the ecological impact of packaging and boost the amount of biodegradable and environmentally friendly materials that are currently available. In place of petrochemicals, which caused the environmental crisis due to their inability to be recycled, biodegradable plastics, also known as eco-friendly bioplastics, are now manufactured from recyclable plant sources like proteins and polysaccharides [41].

Biobased polymers are often derived from high-carbohydrate food crops such as sugarcane or maize. A variety of bioplastics can be made from non-food crops, like lignocellulosic material, by converting them into chemical components. Additionally, animal and plant biomass that is high in protein or oil has been used to make bioplastics. Therefore, the term "bioplastics" refers to new bio-based plastic polymers such as polylactic acid(PLA), polyhydroxyalkanoates (PHA), polyhydroxy butyrate (PHB), and starch blends or microbial polymers such as polypeptides, polynucleotides, and polysaccharides [42].

One of the most versatile materials used in packaging is plastic, which can be readily altered to meet a range of packaging specifications and other needs. Safety, convenience, ergonomics, and ease of use are provided by child-resistant plastic seals and airtight plastic containers for chemicals and medications. Its low weight, along with relative strength, makes it one of the most durable, long-lasting, environmentally friendly, and affordable pharmaceutical materials. The two primary varieties of biodegradable plastics on the market are hydro-biodegradable and oxo-biodegradable. Corn, wheat, and sugarcane are among the agricultural products used to make hydro-biodegradable plastics. Polylactic acid, polyhydroxy alkanoates, polyhydroxy butyrate valerate, and polycaprolactone are a few of the frequently utilised polymers [43].

Paper and Paperboards

The sheet materials known as paper and paperboard, respectively, are made of networks of interwoven cellulose fibres that are very amenable to liquids or moisture because cellulose fibres are hydrophilic. These fibres are highly receptive to liquids and moisture. Materials like plastic as well as aluminium, which have superior water and moisture barriers, are used to circumvent this [44, 45]. (Figure **5**) illustrates the shares of paper/paperboards employed in the USA.

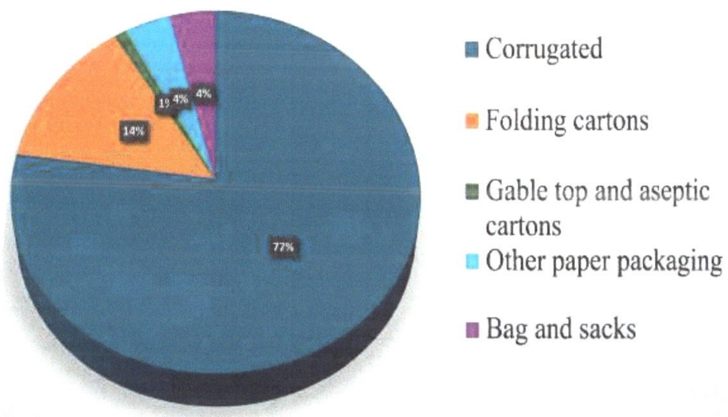

Fig. (5). Shares of paper/paperboards employed in the USA.

Coles and Riley claim that coatings and laminations can be applied to packaging materials to expand their applications and prolong the shelf life of the products they hold [46]. Additionally, the coating improves the paperboard's strength and resistance to chemicals. Polyester (PET), polypropylene (PP), low-density polyethylene (LDPE), as well as high-density polyethylene (HDPE), are some of the polymers that can be coated [47, 48].

Paper is a common packaging material that biodegrades and can be recycled easily. Therefore, they can be used to create pharmaceutical packaging materials that are friendly to the environment. Paper packaging's main advantages include its ease of tearing, resistance to moisture and gases, and lightweight nature. Paperboard comes in a variety of forms, some of which are mentioned below:

- **Chip paperboard -** The outside of a carton is usually composed of chipboard. This paperboard is made from recycled paper. White paperboard is used to line the chipboard, improving its mechanical strength and appearance.
- **White paperboard** - The most common material for white paperboard is chemically bleached paper. White paperboards, which have been laminated, are used for primary packaging. The carton's interior can also be covered with white paperboard.
- **Solid paperboard** – It is composed of several bond layers. Solid paperboards are usually made from bleached sulphate boards. Typically, polyethylene is used to laminate these boards. The covering is given a water-resistant surface by using edible films.
- **Fiber paperboard** - There are two types of fiber-based paperboard: solid and corrugated. Two layers of craft paper are sandwiched between corrugated material to create corrugated paperboard. The fibre paperboard is very resistant to impact. It is frequently used when packaging goods for delivery. The other is made up of two layers: a solid cardboard outer layer and an inner layer. White paperboard makes up the inner layer, while craft paperboard makes up the outer layer. Solid paperboard can be laminated with bioplastics to preserve the product's dry state during packaging.

NEED FOR ECO-FRIENDLY PACKAGING MATERIAL

When it comes to safeguarding goods or contents throughout handling, transportation, and storage, packaging is crucial. Additionally, the product's shelf life is extended and preserved by the packaging. Global environmental problems are made worse by the misuse of raw materials for packaging. Materials have to be recycled to make related products or other potential products in order to ensure sustainable packaging [49].

Packaging materials come in a wide variety, including paper, plastic, metal, and glass. The availability of raw materials, proper recycling procedures, the utilisation of renewable resources, and an effective and practical strategy for product packaging materials are some of the elements that determine the success of the packaging sector. These petroleum-derived polymers have a low recycling rate and are not biodegradable. Therefore, to encourage sustainable plastic-based packaging materials, more research is required than ever before to identify environmentally friendly biodegradable polymers [50].

Second, the increased demand for pharmaceutical products globally has led to an increase in waste from pharmaceutical packaging, which in turn has increased waste production and consequent environmental effects.

THE CURRENT STATE OF RECYCLING: CHALLENGES AND LIMITATIONS

Reducing landfill waste, saving raw materials, and minimising environmental deterioration all depend on recycling. Nevertheless, despite its importance, the global recycling process faces many obstacles that restrict its efficacy and generalizability. The main causes of these issues include insufficient and ineffective recycling infrastructure, contaminated recyclables, troublesome customer behaviour, and the growing complexity of packaging materials. This chapter examines these problems, examining how each affects the overall effectiveness of recycling initiatives and outlining possible ways to make them better [51].

Recycling Infrastructure: Gaps, Inefficiencies, and Limitations

The overall effectiveness of recycling programs is significantly impacted by the infrastructure's durability and accessibility. Unfortunately, many localities still lack adequate or developed recycling infrastructure, especially in rural or less affluent areas. Many recycling systems, even in industrialized countries, are limited in their capacity to efficiently process recyclable materials due to old technology or a lack of financing. The uneven allocation of recycling initiatives is among the most urgent problems. Curbside recycling services are frequently available in urban areas, but they are not available in rural or isolated locations, which leads to notable differences in recycling rates and participation [52]. Furthermore, many recycling operations are underequipped to handle the increasing number of materials, with out-of-date sorting and processing technology that limits their ability to properly separate and process materials. According to a 2016 assessment from the Ellen MacArthur Foundation, only 14% of plastic packaging is properly recycled, revealing how inefficient current recycling processes are. Another major challenge is single-stream recycling, which combines all recyclable materials. While this strategy seeks to simplify the recycling process for customers, it frequently results in contamination since diverse materials cannot be effectively sorted [53]. This raises the possibility that recyclables won't be properly processed and will instead end up in landfills or incinerators. According to a 2017 analysis by the U.S. Environmental Protection

Agency (EPA), single-stream recycling systems are less effective due to their much greater risk of contamination [54].

Packaging Contamination and Its Impact on Recycling Rates

One of the main obstacles to effective recycling is the contamination of recyclable materials. Recyclables need to be clean and devoid of chemicals, food waste, and other impurities to be processed properly. However, food leftovers, liquids, or oils frequently contaminate packaging materials, making them unfit for recycling [55]. For instance, it is frequently not possible to recycle ordinary things like grease-stained pizza boxes, plastic containers containing food scraps, or paper cartons that have absorbed liquids. Because sorting systems are frequently unable to eliminate impurities, even slight contamination can stop the processing of an entire batch of recyclable materials. According to the Recycling Partnership (2022), contamination lowers the effectiveness and profitability of recycling programs and costs the US recycling industry billions of dollars every year [56]. Contaminated materials not only increase operational expenses but also reduce the grade of recycled materials produced. Contamination has serious economic effects since recyclables contaminated with non-recyclable chemicals take more labour and time to treat, increasing prices and diminishing overall recycling effectiveness. A 2022 study conducted by Gupta *et al.* indicated that approximately 25% of materials entering recycling operations are polluted, underlining the need to resolve this issue [57].

The Role of Consumer Behaviour in Recycling Failure

While infrastructure and contamination issues are important, customer conduct has a huge impact on the effectiveness of recycling programs. A huge section of the population lacks basic recycling education, resulting in widespread system inefficiencies. The misapplication of recycling symbols is a serious concern. Many products bear the recycling label, yet they are not recyclable, causing customers to throw them away in the wrong bin. This misconception frequently leads to increased pollution of recycling streams. According to the American Chemistry Council (2022), approximately 45% of U.S. customers are uninformed of the unique recycling rules for their community, contributing to recycling failure. Additionally, inconvenience is a barrier to effective recycling. Many areas lack recycling bins, and sorting can be time-consuming. According to a study conducted by the Natural Resources Defense Council (2022), recycling participation rates decline dramatically when customers struggle to separate recyclables or lack adequate infrastructure to facilitate the process [58]. Complacency and a lack of motivation also contribute to recycling failures. Many consumers do not recycle because they do not consider it an important obligation or believe their efforts will be ineffective. This perspective reduces participation in recycling initiatives, resulting in a lower total recycling rate.

Issues with Multi-Material and Complex Packaging Designs

As packaging designs become more advanced, multi-material packaging has emerged as one of the recycling industry's most complicated challenges. Many current packaging solutions have multiple layers of different materials that are difficult, if not impossible, to separate during the recycling process. Tetra-pack cartons, for example, are made of a combination of paper, plastic, and metal, making them difficult to dismantle using typical recycling techniques. Similarly, chip bags are frequently made up of multiple materials, such as foil, plastic, and paper, making them challenging to process. The growth of composite materials has made recycling much more difficult, as they necessitate specialised sorting gear that is not always available in recycling facilities. Furthermore, many packing materials are coated with protective coatings like plastic films or aluminium laminates, making recycling even more difficult. For example, some beverage cartons may have a thin plastic coating to preserve the contents. However, this layer diminishes the carton's recyclability. These coated materials are frequently rejected in standard recycling systems, adding to the problems connected with packaging waste [59].

CONCLUSION

Finding environmentally friendly materials and state-of-the-art technology to produce sustainable packaging is becoming increasingly crucial. The usage of non-biodegradable as well as non-renewable materials in packaging has brought attention to environmental contamination issues. Bioplastics, a well-known green biomass material, have the potential to progressively replace plastics made from fossil fuels. Bio-based packaging materials have a lot to offer the packaging industry, but the industrial use of these packaging films requires storage tests on packaging equipment. Therefore, before biobased packaging materials are introduced to the market as a stand-alone alternative to conventional packaging materials, a critical assessment is required to enable access to the range of biobased packaging materials. Pharmaceutical companies should focus on creating a single eco-friendly packaging material that takes into account the combined properties of plastic, glass, metal, rubber, and paper.

REFERENCES

[1] Dharmadhikari S. Eco-friendly packaging in supply chain. Int J Sci Case Stud 2012; 1(2): 1-3.

[2] Singh A, Sharma PK, Malviya RJWASJ. Eco friendly pharmaceutical packaging material. World Appl Sci J 2011; 14(11): 1703-6.

[3] Shah K, Singh D, Agrawal R, Garg AJCGC. Eco friendly pharmaceutical packaging. Curr Green Chem 2025; 12(1): 2-14.

[4] Shah S, Matkawala F, Garg S, *et al.* Emerging trend of bioplastics and its impact on society Biocatal Agric Biotechnol 2020; 25: 101614.

[5] Sabee M, Uyen N T T, Ahmad N, *et al.* Plastics packaging for pharmaceutical products Reference Module in Materials Science and Materials Engineering. Amsterdam (NL): Elsevier 2021.

[6] Jenke DJJops. Evaluation of the chemical compatibility of plastic contact materials and pharmaceutical products; safety considerations related to extractables and leachables. J Pharm Sci 2007; 96(10): 2566-81.

[7] Marsh K. Bugusu BJJofs. Food packaging—roles, materials, and environmental issues. J Food Sci 2007; 72(3): R39-55.

[8] Wojnowska-Baryła I, Bernat K, Zaborowska M. Plastic waste degradation in landfill conditions: the problem with microplastics, and their direct and indirect environmental effects Int J Environ Res Public Health 2022; 19(20): 13223.

[9] Hamuyuni J, Tesfaye F, Iloeje C O, Anderson A E. Energy efficiency and low carbon footprint in metals processing JOM 2022; 74(5): 1886-8.
[http://dx.doi.org/10.1007/s11837-022-05253-9]

[10] Nguyen AT, Parker L, Brennan L. Lockrey SJJoCP. A consumer definition of eco-friendly packaging. J Clean Prod., 2020; 252: 119792.

[11] Bikiaris ND, Koumentakou I, Samiotaki C, *et al.* Recent advances in the investigation of poly (lactic acid)(PLA) nanocomposites: incorporation of various nanofillers and their properties and applications. Polymers, 2023; 15(5): 1196.

[12] Rajendran DS, Venkataraman S, Jha SK, Chakrabarty D, Kumar VVJFS. Biotechnology. A review on bio-based polymer polylactic acid potential on sustainable food packaging. Food Sci Biotechnol., 2024; 33(8): 1759-88.

[13] Singha S, Hedenqvist MS. A review on barrier properties of poly (lactic acid)/clay nanocomposites. Polymers, 2020; 12(5): 1095.

[14] Ali W, Ali H, Gillani S, *et al.* Polylactic acid synthesis, biodegradability, conversion to microplastics and toxicity: a review Environ Chem Lett 2023; 21(3): 1761-86.
[http://dx.doi.org/10.1007/s10311-023-01564-8]

[15] Crisafi F, Valentino F, Micolucci F, Denaro R. From Organic Wastes and Hydrocarbons Pollutants to Polyhydroxyalkanoates: Bioconversion by Terrestrial and Marine Bacteria Sustainability 2022; 14(14): 8241.
[http://dx.doi.org/10.3390/su14148241]

[16] Poltronieri P, Kumar P. Polyhydroxyalkanoates (PHAs) in industrial applications. In: Handbook of Ecomaterials. Cham (CH): Springer 2017; pp. 2843-72.

[17] Singh A. Srivastava VJIjohs Production of polyhydroxyalkanoates (PHA) by Pseudomonas from waste products. Int J Health Sci., 2022; 6(S3): 11450-9.

[18] Baranwal J, Barse B, Fais A, Delogu G L, Kumar A. Biopolymer: A sustainable material for food and medical applications. Polymers 2022; 14(5): 983.
[http://dx.doi.org/10.3390/polym14050983]

[19] Ilyas R A, Zuhri M Y M, Aisyah H A, *et al.* Natural Fiber-Reinforced Polylactic Acid, Polylactic Acid Blends and Their Composites for Advanced Applications Polymers 2022; 14(1): 202.
[http://dx.doi.org/10.3390/polym14010202]

[20] Aldowaish A, Kokuryo J, Almazyad O, Goi HCJS. Environmental, social, and governance integration into the business model: Literature review and research agenda. Sustainability, 2022; 14(5): 2959.

[21] Mohammad WMW, Wasiuzzaman SJCES. Environmental, Social and Governance (ESG) disclosure, competitive advantage and performance of firms in Malaysia. Cleaner Environ Syst., 2021; 2: 100015.

[22] Moshood T D, Nawanir G, Mahmud F, *et al.* Sustainability of biodegradable plastics: New problem or solution to solve the global plastic pollution? Curr Res Green Sustain Chem 2022; 5: 100273. [http://dx.doi.org/10.1016/j.crgsc.2022.100273]

[23] Malik S, Muhammad K, Waheed Y. Nanotechnology: a revolution in modern industry. Molecules 2023; 28(2): 661. [http://dx.doi.org/10.3390/molecules28020661]

[24] Schot J, Steinmueller W E. Three frames for innovation policy: R&D, systems of innovation and transformative change. Res Policy 2018; 47(9): 1554-67.

[25] Verma M, Shakya S, Kumar P, *et al.* Trends in packaging material for food products: historical background, current scenario, and future prospects J Food Sci Technol 2021 Nov; 58(11): 4069-82.

[26] Coelho P M, Corona B, ten Klooster R, Worrell E. Sustainability of reusable packaging–Current situation and trends. Resour Conserv Recycl X 2020; 6: 100037. [http://dx.doi.org/10.1016/j.rcrx.2020.100037]

[27] Mohamed S A, El-Sakhawy M, El-Sakhawy M A. Polysaccharides, protein and lipid-based natural edible films in food packaging: a review Carbohydr Polym 2020; 238: 116178. [http://dx.doi.org/10.1016/j.carbpol.2020.116178]

[28] Torres FG, Troncoso OP, Pisani A, Gatto F. Bardi GJIjoms Natural polysaccharide nanomaterials: an overview of their immunological properties. Int J Mol Sci., 2019; 20(20): 5092.

[29] Nechai A, Krvavych A, Konechna R. Prospects for the use of plant materials in creating biodegradable eco-friendly packaging IOP Conf Ser Earth Environ Sci 2021; 915(1): 012015.

[30] Joshi P, Gupta K, Uniyal P, *et al.* Cassava starch-derived aerogels as biodegradable packaging materials Mater Chem Phys 2023; 297: 127282. [http://dx.doi.org/10.1016/j.matchemphys.2022.127282]

[31] Daza LD, Umaña M, Simal S, Váquiro HA. Eim VSJIJoBM Non-conventional starch from cubio tuber (Tropaeolum tuberosum): Physicochemical, structural, morphological, thermal characterization and the evaluation of its potential as a packaging material. Int J Biol Macromol., 2022; 221: 954-64.

[32] Saha T, Hoque ME, Mahbub T. Biopolymers for sustainable packaging in food, cosmetics, and pharmaceuticals Advanced Processing, Properties, and Applications of Starch and Other Bio-Based Polymers. Elsevier 2020; pp. 197-214.

[33] Cinelli P, Coltelli MB, Signori F, Morganti P, Lazzeri AJC. Cosmetic packaging to save the environment: Future perspectives. Cosmetics, 2019; 6(2): 26.

[34] Klemm D, Kramer F, Moritz S, *et al.* Nanocelluloses: a new family of nature-based materials. Angew Chem Int Ed Engl 2011; 50(24): 5438-66. [http://dx.doi.org/10.1002/anie.201001273]

[35] Elfaleh I, Abbassi F, Habibi M, Ahmad F, Guedri M, Nasri M, *et al.* A comprehensive review of natural fibers and their composites: An eco-friendly alternative to conventional materials. Results Eng., 2023; 19: 101271.

[36] De Moura MR, Mattoso LH. Zucolotto VJJoFE Development of cellulose-based bactericidal nanocomposites containing silver nanoparticles and their use as active food packaging. J Food Eng., 2012; 109(3): 520-4.

[37] Rao J, Lv Z, Chen G, Hao X, Guan Y. Peng FJIJoBM Fabrication of flexible composite film based on xylan from pulping process for packaging application. Int J Biol Macromol, 2021; 173: 285-92.

[38] Mellinas C, Valdés A, Ramos M, Burgos N. Active edible films: Current state and future trends. Appl Polym Sci., 2016; 133(2).

[39] Khan A, Riahi Z, Kim JT, Rhim J-WJFH. Chitosan/gelatin-based multifunctional films integrated with sulfur-functionalized chitin for active packaging applications. Food Hydrocolloids, 2024; 149: 109537.

[40] Kumar S. Gupta SKJM-EJoSR. Applications of biodegradable pharmaceutical packaging materials: a review. Middle-East J Sci Res, 2012; 12(5): 699-706.

[41] Brizga J, Hubacek K, Feng K. The unintended side effects of bioplastics: Carbon, land, and water footprints. One Earth 2020; 3(1): 45-53.

[42] Ibrahim NI, Shahar FS, Sultan MTH, Shah AUM, Safri SNA, Mat Yazik MHJC. Overview of bioplastic introduction and its applications in product packaging. Coatings 2021; 11(11): 1423. [http://dx.doi.org/10.3390/coatings11111423]

[43] Dalton B, Bhagabati P, De Micco J, Padamati R B, O'Connor K. A review on biological synthesis of the biodegradable polymers polyhydroxyalkanoates and the development of multiple applications Catalysts 2022 Mar 11; 12(3): 319.

[44] Rhim J W, Lee J H, Hong S I. Increase in water resistance of paperboard by coating with poly(lactide). Packag Technol Sci 2007; 20(6): 393-402.

[45] Lahtinen K, Maydannik P, Johansson P, Kääriäinen T, Cameron D C, Kuusipalo J. Utilisation of continuous atomic layer deposition process for barrier enhancement of extrusion-coated paper. Surf Coat Technol 2011; 205(15): 3916-22. [http://dx.doi.org/10.1016/j.surfcoat.2011.02.009]

[46] Coles R. Paper and paperboard innovations and developments for the packaging of food, beverages and other fast-moving consumer goods. Trends in Packaging of Food, Beverages and Other Fast-Moving Consumer Goods (FMCG). Woodhead Publishing Series in Food Science, Technology and NutritionCambridge: Woodhead Publishing 2013; pp. 187-220.

[47] Riley A. Paper and paperboard packaging. Packaging Technology: Fundamentals, Materials and Processes. Oxford: Elsevier 2012; pp. 178-239.

[48] Ibrahim ID, Hamam Y, Sadiku ER, *et al.* Need for sustainable packaging: an overview. Polymers 2022; 14(20): 4430. [http://dx.doi.org/10.3390/polym14204430]

[49] Nasrollahi M, Beynaghi A, Mohamady F M, Mozafari M. Plastic Packaging, Recycling, and Sustainable Development. In: Leal Filho W, Azul A M, Brandli L, Özuyar P G, Wall T, Eds. Responsible Consumption and Production. Cham: Springer 2020; pp. 605-15.

[50] Etxabide A, Uranga J, Guerrero P, De la Caba KJFH. Development of active gelatin films by means of valorisation of food processing waste. A review. Food Hydrocolloids 2017; 68: 192-8.

[51] Quinto S, Law N, Fletcher C, Le J, Jose S A, Menezes P L. Exploring the E-Waste Crisis: Strategies for sustainable recycling and circular Economy integration. Recycling 2025 Apr 14; 10(2): 72.

[52] Gautam A K, Pingua N, Chandra A, *et al.* Domestic waste management and their utilization In: Arya R K, Verros G D, Verma O P, Eds. From waste to wealth. Singapore: Springer 2024; pp. 1195-210. [http://dx.doi.org/10.1007/978-981-99-7552-5_62]

[53] Haupt M, Zschokke M. How can LCA support the circular economy?—63rd discussion forum on life cycle assessment, Zurich, Switzerland, November 30, 2016. Int J Life Cycle Assess 2017; 22(5): 832-7.

[54] Berardocco C, Delawter H, Putzu T, Wolfe L C, Zhang H. Life cycle sustainability assessment of single stream and multi-stream waste recycling systems. Sustainability 2022 Dec 14; 14(24): 16747.

[55] Srivastava A, Pandey S, Shahwal R, *et al.* Recycling of waste into useful materials and their energy applications. In: Kandasamy S, Shah M P, Subbiah K, Eds. Microbial niche nexus: sustaining environmental biological wastewater and water-energy-environment nexus. Cham (CH): Springer 2025; pp. 251-85. [http://dx.doi.org/10.1007/978-3-031-62660-9_11]

[56] Turner K, Kim YJS. Problems of the US recycling programs: What experienced recycling program managers tell. Sustainability 2024; 16(9): 3539.

[57] Gupta SK, Gupta R. Policies, issues, and major safety operations in the management of hazardous waste . In: Hazardous Waste Management. Elsevier 2022; pp. 117-41.

[58] Zhu R. Trashing the Chasing Arrows: How New York City Can Solve Its Plastics Problem. Urban Law J 2023; 51: 501.

[59] Hui TK, Mohammed B, Donyai P, McCrindle R, Sherratt RSJP. Enhancing pharmaceutical packaging through a technology ecosystem to facilitate the reuse of medicines and reduce medicinal waste Pharmacy 2020; 8(2): 58.
[http://dx.doi.org/10.3390/pharmacy8020058]

CHAPTER 10

Role of Digitalization and Green Technology in Waste Management

Aarti Tiwari[1], **Ajay Kumar Shukla**[1,*], **Rahul Kumar Maurya**[2], **Rama Sankar Dubey**[3], **Shivali Singla**[4] and **Joohee Pradhan**[5]

[1] *Institute of Pharmacy, Dr Rammanohar Lohia Avadh University, Ayodhya, Uttar Pradesh, India*

[2] *National Ayurveda Research Institute for Panchakarma, Cheruthuruthy, Thrissur, Kerala, India*

[3] *Department of Pharmacy, Madan Mohan Malaviya University of Technology, Gorakhpur, Uttar Pradesh, India*

[4] *Department of Anesthesiology & Critical Care Medicine, University of New Mexico School of Medicine, Albuquerque, New Mexico, USA*

[5] *Department of Pharmaceutical Sciences, Mohanlal Sukhadia University, Udaipur, Rajasthan, India*

Abstract: The growing volume of waste generated by industrialization and urbanization poses serious environmental and public health problems. Green technology and digitization have evolved into revolutionary waste management solutions that optimize resources, enhance sustainability, and improve efficiency. The use of smart technologies in waste monitoring, collection, sorting, and recycling, such as blockchain, artificial intelligence (AI), the Internet of Things (IoT), Real-time tracking and predictive modeling are made possible by digital tools such as Geographic Information Systems (GIS), cloud computing, and data analytics, which maximize waste disposal and reduce environmental impacts. Sustainable waste management techniques are also aided by green technologies, including waste-to-energy conversion, biodegradable materials, and circular economy models. Resource recovery is encouraged and reliance on landfills is reduced through digitalization in smart garbage bins, automated segregation systems, and decentralized recycling procedures. Furthermore, legislative frameworks and international case studies demonstrate how well digital and green interventions perform to accomplish sustainable waste management objectives. In order to achieve environmental sustainability, this chapter offers a thorough examination of the advantages, difficulties, and potential applications of digital and green technology in trash management. A cleaner and more effective waste management system is made possible by the combination of these advances, which also aligns with international sustainability goals like the Sustainable Development Goals (SDGs) of the UN.

* **Corresponding author Ajay Kumar Shukla:** Institute of Pharmacy, Dr Rammanohar Lohia Avadh University, Ayodhya, Uttar Pradesh, India; E-mail: ashukla1007@gmail.com

Suman Gautam, Jai Narayan Mishra, Preeti Mishra, Preeti Verma & Sudhanshu Mishra (Eds.)

Keywords: Artificial intelligence, Biodegradable materials, Blockchain, Circular economy models, Internet of things, Sustainable waste management.

INTRODUCTION

Effective waste management is essential for environmental sustainability, public health, and economic development. In recent years, the integration of digitalization and green technology has revolutionized traditional waste management practices. Waste management plays a crucial role in environmental sustainability, public health, and economic development. With increasing global waste production and its adverse effects on ecosystems and human health, there is a need for advanced and effective waste management strategies. In recent years, the integration of digital technologies and green innovations has significantly transformed traditional waste management practices, enhanced their effectiveness, and reduced ecological footprints. Some digitalization and green technologies in waste management are shown in Fig. (**1**).

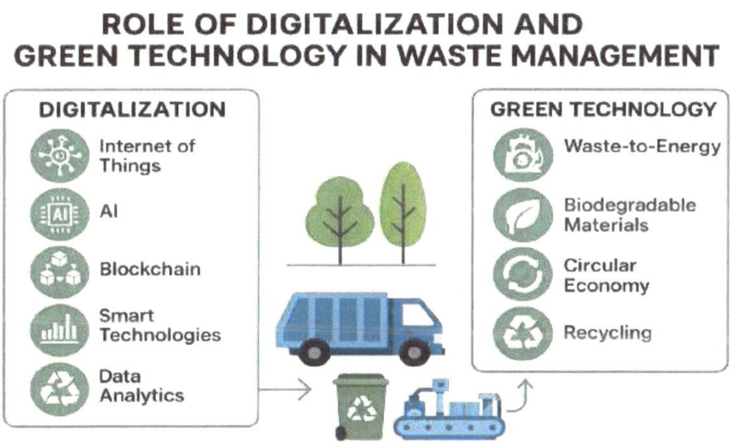

Fig. (1). Role of digitalization and green technologies in waste management.

These innovative approaches not only optimize waste handling processes but also reduce ecological footprints, promote resource efficiency, and enhance overall sustainability [1].

DIGITALIZATION IN WASTE MANAGEMENT

Digitalization refers to the application of digital technologies, data analytics, and smart systems to improve operational efficiency. In the context of waste management, digitalization has significantly transformed how waste is collected, sorted, treated, and disposed of.

Key Applications Include

Smart Bins and IoT Sensors

Smart bins equipped with Internet of Things (IoT) sensors have revolutionized traditional waste management practices. These bins monitor fill levels in real-time and transmit data to centralized systems. The sensors typically use ultrasonic, infrared, or weight-based mechanisms to detect the amount of waste present. Municipalities and waste collection services can analyze this data to optimize collection schedules and routes, thereby reducing operational costs, lowering fuel consumption, and improving environmental performance. Furthermore, smart bins help prevent overflows and enhance hygiene in public spaces [2–4].

Waste Tracking Systems

Modern waste tracking systems utilize Global Positioning System (GPS) and Radio-Frequency Identification (RFID) technologies to monitor waste movement from the point of origin to final disposal. RFID tags can be attached to waste containers or bags, and GPS-enabled vehicles track the route taken during waste collection and transportation. This system ensures transparency, helps authorities combat illegal dumping, and facilitates compliance with waste management regulations. These tracking platforms often feature real-time dashboards that monitor routes, waste types, and disposal statuses [5 - 7].

Data Analytics and Artificial Intelligence (AI)

Predictive analytics and AI technologies play a pivotal role in smart waste management. By analyzing historical and real-time data, these tools can forecast waste generation patterns, enabling municipalities to make data-driven decisions regarding resource allocation, bin placement, and recycling capacity planning. AI-powered algorithms can also detect anomalies, predict maintenance needs, and enhance system efficiency. This approach ensures proactive rather than reactive waste management, significantly reducing operational bottlenecks [8 - 10].

Mobile Applications

Mobile apps have become essential tools in engaging communities in waste management. These applications allow residents to report waste-related issues, schedule waste collection, and receive notifications about recycling programs and educational campaigns. Some advanced apps even offer gamification features to encourage citizen participation and reward eco-friendly behavior. By enabling real-time communication between citizens and service providers, mobile apps significantly improve public responsiveness and civic engagement [11 - 13].

Automation and Robotics

The integration of automation and robotics in waste management introduces smart sorting systems that utilize machine vision, AI, and robotic arms to automatically segregate waste based on material type. These systems can accurately differentiate between recyclable, compostable, and landfill waste, enhancing the efficiency of material recovery facilities (MRFs). Automated sorting minimizes human intervention, reduces contamination rates, and boosts overall recycling yields. Robotics is also being explored for tasks like street sweeping, bin lifting, and hazardous waste handling [14 - 16].

GREEN TECHNOLOGY IN WASTE MANAGEMENT

Green technology, often referred to as environmental or sustainable technology, comprises innovations and systems designed to mitigate environmental degradation and enhance the efficient use of resources. In the context of waste management, green technologies aim to reduce pollution, conserve resources, and support the transition to a circular economy. By minimizing the environmental footprint of waste disposal and encouraging resource recovery, these technologies serve as vital tools in achieving sustainable development goals. Numerous methods under green technology in waste management are shown in Fig. **2**.

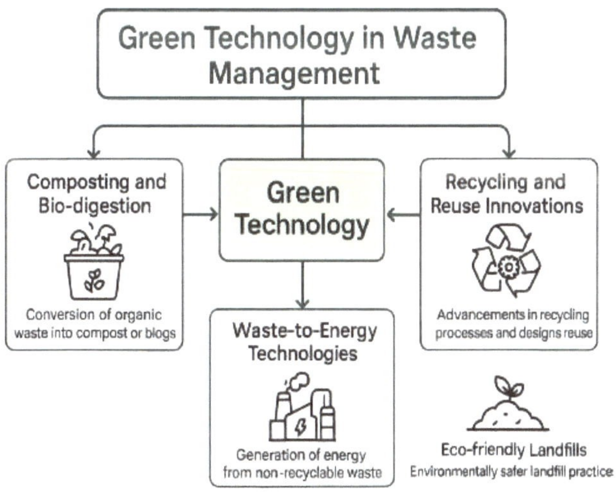
Green Technology in Waste Management
Composting and Bio-digestion
Conversion of organic waste into compost or biogs
Green Technology
Recycling and Reuse Innovations
Advancements in recycling processes and designs reuse
Waste-to-Energy Technologies
Generation of energy from non-recyclable waste
Eco-friendly Landfills
Environmentally safer landfill practice

Fig. (2). Green technology in waste management.

Composting and Bio-digestion

Composting and bio-digestion are biological processes that convert organic waste into valuable products. Composting involves the aerobic decomposition of organic matter, such as food scraps and agricultural residues, into nutrient-rich compost that can be used to improve soil fertility. Bio-digestion, on the other hand, is an anaerobic process where microorganisms break down biodegradable material to produce biogas (a mixture of methane and carbon dioxide) and digestate, a nutrient-rich slurry that can also serve as a fertilizer. These processes reduce the volume of waste directed to landfills, lower greenhouse gas emissions, and provide renewable energy and agricultural inputs. Moreover, they offer decentralized waste treatment options, especially suitable for rural and semi-urban areas [15, 16].

Recycling and Reuse Innovations

Recycling technologies have evolved to manage complex and heterogeneous waste streams. Advanced sorting systems using artificial intelligence (AI), robotics, and sensor-based techniques have significantly improved the efficiency of separating and processing recyclable materials. These innovations are particularly crucial in recycling e-waste, plastics, construction debris, and industrial by-products, which contain valuable yet challenging-to-recover components. Closed-loop recycling systems and the development of reusable product designs are integral in conserving natural resources and minimizing the environmental impact of manufacturing [17]. Encouraging reuse also supports behavioral shifts toward sustainability among both consumers and industries.

Waste-to-Energy (WTE) Technologies

Waste-to-Energy technologies represent a significant advancement in the recovery of resources from non-recyclable waste. These methods include incineration with energy recovery, pyrolysis, and gasification.

Incineration involves burning waste at high temperatures, generating heat that can be converted into electricity or used for district heating.

Pyrolysis thermally decomposes organic material in the absence of oxygen, producing syngas, oil, and char.

Gasification uses limited oxygen to convert carbonaceous materials into syngas, which can be used to produce electricity or synthetic fuels.

WTE technologies not only reduce the volume of solid waste but also generate energy, thereby decreasing dependence on fossil fuels and reducing environmental pollution [18].

Green Packaging and Biodegradable Materials

The rise in environmental awareness has led to the development of green packaging solutions and biodegradable materials. These materials are derived from renewable sources such as starch, cellulose, or polylactic acid (PLA), and they decompose naturally, reducing landfill burden and plastic pollution. Industries are increasingly adopting sustainable packaging alternatives that are compostable, recyclable, or reusable. This shift not only minimizes the ecological footprint of packaging waste but also aligns with eco-labeling and consumer preferences for environmentally responsible products [19 - 21].

Eco-friendly Landfills

Modern landfill design has evolved to include several environmentally protective features. Eco-friendly or engineered landfills incorporate systems such as leachate collection, methane gas capture for energy use, and liner barriers to prevent soil and groundwater contamination.

These landfills are designed to minimize environmental impact, reduce odor and pest issues, and capture landfill gases for energy recovery. Such technologies enable landfills to be safer and more sustainable, especially in regions where other waste treatment options are limited [10]. The integration of green technology in waste management is fundamental to sustainable environmental practices. By transforming waste into valuable resources, minimizing environmental hazards, and encouraging circularity, these technologies pave the way for a cleaner, more resilient future. Continuous innovation and supportive policies are essential to scale up their adoption globally [22 - 24].

INTEGRATION OF DIGITALIZATION AND GREEN TECHNOLOGY

The fusion of digital technologies with green innovations has revolutionized the domain of sustainable waste management. This integration fosters real-time data collection, resource optimization, and informed decision-making, aligning environmental sustainability with the fourth industrial revolution. Below are some significant integrated approaches:

Smart Waste-to-Energy Plants

Smart waste-to-energy (WTE) systems leverage digital technologies such as Artificial Intelligence (AI), the Internet of Things (IoT), and data analytics to improve the efficiency and environmental performance of waste-to-energy generation. AI algorithms support predictive maintenance, real-time emission tracking, and optimal feedstock utilization, thereby minimizing operational costs and ecological impacts. IoT-enabled sensors monitor combustion parameters, waste input, and pollutant outputs, ensuring compliance with environmental regulations while maximizing energy output [25 - 27]. Such digital interventions also facilitate remote monitoring and control, enabling smarter plant management.

Digital Platforms for the Circular Economy

Digital tools are key enablers of the circular economy, particularly in reducing waste, promoting reuse, and enabling recycling. Online platforms and mobile applications now facilitate the exchange of recyclable and reusable materials between producers and consumers. These digital marketplaces not only extend the lifecycle of materials but also create economic incentives for waste segregation and reuse. Furthermore, digital waste auditing systems help businesses assess and optimize their waste generation practices. Blockchain technology, renowned for its transparency and immutability, is increasingly used for tracking the lifecycle of waste, ensuring authenticity, preventing illegal dumping, and building trust in recycling processes [28].

GIS-Based Waste Mapping

Geographic Information Systems (GIS) provide spatial analysis capabilities that are invaluable in strategic waste management planning. GIS technologies help in mapping high-waste generation zones, planning efficient waste collection routes, and siting new treatment and disposal facilities. By integrating demographic, environmental, and logistical data, municipalities can deploy waste resources more efficiently and reduce fuel consumption and emissions associated with transportation. GIS tools also support real-time route optimization and demand forecasting for dynamic resource allocation [29].

AI-Driven Recycling Facilities

Artificial Intelligence plays a transformative role in automating and enhancing recycling processes. Advanced machine learning and computer vision systems enable automated sorting of recyclable materials from mixed waste streams, significantly improving the purity of recovered materials. AI systems can identify and separate plastics, metals, glass, and paper with high accuracy and speed, reducing human error and increasing throughput. This not only increases recycling efficiency but also minimizes contamination, making the output more viable for manufacturers [30]. Some smart recycling facilities now employ robotic arms guided by AI to perform precise, rapid sorting.

The integration of digital and green technologies holds immense promise in modernizing waste management systems. From intelligent energy recovery solutions to blockchain-based waste tracking and AI-enhanced recycling, these innovations contribute significantly to environmental sustainability, economic viability, and operational efficiency. As cities move toward becoming smart and sustainable, such synergistic technologies will be indispensable in achieving global environmental goals [31 - 33]. The Artificial Intelligence plays a transformative role in automating and enhancing recycling processes, as summarized in Fig. (**3**).

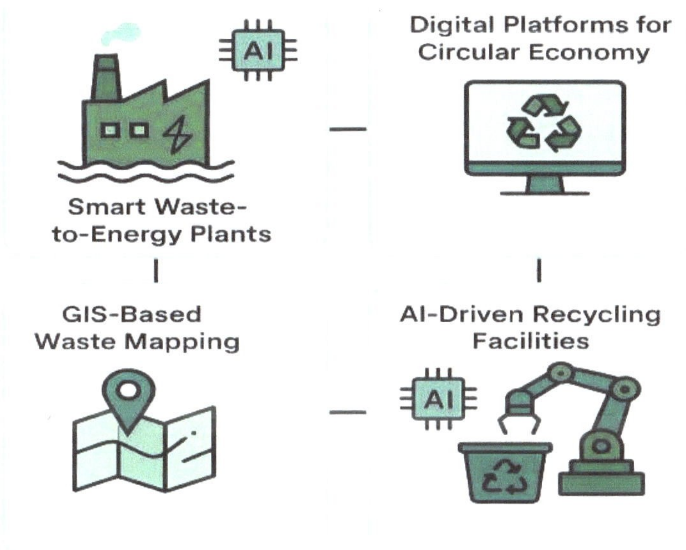

Fig. (3). Artificial Intelligence plays a transformative role in automating and enhancing recycling processes.

BENEFITS AND CHALLENGES

The implementation of advanced technologies, especially in sectors such as waste management, healthcare, and sustainable urban development, offers both a wide array of benefits and distinct challenges. These factors significantly influence the widespread adoption and successful implementation of innovative solutions.

Benefits

Enhanced Efficiency and Cost-effectiveness

Advanced technologies and processes often lead to significant improvements in operational efficiency. Automation and data-driven decision-making streamline workflows, reducing the time and resources required to perform tasks. For instance, in waste management, the use of sensors, IoT (Internet of Things), and AI can enhance route optimization for waste collection, ensuring timely and effective disposal while minimizing fuel consumption. This leads to lower operational costs and the ability to handle larger volumes of waste more effectively. In the context of healthcare, the adoption of telemedicine and AI for diagnosis can reduce the need for physical infrastructure and personnel, thereby decreasing costs associated with healthcare delivery [32].

Reduced Greenhouse Gas Emissions and Environmental Degradation

Technological advancements contribute to lowering environmental impact by reducing greenhouse gas emissions. In urban areas, the use of green technologies such as electric vehicles, renewable energy sources (like solar and wind), and smart waste management systems directly results in lower carbon footprints. Similarly, industries that leverage automated systems for energy management can optimize their energy consumption, reducing emissions and minimizing environmental degradation caused by traditional industrial processes. Moreover, digital solutions in waste management, such as tracking and sorting, help divert waste from landfills, thereby contributing to less environmental pollution [29].

Better Compliance with Regulatory Norms

As governments and international bodies implement more stringent regulations regarding environmental sustainability, digital technologies facilitate compliance through better monitoring, reporting, and management. Automated data collection systems can track emissions, waste disposal, and resource use in real-time, ensuring that industries and organizations adhere to set guidelines. This approach minimizes human error and ensures continuous compliance, which is especially crucial in sectors that are subject to frequent audits and inspections [33 - 35]. Regulatory compliance through automation also helps avoid penalties and improve the reputation of businesses.

Promotion of Sustainable Urban Development

The integration of digital tools and green technologies in urban planning fosters sustainable cities. Smart cities, which utilize IoT, AI, and data analytics, promote energy efficiency, waste reduction, and enhanced transportation systems. By optimizing resource use and improving the quality of life for urban residents, these technologies contribute to creating environmentally friendly, economically viable, and socially inclusive urban spaces [36]. For instance, in waste management, sensor-based waste bins that notify when they are full can optimize collection routes, ensuring timely waste disposal while reducing traffic congestion and fuel consumption [37].

Empowerment of Communities through Awareness and Participation

Advanced technologies, such as mobile apps and online platforms, enable communities to be actively involved in sustainability efforts. These platforms can promote awareness by providing real-time information about waste management, pollution levels, or energy consumption. Additionally, community-driven initiatives, such as crowdfunding for renewable energy projects or waste reduction campaigns, are facilitated by digital technologies, thus empowering local populations to engage directly in environmental preservation [37 - 39]. Furthermore, increased participation in decision-making processes fosters a sense of ownership and responsibility, driving long-term positive outcomes for sustainable development.

Challenges

High Initial Investment and Maintenance Costs

Even though advanced technologies can help save money in the long run, the high initial cost to start using them is often a big challenge. Setting up systems like smart grids, using artificial intelligence in waste management, or shifting to renewable energy requires a large amount of money at the beginning. Also, these systems need regular maintenance and updates, which adds to the ongoing expenses. This is especially difficult in developing countries where financial resources are limited. The costs of things like hardware, software, and trained professionals make the financial burden even heavier [40]. The costs of technology infrastructure, such as hardware, software, and skilled personnel, add to the financial burden.

Need for Technical Expertise and Digital Literacy

The successful implementation and management of advanced technological systems often require specialized knowledge. This includes the technical skills necessary for operating and maintaining complex digital systems, as well as the ability to analyze and interpret data for decision-making. In many parts of the world, especially in rural or underdeveloped regions, there is a lack of skilled professionals who can manage such systems. Moreover, there is a digital literacy gap, where large segments of the population may not have the necessary understanding to utilize technology effectively, hindering the potential for widespread adoption [41 - 43].

Infrastructure Gaps in Developing Regions

One of the primary challenges in implementing advanced technologies, especially in developing regions, is the lack of reliable and robust infrastructure. For example, inadequate internet connectivity, lack of access to electricity, and outdated physical infrastructure can impede the effectiveness of digital solutions. In some areas, the absence of proper waste disposal infrastructure or renewable energy systems limits the application of smart technologies in sectors like waste management and sustainable urban development. Overcoming these gaps requires not only significant investment in physical infrastructure but also policy support and collaboration with local communities [44, 45].

EMERGING FUNGAL DISEASE PREVENTION AND CONTROL

Fungal infections, particularly in immunocompromised populations, are a growing health and environmental concern. Conventional antifungal treatments are facing significant challenges, including toxicity, resistance, and inefficacy. Therefore, there is an urgent need for improved diagnostics, safer antifungal agents, and more sustainable disinfection methods. Recent advancements in green technologies, real-time monitoring, and artificial intelligence (AI)-driven data analysis have shown promise in addressing these challenges. Furthermore, international collaboration and standardization are essential for effective fungal disease management under a One Health framework [46].

DIGITAL IMAGE PROCESSING IN WASTEWATER TREATMENT

The activated sludge system is a cornerstone in domestic wastewater treatment. Traditional methods for monitoring activated sludge are effective but often time-consuming. Digital image processing offers a promising solution by enabling quicker and more insightful analysis. This approach correlates morphological parameters of sludge flocs and filaments with conventional physico-chemical metrics. Advanced techniques, such as z-stacking and image stitching, enhance preprocessing capabilities, making image analysis a valuable tool for real-time monitoring and predictive assessment of the activated sludge processes [47].

IOT-CLOUD SUPPORTED SMART HAND SANITIZER DISPENSER

The COVID-19 pandemic led to a dramatic increase in plastic waste due to the widespread use of disposable personal protective equipment (PPE). A novel approach has been developed to address this issue by converting pandemic-related waste into a valuable energy source. The 3D-printed triboelectric nanogenerator (MG-CS TENG) uses sterilized masks and gloves to harvest mechanical energy, which can then power small electronics and operate a smart hand sanitizer dispenser. Integrated with the Internet of Things (IoT), this system offers real-time monitoring and control, demonstrating a sustainable method for waste management while supporting public health and green energy solutions [47].

NEONICOTINOIDS IN DOMESTIC WASTEWATER TREATMENT

Recent studies have identified the persistent presence of neonicotinoids (NEOs) in domestic wastewater treatment plants (WWTPs) and their receiving environments. Thiamethoxam was found to be the most prevalent compound, with biodegradation playing a key role in its removal. Among the three plants studied, WWTP 2 exhibited the highest removal efficiency, while WWTP 3 showed unintended increases in certain NEO levels. These findings highlight the dual role of WWTPs as both removal sites and sources of NEOs, underscoring the need for targeted pollution control strategies to protect aquatic ecosystems [48 - 50].

TREATMENT OF CONTAMINANTS OF EMERGING CONCERN (CECS) IN WASTEWATER

A study in Guangzhou assessed the effectiveness of a wastewater treatment plant in removing contaminants of emerging concern (CECs), particularly pharmaceuticals, which were the predominant group identified. Using high-resolution mass spectrometry and molecular networking, it was found that 94.5% of the detected compounds were eliminated post-treatment. The study also identified various potential transformation products and varying degrees of removal efficiency, emphasizing the need for ongoing optimization of treatment strategies to better manage CECs [51].

HYBRID DEEP LEARNING TECHNIQUES FOR GHG EMISSIONS PREDICTION

Accurate quantification of greenhouse gas (GHG) emissions from industrial wastewater treatment is essential, especially under varying organic loads. A novel deep learning model, combining Temporal Convolutional Networks (TCN) and attention mechanisms, was developed to predict CO_2, CH_4, and N_2O emissions. The model outperformed traditional approaches and holds significant promise for forecasting GHG emissions and enhancing carbon management strategies in wastewater treatment systems [52].

RESILIENCE OF PARTIAL NITRITATION-ANAMMOX PROCESS UNDER STRESS

The Partial Nitritation-Anammox (PN/A) process plays a key role in nitrogen removal from wastewater. A recent study demonstrated the resilience of this process under sulfamethazine-induced stress in high-ammonia wastewater. Enhanced extracellular polymer production and the upregulation of antibiotic resistance genes were identified as key factors that maintained system stability and nitrogen removal efficiency. These findings provide valuable insights into the adaptive mechanisms of PN/A under antibiotic pressure, supporting its potential for broader wastewater treatment applications [52 - 54].

The integration of advanced technologies, including AI, digital monitoring, and green innovations, is transforming waste management and wastewater treatment practices. These innovations not only optimize waste handling processes but also reduce ecological footprints, promote resource efficiency, and enhance overall sustainability. Ongoing research and international collaboration are essential for addressing the emerging challenges and achieving long-term environmental and public health goals.

DIGITAL TRANSFORMATION IN WASTE MANAGEMENT AND ENERGY SAVING FOR SUSTAINABILITY

The AHP-ANN model serves as a powerful decision-making tool for sustainable waste management by addressing complex, multi-criteria problems and forecasting outcomes. This model combines the Analytic Hierarchy Process (AHP) for multi-criteria decision analysis with Artificial Neural Networks (ANNs) for predictive modeling, facilitating informed decisions on waste management strategies. Construction and demolition waste constitute a significant portion of global landfill content, and managing this waste through recycling and strategies like rethink, reduce, and reuse can contribute to resource conservation. This study demonstrates the effectiveness of combining AHP and ANN to assess solid waste management options, underscoring the AHP-ANN model's value in making informed, sustainable decisions in waste management [55].

In developing countries, green supply chain management plays a critical role in enhancing environmental sustainability and improving firm performance within the manufacturing sector. Practices such as eco-technological innovation, environmental strategies, and collaborative capabilities have been shown to strengthen the positive impacts of green supply initiatives. By adopting these strategies, firms can meet global challenges more effectively while reducing their environmental footprint [56].

Maritime logistics is essential to global trade, but traditional port operations face challenges, including high costs and environmental pollution. The transition to digitalized green ports, as seen in locations like Los Angeles and Long Beach, has the potential to improve efficiency and reduce environmental impact. However, varying levels of digital adoption create communication challenges. Integrated digital solutions across environmental, policy, technological, and managerial domains are crucial for advancing sustainability. Ultimately, digital innovation and intelligent management are pivotal to the future of green ports and maritime logistics [57].

Technological and eco-innovative solutions have transformed solid waste management by viewing waste as a valuable resource. With support from digital tools, government policies, and community engagement, India has made significant strides toward sustainability. These advancements not only promote renewable energy and green business opportunities but also pave the way for improvements in climate action and public health. Continued innovation and the adoption of new technologies are essential for bridging existing gaps and advancing sustainable development in India and similar developing countries [44].

China's green technology transfer plays a significant role in reducing energy intensity in Belt and Road Initiative regions, particularly in developing countries. The transfer of technologies related to alternative energy and waste management has the most substantial impact. Despite some rebound effects, the overall influence remains positive, providing valuable guidance for advancing green technology policies and strategies [45, 58, 59].

Effective management of construction and demolition waste is increasingly critical as global attention on environmental sustainability grows. This study addresses the gap in practical waste estimation tools by introducing a Building Information Modeling (BIM)-based system for accurate planning of demolition and renovation waste. The system enhances waste prediction, supports recycling, aids in transport planning, and estimates costs. A real-world case in Hong Kong demonstrates the potential of this system for wider adoption in future construction practices. Fungal pathogens are a growing health concern, particularly among immunocompromised individuals. Current antifungal treatments and diagnostic methods face significant limitations, including toxicity, resistance, and environmental persistence. There is an urgent need for improved detection methods, safer and more effective antifungal strategies, and eco-friendly disinfection solutions. Embracing digital technologies and a One Health approach will be vital in developing sustainable solutions to reduce the burden of fungal infections [36, 60, 61].

Traditional methods for monitoring activated sludge in wastewater treatment plants are time-consuming and rely heavily on physico-chemical parameters. Digital image processing presents a more efficient alternative by characterizing the current state of sludge and predicting future conditions. This chapter reviews various image acquisition, preprocessing, segmentation, and analysis techniques, highlighting novel methods such as z-stacking and image stitching. The correlation between morphological parameters from image analysis and physico-chemical data demonstrates the potential of image processing to enhance monitoring and prediction in wastewater treatment plants [39].

The development of flow-based microdevices for determining residual free chlorine in water using DPD and OT methods offers a rapid, *in-situ*, and cost-effective solution for monitoring water potability and disinfection efficiency. Optimized procedures provide reliable quantification with low detection limits and high precision. The integration of digital-image colorimetry using smartphone cameras enhances the accessibility and practicality of this tool for field applications, ensuring sustainable and efficient water quality management [62].

Smart city initiatives are crucial for promoting green and sustainable economic growth in China. Based on data from 274 cities, this study confirms that smart city policies contribute significantly to economic green growth by improving energy efficiency and reducing emissions. Through various robustness tests and mechanisms, the study reveals that these cities promote green growth by enhancing economic output while minimizing environmental impact. The positive effects are observed in both large cities and those not reliant on natural resources. This research offers valuable insights for urban development and economic transformation in emerging economies [49, 50, 63].

CONCLUSION

The integration of digitalization and green technology in waste management marks a significant advancement toward achieving sustainable development goals. By enabling data-driven decisions, resource optimization, and environmental protection, these technologies are essential for modernizing waste systems. However, a collaborative approach involving governments, industries, and communities is crucial to harness their full potential and overcome implementation challenges.

REFERENCES

[1] Sharma H, Haque A, Blaabjerg F. Machine learning in wireless sensor networks for smart cities: A survey. 2021; 10(9): 1012.
[http://dx.doi.org/10.3390/electronics10091012]

[2] Uganya G, Rajalakshmi D, Teekaraman Y, Kuppusamy R, Radhakrishnan A. [Retracted] A Novel Strategy for Waste Prediction Using Machine Learning Algorithm with IoT Based Intelligent Waste Management System. Wirel Commun Mob Comput 2022; 2022(1): 2063372.
[http://dx.doi.org/10.1155/2022/2063372]

[3] Khan R, Kumar S, Srivastava AK, *et al.* [Retracted] Machine Learning and IoT-Based Waste Management Model. Comput Intell Neurosci 2021; 2021(1): 5942574.

[http://dx.doi.org/10.1155/2021/5942574] [PMID: 34484322]

[4] Dubey S, Singh P, Yadav P, Singh KK. Household Waste Management System Using IoT and Machine Learning. Proc Comp Sci 2020; 67: 1950-1959.
[http://dx.doi.org/10.1016/j.procs.2020.03.222]

[5] Alnuaimi E, Alsafi M, Alshehhi M, *et al.* Blockchain-based system for tracking and rewarding recyclable plastic waste. Peer-to-Peer Netw Appl 2023; 16(1): 328-46.
[http://dx.doi.org/10.1007/s12083-022-01413-5]

[6] Suvarnamma A, Pradeepkiran JA. SmartBin system with waste tracking and sorting mechanism using IoT. 2021; 5: 100348.
[http://dx.doi.org/10.1016/j.clet.2021.100348]

[7] Bernardo O O, de Souza M T S, Demajorovic J. Innovation in the reverse supply chain of electrical and electronic waste: a study on information systems and tracking technologies. RAE Revista de Administração de Empresas 2020; 60(4): 248-61.

[8] Holmström J. From AI to digital transformation: The AI readiness framework. Bus Horiz 2022; 65(3): 329-39.
[http://dx.doi.org/10.1016/j.bushor.2021.03.006]

[9] Gkinko L, Elbanna A. The appropriation of conversational AI in the workplace: A taxonomy of AI chatbot users. Int J Inf Manage 2023; 69: 102568.
[http://dx.doi.org/10.1016/j.ijinfomgt.2022.102568]

[10] Mikalef P, Conboy K, Lundström JE, Popovič A. Thinking responsibly about responsible AI and 'the dark side' of AI. Eur J Inf Syst 2022; 31(3): 257-68.
[http://dx.doi.org/10.1080/0960085X.2022.2026621]

[11] Southworth J, Migliaccio K, Glover J, *et al.* Developing a model for AI across the curriculum: Transforming the higher education landscape via innovation in AI literacy. Computers and Education: Artificial Intelligence 2023; 4: 100127.

[12] Regona M, Yigitcanlar T, Xia B, Li RYM. Opportunities and Adoption Challenges of AI in the Construction Industry: A PRISMA Review. J Open Innov 2022; 8(1): 45.
[http://dx.doi.org/10.3390/joitmc8010045]

[13] Vaishya R, Javaid M, Khan IH, Haleem A. Artificial Intelligence (AI) applications for COVID-19 pandemic. Diabetes Metab Syndr 2020; 14(4): 337-9.
[http://dx.doi.org/10.1016/j.dsx.2020.04.012] [PMID: 32305024]

[14] Bankins S, Formosa P. The Ethical Implications of Artificial Intelligence (AI) For Meaningful Work. J Bus Ethics 2023; 185(4): 725-40.
[http://dx.doi.org/10.1007/s10551-023-05339-7]

[15] Zhang K, Aslan AB. AI technologies for education: Recent research & future directions. Comp Edu: Arti Intel 2021; 2: 100025.

[16] Minkkinen M, Niukkanen A, Mäntymäki M. What about investors? ESG analyses as tools for ethics-based AI auditing. AI Soc 2024; 39(1): 329-43.
[http://dx.doi.org/10.1007/s00146-022-01415-0]

[17] Haleem A, Javaid M, Qadri M A, Singh R P, Suman R. Artificial intelligence (AI) applications for marketing: A literature-based study. Int J Intell Netw 2022; 3: 119-32.

[18] Wang X, Li L, Tan SC, Yang L, Lei J. Preparing for AI-enhanced education: Conceptualizing and empirically examining teachers' AI readiness. Comput Human Behav 2023; 146: 107798.
[http://dx.doi.org/10.1016/j.chb.2023.107798]

[19] Zhong Y, Godwin P, Jin Y, Xiao H. Biodegradable polymers and green-based antimicrobial packaging materials: A mini-review. Adv Indus Eng Poly Res 2020; 3(1): 27-35.

[20] Wani NR, Dar AH, Dash KK, *et al.* Recent advances in the production of bionanomaterials for

development of sustainable food packaging: A comprehensive review. Environ Res 2023; 237(Pt 1): 116948.
[http://dx.doi.org/10.1016/j.envres.2023.116948] [PMID: 37611789]

[21] Vibha C, Parameswaranpillai J, Krishnasamy S, *et al.* Biodegradable polymers and green-based antimicrobial packaging materials. Biodegradable Polymers, Blends and Composites. Cambridge: Woodhead Publishing 2022; pp. 717-33.

[22] Muliarta I N, Sudita I D N, Situmeang Y P. The effect of eco-enzyme spraying on suwung landfill waste, denpasar, on changes in leachate characteristics. Jurnal Kesehatan Lingkungan 2023; 15(1): 1-8.

[23] Maasarani M, Afify A, Mohsen H, Youssef M. From waste to energy: reuse of landfills to create eco-friendly spaces. BAU Journal - Creative Sustainable Development 2022; 4(1): 1-14.

[24] Anand U, Reddy B, Singh VK, *et al.* Potential environmental and human health risks caused by antibiotic-resistant bacteria (ARB), antibiotic resistance genes (ARGs) and emerging contaminants (ECs) from municipal solid waste (MSW) landfill. Antibiotics (Basel) 2021; 10(4): 374.
[http://dx.doi.org/10.3390/antibiotics10040374] [PMID: 33915892]

[25] Nuvvula RSS, Devaraj E, Madurai Elavarasan R, Iman Taheri S, Irfan M, Teegala KS. Multi-objective mutation-enabled adaptive local attractor quantum behaved particle swarm optimisation based optimal sizing of hybrid renewable energy system for smart cities in India. Sustain Energy Technol Assess 2022; 49: 101689.
[http://dx.doi.org/10.1016/j.seta.2021.101689]

[26] Thomas A, Mishra U. A green energy circular system with carbon capturing and waste minimization in a smart grid power management. Energy Rep 2022; 8: 14102-23.
[http://dx.doi.org/10.1016/j.egyr.2022.10.341]

[27] Johansen K, Werner S. Something is sustainable in the state of Denmark: A review of the Danish district heating sector. Renew Sustain Energy Rev 2022; 158: 112117.
[http://dx.doi.org/10.1016/j.rser.2022.112117]

[28] Kaszycki P, Głodniok M, Petryszak P. Towards a bio-based circular economy in organic waste management and wastewater treatment – The Polish perspective. N Biotechnol 2021; 61: 80-9.
[http://dx.doi.org/10.1016/j.nbt.2020.11.005] [PMID: 33202308]

[29] Ghahramani M, Zhou M, Molter A, Pilla F. IoT-Based Route Recommendation for an Intelligent Waste Management System. IEEE Internet Things J 2022; 9(14): 11883-92.
[http://dx.doi.org/10.1109/JIOT.2021.3132126]

[30] Andeobu L, Wibowo S, Grandhi S. Artificial intelligence applications for sustainable solid waste management practices in Australia: A systematic review. Sci Total Environ 2022; 834: 155389.
[http://dx.doi.org/10.1016/j.scitotenv.2022.155389] [PMID: 35460765]

[31] Dodampegama S, Hou L, Asadi E, Zhang G, Setunge S. Revolutionizing construction and demolition waste sorting: Insights from artificial intelligence and robotic applications. Resour Conserv Recycling 2024; 202: 107375.
[http://dx.doi.org/10.1016/j.resconrec.2023.107375]

[32] Ihsanullah I, Alam G, Jamal A, Shaik F. Recent advances in applications of artificial intelligence in solid waste management: A review. Chemosphere 2022; 309(Pt 1): 136631.
[http://dx.doi.org/10.1016/j.chemosphere.2022.136631] [PMID: 36183887]

[33] Vyas S, Dhakar K, Varjani S, *et al.* Solid waste management techniques powered by *in-silico* approaches with a special focus on municipal solid waste management: Research trends and challenges. Sci Total Environ 2023; 891: 164344.
[http://dx.doi.org/10.1016/j.scitotenv.2023.164344] [PMID: 37244611]

[34] Abioye SO, Oyedele LO, Akanbi L, *et al.* Artificial intelligence in the construction industry: A review of present status, opportunities and future challenges. J Build Eng 2021; 44: 103299.

[http://dx.doi.org/10.1016/j.jobe.2021.103299]

[35] Abdallah M, Abu Talib M, Feroz S, Nasir Q, Abdalla H, Mahfood B. Artificial intelligence applications in solid waste management: A systematic research review. Waste Manag 2020; 109: 231-246.

[36] Cheah CG, Chia WY, Lai SF, Chew KW, Chia SR, Show PL. Innovation designs of industry 4.0 based solid waste management: Machinery and digital circular economy. Environ Res 2022; 213: 113619. [http://dx.doi.org/10.1016/j.envres.2022.113619] [PMID: 35700763]

[37] Javaid M, Haleem A, Khan IH, Suman R. Understanding the potential applications of Artificial Intelligence in Agriculture Sector. 2023; 2(1): 15-30. [http://dx.doi.org/10.1016/j.aac.2022.10.001]

[38] Zhang X, Liu C, Chen Y, Zheng G, Chen Y. Source separation, transportation, pretreatment, and valorization of municipal solid waste: a critical review. Environ Dev Sustain 2022; 24(10): 11471-513. [http://dx.doi.org/10.1007/s10668-021-01932-w] [PMID: 34776765]

[39] Herath HMKKMB, Mittal M. Adoption of artificial intelligence in smart cities: A comprehensive review. 2022; 2(1): 100076.

[40] Sheng TJ, Islam MS, Misran N, *et al.* An Internet of Things Based Smart Waste Management System Using LoRa and Tensorflow Deep Learning Model. IEEE Access 2020; 8: 148793-811. [http://dx.doi.org/10.1109/ACCESS.2020.3016255]

[41] Sivakumar VL, Vickram AS, Krishnan R, Richard T. AI-Enhanced Decision Support Systems for Optimizing Hazardous Waste Handling in Civil Engineering. 2023; 10(11): 1-8.

[42] Kazeem KO, Olawumi TO, Osunsanmi T. Roles of Artificial Intelligence and Machine Learning in Enhancing Construction Processes and Sustainable Communities. 2023; 13(8): 2061. [http://dx.doi.org/10.3390/buildings13082061]

[43] Noman AA, Akter UH, Pranto TH, Haque AKMB. Machine Learning and Artificial Intelligence in Circular Economy: A Bibliometric Analysis and Systematic Literature Review. Annals of Emerging Technologies in Comp 2022; 6(2): 13-40. [http://dx.doi.org/10.33166/AETiC.2022.02.002]

[44] Ugwuanyi E D, Dada M A, Majemite M T, Obaigbena A. AI-driven waste management systems: a comparative review of innovations in the USA and Africa. Eng Sci Technol J 2024; 5(1): 241-55.

[45] Pallathadka H, Mustafa M, Sanchez D T, Sekhar Sajja G, Gour S, Naved M. Impact of machine learning on management, healthcare and agriculture. Materials Today: Proceedings 2023; 80: 2803-6. [http://dx.doi.org/10.1016/j.matpr.2021.07.042]

[46] Solano Meza JK, Orjuela Yepes D, Rodrigo-Ilarri J, Rodrigo-Clavero ME. Comparative Analysis of the Implementation of Support Vector Machines and Long Short-Term Memory Artificial Neural Networks in Municipal Solid Waste Management Models in Megacities. Int J Environ Res Public Health 2023; 20(5): 4256. [http://dx.doi.org/10.3390/ijerph20054256] [PMID: 36901265]

[47] Camaréna S. Artificial Intelligence (AI) for Sustainable Institutional Food Systems: Implementation of AI Tools for School Nutrition Program Management in the United States of America. Front Sustain Food Syst 2022; 6: 743810. [http://dx.doi.org/10.3389/fsufs.2022.743810]

[48] Singh M, Singh M, Singh SK. Tackling municipal solid waste crisis in India: Insights into cutting-edge technologies and risk assessment. Sci Total Environ 2024; 917: 170453. [http://dx.doi.org/10.1016/j.scitotenv.2024.170453] [PMID: 38296084]

[49] Yu KH, Zhang Y, Li D, Montenegro-Marin CE, Kumar PM. Environmental planning based on reduce, reuse, recycle and recover using artificial intelligence. Environ Impact Assess Rev 2021; 86: 106492. [http://dx.doi.org/10.1016/j.eiar.2020.106492]

[50] Joshi LM, Bharti RK, Singh R. Internet of things and machine learning-based approaches in the urban solid waste management: Trends, challenges, and future directions. Expert Syst 2022; 39(5): e12865. [http://dx.doi.org/10.1111/exsy.12865]

[51] Bhardwaj A, Kishore S, Pandey DK. Artificial Intelligence in Biological Sciences. Life (Basel) 2022; 12(9): 1430. [http://dx.doi.org/10.3390/life12091430] [PMID: 36143468]

[52] Ahmed M I B, Alotaibi R B, Al-Qahtani R A, *et al.* Deep learning approach to recyclable products classification: towards sustainable waste management. Sustainability 2023; 15(14): 11138.

[53] Erkinay Ozdemir M, Ali Z, Subeshan B, Asmatulu E. Applying machine learning approach in recycling. J Mater Cycles Waste Manag 2021; 23(3): 855-71. [http://dx.doi.org/10.1007/s10163-021-01182-y]

[54] Hashfi MI, Raharjo T. Exploring the Challenges and Impacts of Artificial Intelligence Implementation in Project Management: A Systematic Literature Review. Int J Adv Comput Sci Appl 2023; 14(9): 366-376. [http://dx.doi.org/10.14569/IJACSA.2023.0140940]

[55] Wang K, Zhao Y, Gangadhari RK, Li Z. Analyzing the adoption challenges of the internet of things (Iot) and artificial intelligence (ai) for smart cities in china. Sustainability 2021; 13(19): 10983. [http://dx.doi.org/10.3390/su131910983]

[56] Rajalakshmi J, Sumangali K, Jayanthi J, Muthulakshmi K. Artificial intelligence with earthworm optimization assisted waste management system for smart cities. Glob NEST J 2023; 25(4): 190-197.

[57] Jiang P, Zhang L, You S, *et al.* Blockchain technology applications in waste management: Overview, challenges and opportunities. J Clean Prod 2023; 421: 138466. [http://dx.doi.org/10.1016/j.jclepro.2023.138466]

[58] Abeygunawardhana A G D T, Shalinda R M M M, Bandara W H M D, Anesta W D S, Kasthurirathna D, Abeysiri L. AI - driven smart bin for waste management. In: ICAC 2020 - 2nd International Conference on Advancements in Computing, Proceedings. New York: IEEE; 2020. p. 110-115.

[59] Fayomi GU, Mini SE, Chisom CM, *et al.* Smart Waste Management for Smart City: Impact on Industrialization. In: IOP Conference Series: Earth Environ. Sci. 2021; 655: 012040.

[60] Bijos JCBF, Queiroz LM, Zanta VM, Oliveira-Esquerre KP. Towards Artificial Intelligence in Urban Waste Management: an early prospect for Latin America. IOP Conf Ser Mater Sci Eng. 2021; 1196; 012030. [http://dx.doi.org/10.1088/1757-899X/1196/1/012030]

[61] Kuok F, Monyrath B, Promentilla M A B. AI application to pollution reduction and waste management toward net zero: a systematic review. Chem Eng Trans 2023; 106: 1333-8.

[62] Pinhal Luqueci Thomaz I, Fernando Mahler C, Pereira Calôba L. Artificial Intelligence (AI) applied to waste management: a contingency measure to fill out the lack of information resulting from restrictions on field sampling. Waste Manag Bull 2023; 1(1): 15-22.

[63] Berroir F, Guernaccini P, Sottet J S. On-site waste management: a use case of lean construction and artificial intelligence synergy. Proceedings of the 31st Annual Conference of the International Group for Lean Construction (IGLC31). Lille: IGLC; 2023. p. 110-121.

CHAPTER 11

Building Partnerships: Government, Industry, and NGOs in Waste Management

Shobhit Raj[1,*], **Prashant Singh**[2], **Priya Rani**[3], **Sonali Dasgupta**[4] and **Neha Srivastava**[5]

[1] *Department of Endocrinology, Kasturba Medical College, Manipal, Manipal Academy of Higher Education, Manipal, Karnataka, India*

[2] *Department of Pharmaceutics, Buddha Institute of Pharmacy, GIDA, Gorakhpur, Uttar Pradesh, India*

[3] *Department of Nephrology, Kasturba Medical College, Manipal, Manipal Academy of Higher Education, Manipal, Karnataka, India*

[4] *Department of Pharmaceutics, Krishak College of Pharmacy, Rajgarh, Mirzapur, Uttar Pradesh, India*

[5] *Department of Pharmacy, Buddha Institute of Pharmacy, GIDA, Gorakhpur, Uttar Pradesh, India*

Abstract: Emphasizing the cooperative roles of government agencies, the pharmaceutical industry, and non-governmental organizations (NGOs), this chapter critically analyses the strategic relevance of tripartite partnerships in pharmaceutical waste management. The study emphasizes how combined approaches, combining strong legislative frameworks, creative waste treatment technology, and proactive public participation, may propel the change toward a circular economy model. While the pharmaceutical sector is acknowledged for its dedication to sustainable practices through careful waste separation, safe storage, and the adoption of eco-friendly technologies, government bodies are shown to establish and enforce comprehensive policies, allocate funding, and ensure rigorous oversight. NGOs are therefore very important in pushing for tighter rules, increasing public awareness, and enabling community-based take-back projects. The chapter critically addresses issues including different stakeholder priorities, budget limits, and communication difficulties, as well as explores successful partnership models and case studies showing observable environmental and financial advantages. The combined approach suggested here provides a reasonable route to improve public health, increase resource recovery, and lower the environmental impact of pharmaceutical waste.

* **Corresponding author Shobhit Raj:** Department of Endocrinology, Kasturba Medical College, Manipal, Manipal Academy of Higher Education, Manipal, Karnataka, India;
E-mail: shobhit.kmcmpl2024@learner.manipal.edu

Suman Gautam, Jai Narayan Mishra, Preeti Mishra, Preeti Verma & Sudhanshu Mishra (Eds.)

Keywords: Circular economy, Community engagement, Eco-friendly technologies, Environmental contamination, Environmental stewardship, Extended producer responsibility.

INTRODUCTION

The major environmental, health, and economic consequences of improper waste management have made the problem of pharmaceutical waste management more and more pressing. Improper disposal of pharmaceutical chemicals can pollute soil and water, endangering human health as well as ecological balance [1]. The need for strategic and sustainable methods for pharmaceutical waste management, including recycling where possible, becomes critical as awareness of these effects increases. Effectively tackling this difficult issue calls for the coordinated efforts and active participation of many different stakeholders, especially government agencies, the pharmaceutical sector, and non-governmental organisations (NGOs). The multifaceted nature of pharmaceutical waste, including complex regulatory environments, diverse industrial practices, and the need for widespread public involvement, calls for a coordinated effort across all three sectors to develop and implement solutions that are both efficient and sustainable [2]. A unified approach cannot be created or carried out in isolation; rather, it requires a shared awareness of responsibilities and a dedication to cooperating toward shared objectives. Distinct roles of each of these stakeholder groups will be discussed in this chapter, along with successful models of their cooperation, obstacles impeding efficient partnerships will be identified, and significant advantages resulting from a unified approach to pharmaceutical waste management will be underlined.

DISMANTLING THE FUNCTIONS: DUTIES OF GOVERNMENT, BUSINESS, AND NONPROFITS

Government: Regulatory Framework, Policy Implementation, and Monitoring

Local, regional, national, and even international government agencies play a fundamental role in creating and enforcing the comprehensive rules and standards that govern the entire lifecycle of pharmaceutical waste management [3]. This includes the vital work of classifying pharmaceutical waste into several categories, including hazardous versus non-hazardous waste and controlled substances, which determines the suitable handling, treatment, and disposal techniques. Agencies that specify acceptable treatment and disposal technologies include the Federal Environmental Protection Agency and state environmental and health departments. These might include chemical disinfection, autoclaving, incineration, and other techniques intended to reduce health hazards and environmental impacts [4]. The government's main duty, thus, is to build the basic legal and regulatory infrastructure, establishing the baseline for safe and environmentally sound pharmaceutical waste management techniques for all stakeholders. Without these clearly defined criteria, there would be inconsistency and a lack of responsibility in the management of pharmaceutical waste. Regulations provide the required framework for action, therefore guaranteeing that every person follows a shared set of rules meant to safeguard the environment and public health.

Apart from establishing the policies, government agencies have a major duty of monitoring various means of monitoring adherence to these set rules, which helps government agencies to fulfil their critical role [5].

Regular inspections and audits of treatment facilities, pharmaceutical manufacturing plants, healthcare institutions, disposal sites, and treatment facilities are vital to guarantee that rules are being followed in practice. Moreover, governments sometimes penalise facilities that do not follow waste management rules; the effects might be monetary fines or operating license suspensions [6]. To promote openness and support following high standards, facilities might also have to disclose their waste management policies.

Effective monitoring and enforcement are vital to guarantee that the rules are not only theoretical but also really implemented and followed by all relevant organisations, to preserve the environment and public health. Though well-designed, rules are not effective in the case of no supervision. Audits guarantee responsibility and stop malpractices that might have negative effects, including the release of untreated pharmaceutical waste into the environment or its diversion for illegal purposes.

Government agencies also play a key part in designating funds and resources to assist projects in the management of pharmaceutical waste. This can be in the shape of grants and subsidies given to waste management businesses and healthcare institutions to help invest in advanced technologies and the development of required infrastructure for the safe and efficient treatment and disposal of pharmaceutical waste [6]. For example, programs offered by the USDA for solid waste management can offer financial assistance for related initiatives [7]. A key catalyst is government funding, which helps especially with the rapid adoption of required but possibly costly technologies and infrastructure for smaller companies or in areas with limited financial resources.

Investing public money in appropriate waste management infrastructure and research shows a dedication to environmental protection and public health, and can drive sector innovation. This financial help can help overcome economic obstacles that might otherwise stop the application of best practices in pharmaceutical waste management.

Moreover, governments play a key role in creating and carrying out plans to handle new issues in the sector, such as efficiently controlling surges in medical waste during public health crises [8]. They also help promote sustainable methods in pharmaceutical waste management, such as promoting waste reduction at the source, boosting recycling rates where practical, and supporting the evolution and use of environmentally friendly treatment techniques. Rules include the ban on flushing hazardous waste pharmaceuticals down the toilet or drain, as required by the Resource Conservation and Recovery Act (RCRA) and adopted by states such as Florida, showing this dedication to avoiding environmental pollution [9], anticipating future difficulties, and in governments pushing the change toward a more sustainable attitude to pharmaceutical waste. Establishing long-term objectives and encouraging environmentally friendly behaviours help to drive the shift toward a more sustainable approach to pharmaceutical waste management [10]. This proactive approach guarantees resilient and adaptable waste management systems. Future requirements and environmental effects are reduced over time, therefore supporting a healthier and more sustainable future for all.

Companies: Sustainable Practices, Innovation, and Extended Producer Responsibility

The pharmaceutical sector has a major ethical and operational duty in developing and strictly following thorough and sustainable waste management policies along its whole production chain, including research and development, protocols, manufacturing techniques, and distribution systems. A fundamental component of this duty is waste segregation at the point of generation. This calls for careful separation of hazardous and non-hazardous waste streams to guarantee suitable handling and disposal, as well as correct labelling of every waste container with unambiguous information on the kind of waste and any related hazards [11]. The industry also must make sure all pharmaceutical waste is securely stored in designated, suitably built containers to avoid unintentional exposure, possible abuse, or any kind of environmental contamination. Since they are the main manufacturers of pharmaceutical products and, hence, major waste producers, the industry has a basic responsibility to include sustainable waste management strategies in its main operations. Minimising the environmental impact of the industry depends on this proactive attitude and maintaining the tenets of product stewardship, guaranteeing that items are managed sensibly throughout their lifetime.

The pharmaceutical sector is also quite important in funding research, development, as well as the acceptance of creative technologies and practices meant to lower the generation of pharmaceutical waste, improving recycling possibilities for kinds of waste, and strengthening the efficacy of treatment techniques for the waste generated [12]. This covers developments in the design of pharmaceutical packaging. For instance, the use of blister packs for single doses can help to limit over-prescribing and lower the number of unused drugs that finally turn into waste [13]. Moreover, the evolution of smart packaging fitted with sensors offering real-time data on storage conditions and expiration dates helps to cut waste as well by guaranteeing that medications are used before they expire [14].

The industry can also invest in and use sophisticated waste treatment technologies, including biological treatment techniques, chemical neutralisation for liquid waste streams, and incineration with energy recovery, which are scientifically appropriate and environmentally sound [15]. The technical expertise of the industry and significant financial resources qualify it as a major innovator in pharmaceutical waste management, which helps to create more efficient, cost-effective, environmentally responsible solutions that can help the whole industry and society in general.

Other than the protocol-based strategies, companies should provide education to the specialists working under the company and take their feedback regarding the problems they are facing to truly understand the issue and find a solution that is safe for the workers and the environment. Since the workers are the frontline who manage the waste, they should be provided with a voice and listened to their perspective to build strategies. One important trend in pharmaceutical waste management is the increasing use of the Extended Producer Responsibility (EPR) concept, which is a major trend in pharmaceutical waste management. EPR allows pharmaceutical companies to assume more operational and financial responsibility for the management of their products post-consumer, especially regarding the collection and correct disposal of expired or unused drugs.

Successful EPR initiatives have been implemented at the state level in the United States, such as California's industry-run statewide stewardship programs, and in several European nations, showing the practicality and efficacy of this method [16]. These are being found effective in safeguarding the environment by spreading awareness and building requisite convenient technologies for the smooth application of the policies. Often, these programs offer consumers no-cost disposal choices by means of the creation of take-back sites, other easily reachable collection methods, mail-back programs, and pharmacies, which will help to shape these projects [17]. Another way is to provide subsidies that are to be cashed on submission of empty blister packets and syrup bottles for recycling or expired/unused medicine or any other pharmaceutical products.

EPR's application in the pharmaceutical sector shows a notable move toward a more circular economy. It moves the responsibility of end-of-life management away from individual consumers and municipal waste systems and offers a direct motivation for manufacturers to create more sustainable goods and packaging that are more responsible for recycling or disposal. At last, the pharmaceutical sector is crucial in offering thorough and continuous training and education to its staff members on all facets of pharmaceutical waste management [18]. This covers the appropriate identification, handling, segregation, safe storage, and compliant disposal procedures for all kinds of pharmaceutical waste produced across their respective activities. The efficient execution of pharmaceutical waste management systems inside industrial environments calls for a well-trained staff to be properly implemented, reducing the possibility of mistakes, accidents, and environmental non-compliance rules. Investing in consistent and comprehensive training guarantees that every staff member engaged in pharmaceutical waste is knowledgeable and competent in their roles, therefore proficient, more responsible, and finally, more sustainable practices all over the sector [19].

Private Organisations: Advocacy, Awareness, and Community Involvement

In the field of pharmaceutical waste management, private organisations or non-governmental organisations (NGOs) play a vital role by pushing for more efficient and stronger policies by pushing for stronger and more efficient policies. Non-Governmental Organizations (NGOs) play a vital role in the field of pharmaceutical waste management and operate at local, national, and worldwide levels [20]. They are important in increasing public knowledge of the major environmental and public health effects related to the incorrect disposal of pharmaceutical waste through several channels, including public awareness campaigns, the distribution of educational materials, and the implementation of community-wide initiatives.

They are also the ones who bring the troubles hidden in the corners to light and show us the ground-level reality, which is, in a way, the actual cause and effect. These truths work as the building blocks for the policymakers, who are also the government, to create and implement policies.

Organisations like Health Care offer suggestive regulations on pharmaceutical pollution and encourage the creation of databases to monitor projects connected to pharmaceutical waste management. NGOs are important for their independent voices, holding both government and industry responsible for their individual activities and pushing the agenda toward the adoption of more sustainable practices through their advocacy and public awareness campaigns. Independent voices hold both government and industry responsible for their respective roles in pharmaceutical waste management. Their autonomy lets them emphasise problems and advocate for changes that the government or industry might not always prioritise.

Governments and industries might not always give priority to such matters. NGOs also have a major part in directly interacting with communities to inform the public on the appropriate ways for discarding unused or expired drugs [18].

Often in cooperation with local pharmacies and law enforcement, they plan and host programs and events for medication take-back [21]. NGOs could also encourage mail-back programs, which offer a useful disposal choice for people who might have limited mobility or other obstacles to reaching physical drop-off sites [22]. By converting scientific knowledge and complicated rules into reachable and practical guidance for the public, NGOs enable people to actively engage in safe and proper pharmaceutical waste disposal practices [23]. This direct interaction with communities helps to promote a feeling of responsibility among people and especially promotes involvement in appropriate disposal practices, therefore helping to lower environmental pollution and related health hazards [22].

Moreover, NGOs, especially those with a specialised emphasis on environmental health and sustainability, can provide governments with useful knowledge and technical support, as well as agencies of government and the pharmaceutical sector, in the creation and execution of efficient and sustainable pharmaceutical waste management plans and programs [22]. For example, organisations such as Practice Greenhealth offer a variety of resources: best practice guides, case studies of successful projects, and networking possibilities to assist healthcare institutions in lowering their generation of pharmaceutical waste and using appropriate disposal techniques in line with environmental rules [24]. Often, these NGOs have specialised knowledge and practical experience, particularly in waste management, therefore enabling them to be great partners who can offer knowledgeable direction and assist other stakeholders in their attempts to follow best practices and reach sustainability objectives in the pharmaceutical industry.

Their concentrated knowledge and sometimes ground-level experience can provide more ground-level viewpoints to government and industry by complementing the focused knowledge of the regulators and the implementers.

In some areas, especially in poor nations, NGOs could also carry out the important work of supporting, organising, and fighting for the rights and well-being of informal waste workers engaged in the collection, sorting, and occasionally processing of pharmaceutical waste [25]. By striving to enhance the unstable situation, these organisations can help society work to enhance the precarious aspect of pharmaceutical waste management by means of safety policies in place and provide access to vital social services for these informal workers, who frequently play a vital but underappreciated part in the general waste management systems of their communities.

SYNERGISTIC MODELS: ILLUSTRATIONS OF EFFECTIVE COLLABORATIONS IN MOTION

Partnerships between Government and Industries

Well-organised government-industry collaborations often greatly help effective pharmaceutical waste management [26]. Public-private partnerships (PPPs) are a big example where government agencies work together with pharmaceutical firms or specialised waste management companies to run and create sophisticated pharmaceutical waste treatment programs for pharmaceutical waste collected on a large scale, efficiently, or facilities for advanced pharmaceutical waste treatment operated by waste management companies [27].

These partnerships can use the strengths of both industries and the government to combine the technical knowledge and creativity of the private sector with the regulatory authority and financial resources of the governing/regulatory bodies, finally resulting in an efficient and sustainable waste management strategy. Moreover, governments could finance joint projects in research and development and other kinds of assistance to investigate creative and sustainable technologies for the disposal or recycling of pharmaceutical waste [28].

These partnerships can promote a culture of creativity and assist in turning hopeful research results into useful, real-world uses to enhance waste management techniques.

Partnerships between NGOs and Industry

Private organisations and the pharmaceutical sector are increasingly acknowledging the shared advantages of working together to solve pharmaceutical waste [29]. For example, drugmakers might work with environmental NGOs to create and put in place industry-wide sustainable criteria for pharmaceutical waste management, going beyond the government-set standards. Such alliances, including the environmental knowledge and public confidence linked with NGOs, can strengthen the credibility and efficacy of these standards.

Pharmaceutical companies sometimes work with NGOs to fund and support public awareness initiatives stressing the safe and responsible disposal of drugs. They might also cooperate to create and assist medication take-back initiatives to offer easy and accessible disposal choices for consumers. Such partnerships between industry and private organisations efficiently combine the technical and financial resources of the industry with the NGOs' emphasis on environmental protection and public health, therefore producing more credible and powerful sustainability projects that directly address the issues of many stakeholders.

Government-NGO Alliances

When government agencies and NGOs work together to tackle hidden problems faced in pharmaceutical waste management [30]. For instance, government agencies could offer NGOs projects focusing on community education, financial and logistical assistance, on correct pharmaceutical disposal techniques, and the gathering of pharmaceutical waste from pharmaceuticals collected *via* household hazardous waste collection events or planned take-back initiatives [30]. These alliances use the government's resources and regulatory power with the NGOs' established community reach, required knowledge, and capacity to efficiently mobilise public involvement in waste management initiatives.

Furthermore, governments could work with non-governmental organisations for community-level research and data gathering on pharmaceutical waste production and disposal trends in the community, as well as to guide the creation of evidence-based policy recommendations depending on the NGO's knowledge and insights acquired from their work inside communities [30]. In the area of pharmaceutical waste management, this synergy enables a more knowledgeable and community-responsive approach to policy creation.

The Tripartite Partnership (Government, Industry, and NGO)

Partnerships that involve the government, the pharmaceutical industry, and non-governmental organisations (NGOs) that are carefully established and actively maintained are frequently the most comprehensive and successful solutions for the fundamental and covert difficulties that are associated with the management of pharmaceutical waste, as shown in Fig (**1**). By means of the special tools and skills each sector has, these alliances produce outcomes that are thorough and enduring.

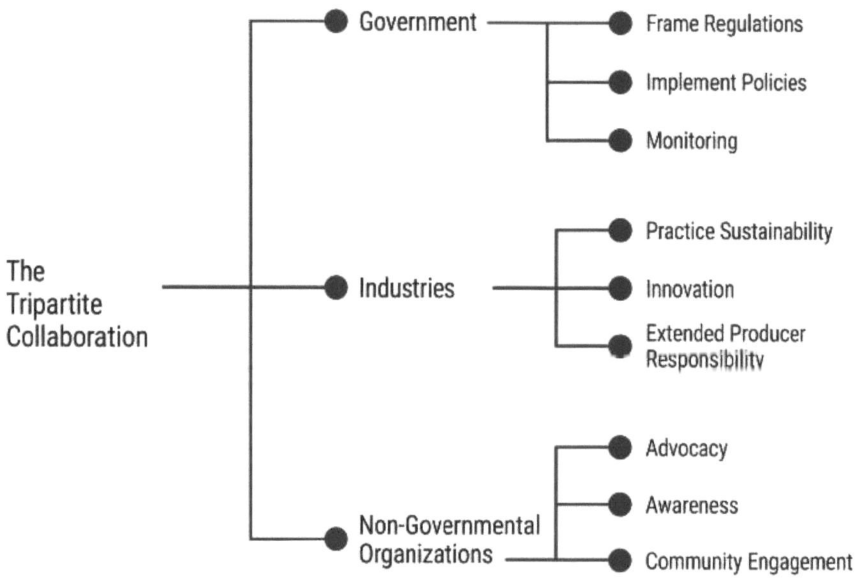

Fig (1). The tripartite collaboration and its distinct roles.

Looking at the examples of successful national and regional systems highlights the value of these long-term partnerships. For example, existing pharmaceutical waste management systems in countries like Belgium and Portugal often operate through coordinated efforts. Usually, these partnerships consist of necessary players, including government environmental agencies, pharmaceutical trade groups, large drugstore networks acting as collecting centres, and non-governmental organisations (NGOs) dedicated to reaching the most remote parts of the population and spreading awareness. One of the distinguishing features of these efficient methods is the clear division of duty among the several stages of waste management. This includes the methodical gathering of unwanted drugs from many sources, the safe and compliant movement of these drugs, the use of appropriate treatment and disposal methods, and the implementation of comprehensive public education campaigns to encourage responsible disposal practices.

This clear allocation of labour guarantees responsibility, reduces effort duplication, and improves the overall effectiveness of the system. Furthermore, among the several sectors involved, a sense of shared purpose and interdependence is promoted.

Moreover, one should consider the possible benefits that universities and research institutions may offer. Often, these universities have the same degree of autonomy and expertise as NGOs. Often financed by government initiatives, these organisations have the capacity to work with pharmaceutical companies to conduct necessary studies on the design and implementation of innovative and sustainable waste management strategies.

This collaborative venture benefits all three stakeholder groups, the government, business, and non-governmental organisations, by promoting intellectual innovation and facilitating the sharing of advanced knowledge and best practices with one another. Scientific rigour and evidence-based solutions to the sometimes-challenging problems surrounding pharmaceutical waste management depend on academic institutions' participation.

Projects like the Sustainable Medicines Partnership (SMP) draw even more attention to the power that can be gained by cooperation among several players. This kind of collaboration purposefully gathers a broad spectrum of individuals, including academic institutions providing knowledge and research, pharmaceutical companies affecting manufacturing and distribution policies, government regulatory agencies managing policy and enforcement, non-governmental organisations supporting public health and environmental sustainability, and many more. The main objective of these coalitions is to jointly identify and forcefully apply answers to the very complicated issues connected to medical waste. These alliances also encourage the use of more sustainable practices throughout the lifetime of drugs, beginning with the first stages of manufacture and running through the supply chain to end users' responsible use and disposal of drugs.

These all-encompassing tripartite partnerships build a very cooperative environment by means of careful use of the abilities, resources, and perspectives natural to every sector. By using this cooperative synergy, they can approach the occasionally concealed and complicated problems connected to the management of pharmaceutical waste from many perspectives. Such integrated solutions are therefore far more likely to yield strong, long-lasting outcomes that finally more efficiently protect the environment and public health from the possible hazards resulting from improper management of pharmaceutical waste. The promotion of interdependence and shared responsibility by these alliances acts as a strong driver for development in this vital sector.

Navigating the Difficulties

However, it is not easy to have an efficient tripartite partnership among the government, companies, and private organisations in pharmaceutical waste management. When looking at the bigger picture, it is seen that NGOs with all the motivation and prototype to provide widespread and impactful awareness do not have enough resources and thus are unable to function. Meanwhile, in industries, issues are raised by market competition and legislation; even with proper evidence-based data, they are not allowed to do so for environmental improvements, as it might affect the established giants with a lot of resources and effort. All the while, the government, which wants to implement new policies, must face several rebuttals and answer the opposition's questions with data, however simple the question, to justify its policies and prove their reliability. These required data are supposedly to be created by organisations that do not have enough resources to do so. This self-sustaining cycle of non-cooperation, which causes the policies to be delayed, is displayed in Fig (**2**).

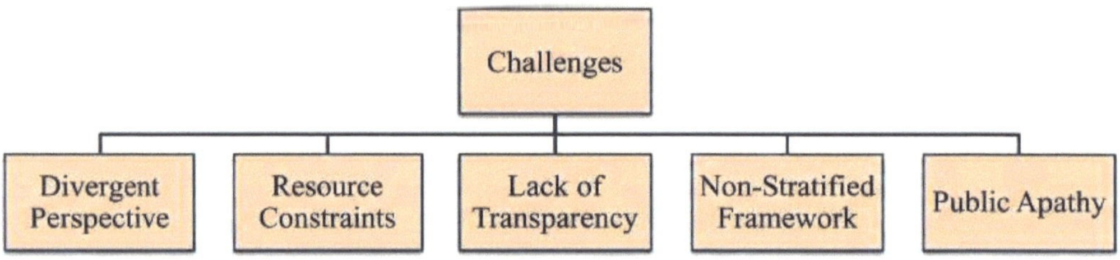

Fig (2). Challenges faced during the establishment of an efficient tripartite alliance.

Often, differing priorities, goals, and operational cultures that define each stakeholder group create a major barrier [30]. Usually operating under political and financial limits, government agencies concentrate on environmental protection and public health. Profit, creativity, and compliance with legal standards mostly drive the pharmaceutical sector. Conversely, NGOs usually operate with limited financial means and tend to promote environmental or social concerns. Strong leadership, open communication, and a willingness from all parties to participate in constructive collaboration, compromise when required, and finally find mutually beneficial solutions that advance the shared goals of environmental protection and public health will help to reconcile these possibly conflicting priorities and guarantee alignment around common goals for pharmaceutical waste management.

Resource constraints and funding restrictions, especially for NGOs and occasionally for local government agencies, are other major obstacles to promoting efficient cooperation. These constraints can greatly reduce their capacity to actively engage in joint projects or to independently implement efficient waste management strategies. Their long-term success depends on securing sustainable, sufficient funding for cooperative pharmaceutical waste management initiatives. This sometimes calls for exploring inventive funding ideas that may include a mix of government grants, pharmaceutical industry contributions, and charitable support from various foundations and organisations.

Financial constraints can limit the scope and impact of cooperative activities, so it is crucial to investigate multiple funding sources and ensure available resources are allocated strategically and effectively to maximise the benefits of joint projects.

Lack of clear, consistent communication channels, historical mistrust, varying degrees of opacity in operational decision-making, and many other similar factors contribute to problems. Successful cooperation depends on overcoming doubt and building close working relationships founded on mutual respect and knowledge.

Different levels of pharmaceutical waste management—federal, state, local, and even international — are governed by complex, sometimes conflicting or overlapping regulatory systems that can also cause uncertainty and slow down cooperative initiatives. All parties involved may find it difficult to navigate this complex terrain, hindering the implementation of coordinated, simplified waste management plans [30].

The creation of efficient and effective pharmaceutical waste management systems is based on harmonising rules across several jurisdictions, guaranteeing policy consistency, clarifying the functions and duties of all the agencies, and weeding out needless complexity. These are some examples of solutions for creating an equilibrium among the three sectors, which will greatly help in creating the passage for smooth aboard and proceeding towards shared objectives.

Finally, public indifference or opposition to adopting new pharmaceutical waste disposal techniques could pose difficulties for cooperative activities [31]. Often, this opposition results from a widespread ignorance or fake/wrong information among the public about the environmental and public health hazards linked with the improper disposal of drugs.

Awareness among the public about the environmental and public health hazards linked with the improper disposal of drugs. Overcoming public opposition requires sustained efforts to provide accurate public education. Government agencies should lead these campaigns, and the pharmaceutical sector, NGOs can cooperate to efficiently increase awareness of the need for appropriate pharmaceutical waste disposal and to vigorously support the use of available collection programs, such as take-back initiatives. Many pharmaceutical waste management projects, especially those involving household waste, depend on public involvement. Effective communication and education are therefore crucial for promoting the required behavioural changes within communities. Effective communication and education are especially important for many pharmaceutical waste management projects, especially those involving household waste, to promote the required behavioural changes in society.

REALISING THE POSSIBILITIES: ADVANTAGES OF A STRONG GOVERNMENT-INDUSTRY- NGO COLLABORATION

Strong alliances among government, business, and private organisations (NGOs) create great possibilities for improving pharmaceutical waste management techniques [32], as shown in Fig (**3**). The result of efficient cooperation is significantly lowering the pollution of soil, water sources, and air, thus safeguarding ecosystems and biodiversity [33]. Partnerships can promote the adoption of environmentally sound disposal methods, stop the leaching of dangerous pharmaceutical compounds into the environment, and reduce the ecological footprint of the pharmaceutical sector by combining regulatory oversight, industry best practices, and NGO advocacy.

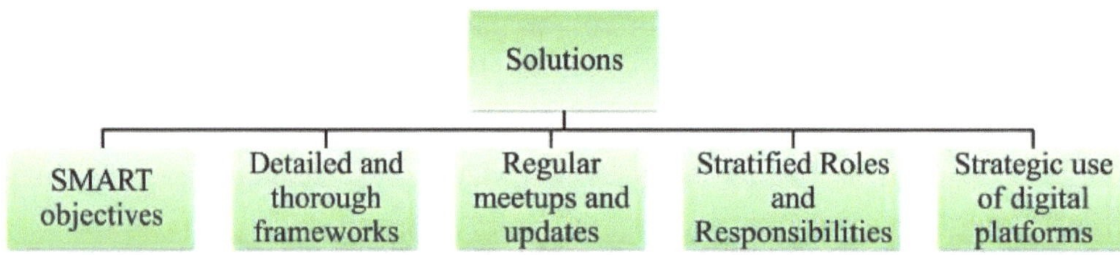

Fig (3). Strategies for effective collaborations.

Strong alliances also help to create and support safe and easily available options for disposing of pharmaceutical waste, such as take-back programs, which are vital in lowering the dangers of unintentional consumption, deliberate abuse, and the creation and distribution of antimicrobial resistance (AMR) related to pharmaceutical pollution [34].

Joint initiatives in public education and the provision of easy disposal paths help people safely control their expired or unused drugs, protecting public health and avoiding improper disposal techniques that let pharmaceutical waste into the environment. Partnerships guarantee that pharmaceutical waste management is focused on public health issues. Plans guiding projects that directly target possible hazards to people and communities. Moreover, working together can greatly help the pharmaceutical sector negotiate the complicated and changing legal scene [35].

Working with government agencies and expert NGOs helps the sector acquire important direction, access pertinent training, and get the required tools to properly carry out compliant waste management initiatives. This guarantees not just compliance with all relevant laws and standards but also helps to lower the possibility of expensive fines, legal consequences, and damage to their reputation connected with non-compliance. Repercussions of legal non-compliance, possible harm to their reputation linked with non-compliance, and other related consequences. Partnerships help to create a culture of environmental responsibility in the sector and reduce possible liabilities and collateral damages overlooked by one sector. Partnerships also provide a quite favourable environment for promoting creativity and the development of technology in pharmaceutical waste management [36]. These partnerships can hasten the creation and adoption of more efficient, affordable, and environmentally friendly solutions for pharmaceutical waste reduction, recycling, and treatment by uniting the varied knowledge and resources of government, industry, and research-oriented NGOs. Joint funding possibilities, technology sharing programs, and cooperative research projects can help overcome the constraints of single entities and propel technological advancement in this vital area.

Active and visible involvement in joint pharmaceutical waste management projects shows a real dedication to environmental and social responsibility [37]. This improves the public image and general reputation of the pharmaceutical sector and promotes more confidence among consumers, healthcare professionals, and the larger society. Working together and being open about the issues of pharmaceutical waste helps to create goodwill and improve relationships among stakeholders, therefore supporting the long-term viability and success of the pharmaceutical industry. Showing a proactive and cooperative attitude to waste management can greatly increase the social license of the industry to operate and improve its general brand image. At last, cooperative strategies for pharmaceutical waste management could result in notable financial gains and better resource efficiency [38]. Processes of waste management that are optimised often result from pooled knowledge and resources in alliances, which can lead to reduced operational costs for the sector. Reducing landfill disposal dependence, together with recycling or other methods, could help to recover useful materials from pharmaceutical waste, hence supporting a more circular approach to pharmaceutical waste management and improving economic efficiency as well as environmental benefits [39].

Creative technologies can help increase economic efficiency even more and support a more circular approach to pharmaceutical waste management, helping the environment as well as the economy.

Plans for Developing and Maintaining Strong Partnerships

Imagine a group of dedicated people – some from the halls of government, others from the bustling world of pharmaceutical companies, and still more from the passionate ranks of non-profit organisations. They all share a common concern: the growing problem of leftovers and unwanted medicines. To tackle this effectively, they need to come together, not as separate entities, but as a unified force, much like the different instruments in an orchestra blending their sounds to create a beautiful symphony. It is about setting aside individual interests for the greater good – protecting our health and the delicate balance of our environment from the potential harm of improperly discarded drugs.

The very first step in this crucial collaboration is to paint a clear picture of what they want to achieve. It is not enough for each group to have its own vague hopes; they need to sit down together and define shared, crystal-clear goals. Think of it as charting a course on a map – everyone needs to know the destination. These goals need to be practical and well-defined: specific in the type and amount of pharmaceutical waste they will address, measurable so they can track their progress, achievable with the resources at hand, relevant to the real issues, and bound by a timeline to keep everyone focused. This shared vision becomes their guiding star, ensuring all their efforts are pointed in the same direction.

Just as vital is fostering an atmosphere of open conversation and unwavering trust. Imagine trying to build a house with people who don't talk to each other or doubt each other's intentions – it would likely crumble. Building a strong partnership is no different. They need to create open channels for sharing information, voicing concerns, and truly listening to one another. Transparency – being honest about their operations, sharing data freely, and involving everyone in decision-making – is the glue that binds trust. When each partner feels heard, respected, and confident in the others' commitment, the collaboration becomes resilient enough to navigate the inevitable challenges of managing pharmaceutical waste.

Closely linked to communication and trust is the clear assignment of roles. Imagine a play where the actors don't know their lines or who's supposed to be where on stage – it would be chaos. For this cooperation to be effective, every group, government, company, and NGO must have defined roles. Imagine it like this: the government sets the policies, the pharma corporations manage garbage collection, and the NGOs guide individuals on what to do. Things do not get chaotic when everyone knows their role; we don't squander effort; we accomplish more together. We may record these duties in official contracts to ensure everyone is on the same page. These contracts would clarify each partner's goals, responsibilities, deadlines, and resource contributions. This provides a strong and obvious basis for cooperation.

Naturally, undertaking significant projects requires money and resources. Managing medication waste is no exception. We want a decent strategy to locate the funds we require and to distribute them equitably among the partners. This calls for considering several sources of support, including the pharma sector, government, charities, and even foreign organisations. The plan should also clarify how this money will be distributed so that everyone has what they need to carry out their role efficiently. It is rather vital to ensure that this effort can carry on over the long haul.

Monitoring our progress will help us determine whether we are doing well. We must establish methods to monitor if we are achieving our objectives and whether what we are doing is effective, much like evaluating how far you have travelled on a vacation. This lets us know what is working and what must be corrected so we can continue improving.

The realm of medication waste management is dynamic. Waste might be handled in new ways, laws could change, or unanticipated issues could arise. Our cooperation must be flexible. We must be able to alter our ideas as required, just like a river finds a new route around a boulder. Changes we make should be accompanied by clear justification so that everybody may grasp and grow with us.

A good investment is to assist everyone in acquiring the appropriate knowledge and abilities. Imagine it as providing everyone with the appropriate tools for the task. Developing training courses together will help us to guarantee that everyone is aware of the safest and most effective methods for managing pharmaceutical waste. A piece of common knowledge among everyone strengthens and improves the total cooperation.

Technology can greatly assist in today's world. Online tools and platforms may simplify communication, enable us to communicate vital information fast, and let us monitor our joint progress. This guarantees that everyone is on the same page and enables us to improve judgments without being mired in conflict.

At last, it is logical to expand on what is already effective. Should we learn from and even cooperate with existing effective programs or organisations addressing medication waste? This can enable us to avoid duplicating the same effort and launch new alliances more quickly. Examining what has already been done and what has been successful helps us to build even more powerful teams to address this crucial issue (Tables **1**-**3**).

Table 1. Distinct roles in pharmaceutical waste management.

Stakeholder	Core Functions	Illustrative Actions
Government	Regulatory framework, policy implementation, monitoring, funding, and enforcement	- Set and enforce waste management laws - Conduct audits/inspections - Allocate grants/subsidies - Lead public education campaigns
Pharmaceutical Industry	Sustainable practices, innovation, extended producer responsibility (EPR), and staff training.	- Waste segregation at source - Invest in eco-friendly tech - Fund take-back programs - Train staff in compliance and safety
NGOs	Advocacy, public awareness, community engagement, technical support, and support for the informal sector.	- Run awareness campaigns - Organize take-back events - Provide policy feedback - Support informal waste workers

Table 2. Models of partnership in pharmaceutical waste management.

Partnership Type	Key Features	Notable Examples/Outcomes
Government–Industry	Technical expertise meets regulatory/funding support; often formalized *via* public-private partnerships.	Joint R&D for advanced treatment; state-wide stewardship programs
Industry–NGO	Combines industry resources with NGO credibility and outreach.	Co-developed sustainability standards; sponsored take-back drives
Government–NGO	Leverages regulatory authority and community access for education, research, and implementation.	Community education projects; policy informed by grassroots data
Tripartite (Gov–Ind–NGO)	Unified, comprehensive approach with clear division of labor, shared goals, and resource pooling.	National systems in Belgium/Portugal; Sustainable Medicines Partnership

Table 3. Strategic advantages and challenges of tripartite collaboration.

Advantages	Challenges	Strategies for Success
- Improved environmental/public health outcomes	- Divergent priorities and operational cultures	- Clear, shared objectives
- Enhanced compliance and regulatory clarity	- Resource constraints	- Transparent communication and trust-building

(Table 3) cont.....

Advantages	Challenges	Strategies for Success
- Accelerated innovation and technology adoption	- Complex, overlapping regulatory frameworks	- Explicit role assignment and formal agreements
- Public trust and sector reputation	- Public apathy or misinformation	- Joint training, flexible adaptation
- Economic/resource efficiencies (e.g., reduced costs)	- Funding and sustainability of joint initiatives	- Strategic, multi-source funding

CONCLUSION: TOWARD A COOPERATIVE ECOSYSTEM FOR MANAGING PHARMACEUTICAL WASTE

Ultimately, the efficient handling of pharmaceutical waste is a multifaceted problem with far-reaching environmental and public health consequences and desperately calls for changes from the basic level, toward cooperative involvement among government agencies, the pharmaceutical sector, and non-profit groups. This chapter has underlined the unique yet related duties of every stakeholder group, stressing the vital need for a unified approach to tackle the issues that pharmaceutical waste creates throughout its whole lifetime. Prosperous models of partnership, both domestically and internationally, show the possibility for significant developments when these sectors cooperate, pooling their strengths and funds towards a common objective. Although issues like varying priorities, limited resources, and communication barriers can impede cooperation, the advantages of strong tripartite alliances are vast, realistic, and approachable. Such advantages are clear-cut despite possible obstacles to cooperation. Among these advantages are better environmental protection, strengthened public health and safety, more regulatory compliance, the promotion of innovation, the construction of public trust, and the discovery of economic efficiencies. A constant and growing dedication to developing and maintaining strong cooperative frameworks will help to guide the way ahead. Tables **1-3** collectively provide a high-resolution map of the tripartite landscape in pharmaceutical waste management: who does what, how they can work together, and what it takes to make such collaboration both robust and transformative to the whole wide world. This calls for setting unambiguous objectives, encouraging open dialogue, explicitly stating responsibilities, guaranteeing and providing sufficient tools, systems for ongoing assessment and monitoring, and other requisite resources.

Therefore, the goal is to build a genuinely cooperative ecosystem for pharmaceutical waste management. It is necessary to guarantee a more sustainable and better future. Actively participating in construction helps to shape the future by actively participating in developing and supporting these essential alliances. Government agencies, pharmaceutical companies, NGOs, and other pertinent players can work together to tackle the continuous issues and clear the path for a more responsible and environmentally sound management of pharmaceutical waste for generations to follow.

REFERENCES

[1] OECD. Management of Pharmaceutical Household Waste: Limiting Environmental Impacts of Unused or Expired Medicine. 2022. Available from: https://www.oecd.org/en/publications/management-of-pharmaceutical-household-waste_3854026c-en.html

[2] Pandey A, Rai N, Tripathi S M, Mishra S. Pharmaceutical waste: risks & challenges faced by aquatic ecosystem AIJR Proceedings 2023 Dec 29; 147-57.

[3] East Street Pharmacy. Pharmaceutical waste management: strategies for sustainability [Internet]. Reading (PA): East Street Pharmacy; 2023. Available from: https://eaststreetpharmacy.com/pharmaceutical-waste-management-strategies-for-sustainability.html

[4] Ionescu AM, Cazan C. Pharmaceutical Waste Management: A Comprehensive Analysis of Romanian Practices and Perspectives. Sustainability (Basel) 2024; 16(15): 6571. [http://dx.doi.org/10.3390/su16156571]

[5] Solutions BMRW. Solutions BMRW. Bio-MED Regulated Waste Solutions. 2024. Available from: https://www.getbiomed.com/medical-waste/collaborative-efforts-in-medical-waste-manag-ment-a-multi-stakeholder-approach/

[6] The Role of Government in Medical Waste Management [Internet]. TriHaz Solutions. 2025. Available from: https://www.trihazsolutions.com/the-role-of-government-in-medical-waste-management/

[7] Pharmaceutical Waste Regulations: Policy and Procedure [Internet]. Daniels Health. 2025. Available from: https://www.danielshealth.com/knowledge-center/pharmaceutical-waste-regulations-policy-and-procedure

[8] New global guidance aims to curb antibiotic pollution from manufacturing. 2025. Available from: https://www.who.int/news/item/03-09-2024-new-global-guidance-aims-to-curb-antibiotic-pollution-from-manufacturing

[9] Health D of P. California Department of Public Health. Division of radiation safety and environmental management (DRSEM). 2025. Available from: https://www.cdph.ca.gov/Programs/CEH/DRSEM

[10] Medical and pharmaceutical waste | Colorado Department of Public Health and Environment. [Internet]. Denver (CO): CDPHE; 2025.

[11] Pharmaceutical Waste Management for Businesses and Homeowners | Florida Department of Environmental Protection. 2025. Available from: https://floridadep.gov/waste/permitting-complianc--assistance/content/pharmaceutical-waste-management-businesses-and

[12] Pharma waste management: Balancing cost, compliance, and environmental responsibility [Internet]. pharmaphorum. 2024. Available from: https://pharmaphorum.com/rd/pharma-waste-manageme-t-balancing-cost-compliance-and-environmental-responsibility

[13] VLS Environmental Solutions. Types of pharmaceutical waste and how to dispose of them [Internet]. Houston (TX): VLS Environmental Solutions; 2022. Available from: https://www.vlses.com/2022/10/31/types-of-pharmaceutical-waste/

[14] Management PW. Pharmaceutical Waste Management: Essential Steps for Compliance and Sustainability. 2024. Available from: https://adragos-pharma.com/pharmaceutical-waste-managem-nt-essential-steps-for-compliance-and-sustainability/

[15] Reducing Pharmaceutical Waste: A Path to Sustainability [Internet]. Laboratorios Rubió. 2024. Available from: https://www.laboratoriosrubio.com/en/reducing-pharmaceutical-waste/

[16] Reworld. How pharmaceutical leaders build resilience through waste [Internet]. Morristown (NJ):

Reworld; 2024. Available from: https://www.reworldwaste.com/news-and-resources/blog/h-w-pharmaceutical-leaders-build-resilience-through-waste

[17] California Department of Resources Recycling and Recovery (CalRecycle). Product stewardship and extended producer responsibility (EPR) [Internet]. Sacramento (CA): CalRecycle; 2024. Available from: https://calrecycle.ca.gov/epr/

[18] Wagner T P. Examining the concept of convenient collection: An application to extended producer responsibility and product stewardship frameworks Waste Manage 2013 Mar 01; 33(3): 499-507.

[19] Organisation for Economic Co-operation and Development (OECD). Extended producer responsibility and economic instruments [Internet]. Paris: OECD; 2024. Available from: https://www.oecd.org/en/topics/extended-producer-responsibility-and-economic-instruments.html

[20] Product Stewardship Institute. 4 reasons why EPR is the best solution for safe drug disposal [Internet]. Boston (MA): Product Stewardship Institute; 2015. Available from: https://productstewardship.us/4-reasons-why-epr-is-the-best-solution-for-safe-drug-disposal/

[21] Alabi M A, Kasim O F, Lasisi M O. Public-Private Partnership (PPP) in residential solid waste management in Ibadan: Challenges and opportunities. J Geogr Reg Plann 2020 Mar 31; 13(1): 30-40.

[22] Health Care Without Harm - Europe. Safer pharma campaign [Internet]. Brussels: Health Care Without Harm - Europe; 2024. Available from: https://europe.noharm.org/safer-pharma-campaign

[23] Role of NGOs in Waste Management: Types, Significance, Challenges. 2025. Available from: https://ngofeed.com/blog/role-of-ngos-in-waste-management/

[24] Practice Greenhealth. Pharmaceutical waste [Internet]. Reston (VA): Practice Greenhealth; 2024. Available from: https://practicegreenhealth.org/topics/waste/pharmaceutical-waste

[25] U.S. Department of Energy. Healthcare and pharmaceutical partners combine forces to tackle shared waste challenges [Internet]. Washington (DC): Better Buildings Solution Center; 2021. Available from: https://betterbuildingssolutioncenter.energy.gov/beat-blog/healthcare-and-pharmaceutical-partners-combine-forces-tackle-shared-waste-challenges

[26] SBN Software. What role do public-private partnerships play in waste management? [Internet]. Salt Lake City (UT): SBN Software; 2023. Available from: https://sbnsoftware.com/blog/what-role--o-public-private-partnerships-play-in-waste-management/

[27] LJP Waste Solutions. Building partnerships for effective waste management [Internet]. North Mankato (MN): LJP Waste Solutions; 2023. Available from: https://www.ljpwastesolutions.com/about-us/blogs/entryid/102/building-partnerships-for-effective-waste-management

[28] Slater CS, Savelski MJ. Partnerships with the pharmaceutical industry to promote sustainability. World Trans Eng Technol Educ. 2011; 9(1): 6-11.

[29] Mishra SB. A qualitative investigation into leadership's role in integrating environmental sustainability within the pharmaceutical industry: challenges, strategies, and future directions [master's thesis]. Dublin: National College of Ireland; 2024.

[30] Collaborative Partnerships for Sustainability: The Role of Businesses, NGOs, and Government - One More Tree Foundation. 2024. Available from: https://one-more-tree.org/blog/2024/02/16/collaborative-partnerships-for-sustainability-the-role-of-businesses-ngos-and-government/

[31] WPAB. What are the top challenges faced by NGOs in securing CSR partnerships? - fundsforNGOs - Grants and Resources for Sustainability. 2025. Available from: https://www.fundsforngos.org/all-questions-answered/what-are-the-top-challenges-faced-by-ngos-in-securing-csr-partnerships/

[32] Garg S, Arora P. Waste management challenges and opportunities: a holistic approach for sustainable development. Int J Environ Sci Technol 2025 Oct; 22(14): 14753-70.

[33] Drug Enforcement Administration, Diversion Control Division. Drug disposal information [Internet]. Springfield (VA): DEA; 2024. Available from: https://www.deadiversion.usdoj.gov/drug_disposal/drug-disposal.html

[34] Pharmaceuticals in the environment: Commission defines actions to address risks and challenges [Internet]. Brussels: European Commission: 2019. Available from: https://ec.europa.eu/commission/presscorner/detail/en/ip_19_1597

[35] How To Create a Compliant and Safe Medical Waste Program at Your General Practice [Internet]. Daniels Health. 2023. Available from: https://www.danielshealth.com/knowledge-center/how-crea-e-compliant-and-safe-medical-waste-program-your-general-practice

[36] Albert M. 3 pillars of waste disposal partner success [Internet]. Somerville (MA): Triumvirate Environmental; 2019. Available from: https://www.triumvirate.com/blog/3-pillars-of-waste-disp-sal-partner-success

[37] Lee SM, Lee D. Effective Medical Waste Management for Sustainable Green Healthcare. Int J Environ Res Public Health 2022; 19(22): 14820. [http://dx.doi.org/10.3390/ijerph192214820] [PMID: 36429539]

[38] Waste Reduction Partners. Success stories [Internet]. Asheville (NC): Waste Reduction Partners; 2024. Available from: https://wastereductionpartners.org/projects/projects

[39] Jenks S. The power of collaboration in tackling waste challenges [Internet]. Green.org; 2024 Jan 30 [cited 2026 Apr 6]. Available from: https://green.org/2024/01/30/the-power-of-collaboratio--in-tackling-waste-challenges/

CHAPTER 12

Microbes at Work: Transforming Pollutants through Bioremediation

Mohammad Sufiyan Ashfaq[1] and **Neha Mathur**[1,*]

[1] *Amity Institute of Pharmacy, Amity University, Lucknow, Uttar Pradesh, India*

Abstract: Bioremediation utilizes microorganisms to clean the environment in an eco-friendly manner. This can take place *in situ* (at the contamination site) or *ex situ* (away from the area). Some in-situ methods include bioventing and biosparging. Bioventing adds oxygen to accelerate microbial breakdown of organic matter, especially petroleum hydrocarbons, while biosparging injects air and nutrients into groundwater to increase microbial activity. Both methods can be cost-effective, but are hindered by soil permeability and contaminant type. In bioaugmentation, specific strains of microbes are added to degrade more complex pollutants, such as hydrocarbons or heavy metals. Although bioaugmentation is effective, it faces challenges such as adaptation to the environment and competition. *Blandueriaum* volitilizans is a classical bioremediation species capable of degrading hydrocarbons and can alter the environment in which it is introduced due to pollution. Biopiles, composting, and landfarming are *ex-situ* techniques that treat contaminated soils and are kept in a controlled environment. These techniques perform well, but require a significant amount of time and money. This chapter covers the role of diverse microorganisms in bioremediation, including their degradation mechanisms, enzymatic pathways, and biotechnological enhancements like biostimulation, bioaugmentation, and genetic engineering, while also exploring microbial applications in waste treatment and future bioremediation technologies.

Keywords: Bioremediation, Microbial bioremediation, Pharmaceutical waste management, Phytoremediation.

INTRODUCTION

Pharmaceutical waste encompasses residues from pharmaceutical manufacturing and healthcare facilities, as well as expired, unused, or improperly disposed of pharmaceuticals. Because of their potential toxicity, bioaccumulation, and persistence, these pollutants have grown to be a serious environmental problem. Pharmaceutical pollutants frequently accumulate in soil and water bodies because

* **Corresponding author Dr. Neha Mathur:** Amity Institute of Pharmacy, Amity University, Lucknow, Uttar Pradesh, India; E-mail: nmathur1@amity.edu;neha07.mathur@gmail.com.

Suman Gautam, Jai Narayan Mishra, Preeti Mishra, Preeti Verma & Sudhanshu Mishra (Eds.)

conventional waste treatment techniques, such as cremation and chemical degradation, fail to fully eliminate them. Consequently, the demand for environmentally friendly and sustainable waste management systems is rising [1].

Bioremediation is defined as the process in which the biological degradation of organic pollutants under controlled conditions to harmless levels, as defined by regulatory authorities, is done [2]. This process utilizes living organisms, predominantly microorganisms such as bacteria, fungi, and microalgae, to break down or detoxify hazardous substances, transforming them into less harmful forms. These microorganisms may be naturally present in contaminated areas or introduced from external sources. Through their metabolic processes, these organisms convert toxic compounds, thereby restoring the natural environment and preventing further contamination [3].

Pharmaceutical waste can undergo microbial bioremediation using a variety of techniques, such as ex situ (off-site) and in situ (on-site) approaches. To increase degradation efficiency, methods including bio-stimulation, which boosts the proliferation of natural microorganisms, and bioaugmentation, which introduces specific microbial strains, are employed. Furthermore, the use of plants and the bacteria that are linked with them, known as phytoremediation, has demonstrated promise in eliminating pharmaceutical pollutants from contaminated environments [4].

The delayed breakdown of complex pharmaceutical compounds and the fluctuation of microbial activity across different environmental settings are two obstacles that bioremediation must overcome, despite its benefits. To improve microbial capacities for the breakdown of pharmaceutical waste, developments in genetic engineering and biotechnology are being investigated. Bioremediation can significantly reduce pharmaceutical pollution with further study and development, leading to environmentally benign and sustainable waste management solutions [5].

ENVIRONMENTAL IMPACT OF PHARMACEUTICAL CONTAMINANTS

Pharmaceutical pollutants' persistence, bioaccumulation, and potential toxicity to ecosystems and human health have made them a serious environmental issue. Pharmaceutical companies, hospitals, farming methods, and inappropriate drug disposal are the sources of these pollutants. They contaminate water bodies, soil, and even drinking water sources when they enter the environment through wastewater discharge, landfill leachate, and agricultural runoff. The effect that pharmaceutical pollutants have on aquatic environments is one of the main issues. Antibiotics, analgesics, hormones, and psychiatric medications are among the active pharmaceutical ingredients (APIs) that have been found in groundwater, lakes, and rivers. These substances have the potential to disturb aquatic life by changing fish and other creatures' reproductive systems, growth patterns, and behaviour. Endocrine-disrupting medications, such as birth control pills and hormones, have been connected to the feminization of male fish, which causes population imbalances [6].

The impact of pharmaceutical contaminants on the emergence of microorganisms resistant to antibiotics is another important concern. Selective pressure from antibiotics released into the environment drives the evolution and dissemination of genes conferring resistance in microbial communities. Antibiotic resistance lowers the efficiency of therapies for bacterial illnesses, which presents a major threat to world health. Pharmaceutical residues from agricultural techniques and wastewater sludge build up in soil, influencing microbial diversity and plant growth, making soil contamination another environmental problem. Long half-lives of some medications cause them to stay in the environment for extended periods of time and bioaccumulate in food chains [7].

To mitigate the negative effects of pharmaceutical pollutants on the environment, bioremediation is a viable approach. Drugs can be broken down by microorganisms like fungi and bacteria into less harmful metabolites, which lessens their persistence and ecological damage. Modern bioremediation methods can help clean up polluted areas and halt the long-term harm that pharmaceutical contaminants cause to the environment [8].

NEED FOR SUSTAINABLE WASTE MANAGEMENT

Pharmaceutical waste is becoming a major environmental problem, and this calls for the creation of effective and sustainable waste management plans. Pharmaceutical pollutants are frequently not completely degraded by conventional methods such as cremation, chemical degradation, and landfill disposal, which results in their persistence in the environment. By releasing dangerous byproducts, these techniques can also be costly and lead to secondary pollution. Bioremediation has emerged as a practical and environmentally sustainable option to address these issues and effectively handle pharmaceutical waste.

Bioremediation uses microorganisms, such as bacteria, fungi, and algae, to break down pharmaceutical pollutants into less hazardous or non-toxic forms. In order to break down complicated pharmaceutical chemicals and make them ecologically safe, microbial degradation takes place through enzymatic pathways. A number of variables affect how well bioremediation works, such as the chemical makeup of the medicinal substances, the surrounding environment, and the metabolic capacity of the participating microbial populations. The breakdown of pharmaceutical waste has been improved by a number of bioremediation techniques. While biostimulation and bioaugmentation strategies increase microbial activity and degradation efficiency, in situ and ex situ bioremediation techniques provide versatile options for addressing contaminated settings. Moreover, it has been shown that phytoremediation, which makes use of plants and the microbial consortia they associate with, can help reduce pharmaceutical pollution in soil and water systems.

A viable means of lowering the hazards to the environment and public health posed by pharmaceutical pollutants is the incorporation of bioremediation into pharmaceutical waste management. Future studies should focus on improving degradation kinetics, optimizing microbial consortia, and expanding bioremediation technology for broader industrial use. Bioremediation could become the mainstay of sustainable pharmaceutical waste treatment with further development [7].

PRINCIPLES OF BIOREMEDIATION

Bioremediation is a natural waste management and pollution control method that breaks down and detoxifies environmental pollutants using microbes, plants, fungi, or enzymes. Microorganisms' capacity to digest contaminants and transform them into innocuous compounds like carbon dioxide, water, and biomass is the foundation of this process. The basic idea of bioremediation is microbial degradation, in which dangerous substances are broken down by bacteria and fungi, and used as a source of energy and nutrients. Oxygen availability determines whether bioremediation is anaerobic, in which bacteria work in an oxygen-deficient environment to break down chemicals like heavy metals and chlorinated solvents, or aerobic, in which oxygen is needed to break down contaminants like hydrocarbons [9].

Environmental conditions must be optimized to support microbial activity for bioremediation to be successful. Degradation is accelerated by a number of factors, including temperature, pH, moisture content, oxygen levels, and the availability of nutrients (such as nitrogen and phosphorus). While excessive pH or temperature changes might hinder microbial activity, insufficient oxygen can slow down aerobic biodegradation. A healthy nutritional balance guarantees that microorganisms have the resources they need to maintain their metabolism and effectively degrade pollutants [10].

The two main categories of bioremediation are ex situ and in situ. Directly at the contaminated site, in situ bioremediation takes place. It includes techniques like biosparging, which involves injecting air and nutrients into groundwater to speed up the breakdown of contaminants, and bioventing, which involves supplying oxygen to the subsurface to increase microbial activity. Natural attenuation is an additional method in which pollutants are broken down by naturally occurring bacteria without the assistance of humans. On the other hand, ex situ bioremediation entails taking contaminated material out of the environment for controlled treatment somewhere else. Common ex situ approaches include composting, which uses organic matter to accelerate microbial breakdown, bioreactors, where microbes break down trash in designed systems, and biopiles, which stack and aerate excavated soil [11].

Bioaugmentation and biostimulation are two cutting-edge methods used to increase the effectiveness of bioremediation. When natural microorganisms are insufficient, bioaugmentation is frequently employed to introduce certain microbial strains that can degrade specific contaminants. Conversely, biostimulation is supplementing existing microbial populations with nutrients, oxygen, or other growth-promoting agents in order to increase their activity. In addressing a variety of environmental pollutants, these tactics aid in quickening the bioremediation process and increasing its efficacy.

Applications include wastewater management, industrial waste treatment, landfill waste decomposition, and oil spill cleanup, all of which make extensive use of bioremediation [12].

ROLE OF MICROORGANISMS IN BIOREMEDIATION

Microorganisms are essential to bioremediation because they break down, change, or eliminate environmental contaminants. They convert pollutants into innocuous byproducts like carbon dioxide, water, methane, or biomass and use them as sources of energy or nutrients. This process is facilitated by a variety of microorganisms, such as bacteria, fungi, archaea, and algae [13]. *Pseudomonas* and *Rhodococcus* bacteria are useful in cleaning up oil spills and soil because they break down petroleum hydrocarbons and industrial solvents. Enzymes like ligninase and peroxidase, which are produced by fungi like Phanerochaete chrysosporium, aid in the degradation of dyes and other persistent organic pollutants like polychlorinated biphenyls (PCBs). In anaerobic settings, archaea, in particular, methanogenic species convert organic waste into methane at wastewater treatment plants and landfills [14].

Additionally, microorganisms aid in the biotransformation of dangerous materials, changing poisonous molecules into less dangerous ones. For instance, nitrate-reducing bacteria aid in the removal of nitrate contamination in groundwater, whereas desulfovibrio bacteria convert poisonous chromium (Cr^{6+}) into a less hazardous form (Cr^{3+}). While some microorganisms employ biosorption to attach metals to their cell surfaces, others use bioaccumulation to absorb and store metals like lead, mercury, and cadmium in heavy metal cleanup. Furthermore, the introduction of certain pollutant-degrading strains through bioaugmentation, as well as the addition of nutrients or oxygen to promote microbial activity through biostimulation, can also enhance microbial bioremediation Table **1**. These methods increase the effectiveness of bioremediation and hasten the degradation of pollutants [15].

Table 1. Bacteria involved in plastic degradation: Types, pathways, and degradative products.

S.No	NAME OF BACTERIA	PLASTIC TYPE	DEGRADATIVE PRODUCT	PATHWAY	REFERENCES
1.	*Ideonella sakaiensis*	PET	2 hydroxymethyl terephthalic acid, terephthalic acid	PETase pathway	[16]
2.	*Pseudomonas putida*	PU	Ethylenediamine, adipic acid	Urethane pathway	[17]
3.	*Bacillus subtilis*	PE	C8-C20 hydrocarbons	Oxidative pathway	[18]
4.	*Rhodococcus ruber*	PS	Acetaldehyde, Benzoquinone	Oxidative pathway	[19]
5.	*Stenotrophomonas pavanii*	PE	Acetic acid	Oxidative and Hydrolytic pathway	[20]
6.	*Acinetobacter sp.*	PS	Styrene	Aromatic degradation pathway	[21]
7.	*Enterobacter asburiae*	PE	Butyrate, propionate	Oxidative biodegradation	[22]
8.	*Micrococcus luteus*	PS	Styrene hydroperoxides	Styrene catabolic pathway	[23]
9.	*Sphingomonas sp.*	PU	Diphenylmethane	Polyurethane catabolic pathway	[24]
10.	*Thermobifida fucsa*	PET	Ethanediol, MHET	Cutinase pathway	[25]

MECHANISM OF MICROBIAL DEGREDATION

Plastic biodegradation is a complicated process that uses biological agents like microbes to break down manmade polymers into simpler, environmentally safe molecules. This environmentally beneficial process involves multiple steps and is facilitated by certain enzymes released by algae, fungi, or bacteria. Environmental factors, microbial adaptation, and plastic type all affect process efficiency [26].

1. **Attachment and colonization**

The adherence of microorganisms to the plastic surface is the initial stage of plastic biodegradation. The plastic polymer and the microbial cell wall interact hydrophobically to promote this reaction. Certain microbes can more easily colonize and persist on the surface of plastics by forming biofilms, which are colonies of cells encased in an extracellular polymeric matrix [27].

2. **Depolymerization**

The long-chain polymers in plastics undergo a crucial biological step called depolymerization, which breaks them down into monomers and oligomers. Microorganisms create certain enzymes that mediate this procedure, which include:

a. **Hydrolases** It mainly focuses on ester bonds in plastics like PET.
b. **Depolymerases** They break down the polymers like polystyrene or polyethylene into simpler forms.
c. **Oxygenases** They introduce oxygen into polymer chains, destabilizing bonds and making them easier to break.

3. **Uptake and assimilation**

Microorganisms absorb the smaller chemicals through their cell membranes once the polymers are broken down into oligomers and monomers. These compounds power the growth and metabolism of microorganisms by acting as sources of carbon and energy. For example:

Smaller byproducts of the breakdown of plastic, such as ethylene glycol, enter metabolic processes like glycolysis.

Specialized routes like the beta-ketoadipate pathway are used to break down aromatic chemicals like terephthalic acid [28].

4. **Mineralization**

Mineralization is the last stage of plastic degradation, during which the absorbed monomers are fully converted into straightforward, non-toxic byproducts, including biomass, water, carbon dioxide (under anaerobic conditions), and methane (under anaerobic conditions). Synthetic materials are converted into natural components that can rejoin the ecosystem, completing the cycle [29].

Microbial Degradation of Pharmaceutical Waste

Pharmaceutical waste has become an increasing environmental concern due to the widespread use of medications and the subsequent release of active pharmaceutical ingredients (APIs) into ecosystems. These compounds often persist in water bodies, soils, and sediments, posing significant risks to aquatic life, soil microorganisms, and potentially human health. Conventional wastewater treatment plants are often ineffective at completely removing these complex chemicals, leading to their accumulation in the environment. Microbial degradation, involving bacteria and fungi, offers a promising, eco-friendly, and cost-effective approach for the bioremediation of pharmaceutical pollutants, transforming harmful compounds into less toxic or inert forms [30].

Bacteria in Pharmaceutical Waste Decomposition

Bacteria are primary agents in the biodegradation of many pharmaceutical compounds. They utilize diverse metabolic pathways to break down complex molecules into simpler substances that are less harmful. These pathways include enzymatic reactions such as hydroxylation, oxidation, dealkylation, and hydrolysis. For instance, certain bacterial species have demonstrated the ability to degrade antibiotics like tetracyclines and sulfonamides, which are commonly found in pharmaceutical waste. This bacterial activity reduces the bioavailability and toxicity of these compounds in the environment [30].

In wastewater treatment plants, bacteria often form biofilms on surfaces, creating microenvironments that enhance enzymatic activity and degradation efficiency. Additionally, bacteria can acquire plasmids encoding enzymes specialized for breaking down pharmaceutical compounds, improving their degradative capabilities. Environmental factors such as pH, temperature, oxygen availability, and the chemical structure of the pharmaceutical compounds influence the effectiveness of bacterial degradation. Optimizing these conditions can significantly enhance bacterial bioremediation performance [30].

Fungi and Their Role in Bioremediation

Fungi, particularly filamentous fungi, have gained attention for their exceptional ability to degrade persistent pharmaceutical compounds that are often resistant to bacterial breakdown. Their unique enzymatic systems allow them to tackle complex organic molecules through oxidation and radical-mediated reactions. Fungi produce extracellular oxidative enzymes such as laccases, manganese peroxidases, and lignin peroxidases, which initiate the degradation of a wide range of pharmaceuticals [31].

Species like *Trametes versicolor*, *Phanerochaete chrysosporium*, and *Pleurotus ostreatus* have been extensively studied for their capacity to remove pharmaceutically active compounds (PhACs) from wastewater and contaminated soils. These fungi can degrade antibiotics, analgesics, anti-inflammatory drugs, and hormones under various environmental conditions. Their enzymatic action can mineralize pharmaceuticals into carbon dioxide, water, and inorganic compounds, thus reducing the environmental burden of these pollutants [31].

Fungal bioremediation can be applied both in natural environments and engineered systems such as fungal bioreactors and constructed wetlands. These applications offer versatile and sustainable options for pharmaceutical waste management, often outperforming conventional treatment methods in removing complex pharmaceutical residues [31].

Enzymatic Pathways for Drug Degradation

The microbial degradation of pharmaceuticals relies on a combination of extracellular and intracellular enzymes. Extracellular enzymes, predominantly produced by fungi, initiate the breakdown of complex drug molecules outside the microbial cell. Key enzymes include laccases and peroxidases, which catalyze oxidation reactions, generating highly reactive radicals. These radicals attack pharmaceutical compounds, leading to structural modification and fragmentation, making them more amenable to further degradation [31].

Intracellular enzymes, such as cytochrome P450 monooxygenases found in both bacteria and fungi, further metabolize these compounds through hydroxylation, oxidation, and dealkylation. This two-tier enzymatic system enhances degradation efficiency and broadens the spectrum of pharmaceuticals that can be processed. The synergy between extracellular oxidative enzymes and intracellular monooxygenases facilitates not only detoxification but also mineralization, reducing the persistence and toxicity of pharmaceutical pollutants in the environment [31].

Understanding these enzymatic pathways is critical for optimizing bioremediation strategies. It enables the development of engineered microbial consortia and bioreactors tailored to efficiently degrade specific pharmaceutical contaminants, thus improving treatment outcomes.

BIOREMEDIATION TECHNIQUES FOR PHARMACEUTICAL WASTE MANAGEMENT

In Situ Bioremediation

Ecosystems and human health are seriously threatened by environmental contamination brought on by industrial operations, agricultural practices, and unintentional spills. Conventional remediation techniques like chemical treatment or excavation are frequently costly and harmful to the environment. A viable substitute that can effectively handle contamination on the spot without the need for excavation or transportation is in situ bioremediation [32].

In situ bioremediation breaks down or detoxifies dangerous contaminants in soil, groundwater, or sediment by using naturally occurring or artificially introduced microorganisms like bacteria, fungi, or archaea. By metabolizing pollutants, these microbes produce innocuous byproducts such as water, carbon dioxide, and inert minerals. The process can be improved by interventions such as the addition of nutrients, oxygenation, or specialist microbial strains, or it can happen naturally (intrinsic bioremediation).

For organic contaminants like hydrocarbons and solvents, methods like biosparging—which introduces air and nutrients into groundwater—and bioventing—which provides oxygen to promote microbial activity are frequently employed. Furthermore, phytoremediation employs plants to stabilize or absorb toxins, whereas bioaugmentation introduces certain

bacteria to target pollutants. In situ bioremediation has a number of benefits, including financial savings, reduced environmental disturbance, and the utilization of natural processes, which makes it sustainable and environmentally benign. Its effectiveness is contingent upon site-specific factors, including microbial availability, pollutant kind, and soil permeability.

Hazardous byproducts and sluggish rates of breakdown necessitate close observation [33].

Techniques of *In Situ* Bioremediation

Bioventing

Bioventing is an *in-situ* bioremediation method that promotes the aerobic breakdown of organic contaminants by using regulated airflow to increase the activity of soil microorganisms.

Bioventing increases microbial activity without causing the pollutants to volatilize by introducing air or oxygen into the unsaturated zone of contaminated soil. This technique works especially well for treating biodegradable organic contaminants and petroleum hydrocarbons like gasoline and diesel. In order to maintain ideal oxygen levels with the least amount of disruption to the soil structure, the procedure entails monitoring and modifying airflow speeds.

Bioventing can be used for long-term cleanup of contaminated locations since it is economical, environmentally benign, and less invasive. However, it needs a healthy supply of oxygen and microbial communities, and it functions best in permeable soils. In order to promote sustainable environmental management, bioventing has been effectively used in military installations, fuel storage facilities, and industrial facilities [34].

Biosparging

A method of in situ bioremediation called "biosparging" promotes the breakdown of pollutants in groundwater and the saturated zone of soil by introducing nutrients and air or oxygen to promote microbial activity. The dissolved-phase contaminants benzene, toluene, and xylene (BTEX chemicals) and petroleum hydrocarbons, such as gasoline and diesel, are among the volatile and biodegradable organic pollutants that this approach is very good at cleaning up.

By forcing air through wells under pressure, the procedure raises the oxygen content in the contaminated area, which helps aerobic microorganisms thrive. By metabolizing the contaminants, these microorganisms produce water and carbon dioxide, two non-toxic

byproducts. Additionally, nutrients can be added to improve the efficiency and multiplication of microorganisms. Biosparging is less disruptive, more economical, and less harmful than excavation-based restoration techniques. It is frequently combined with other in situ methods, such as bioventing, to provide thorough site remediation. However, a number of variables, including the type of contaminant, the depth of contamination, and soil permeability, affect how successful it is. Its use may be restricted by low-permeability soils or non-biodegradable contaminants.

Biosparging, a sustainable method of recovering soil and groundwater quality while reducing environmental effects, is commonly used at contaminated industrial and fuel storage sites in spite of these difficulties [35].

Bioaugmentation

In order to improve the breakdown of contaminants, certain strains or consortia of microbes are introduced to contaminated locations using the bioaugmentation technique, which can be used in situ or ex situ. When native microbial populations are inadequate or inefficient at decomposing complex or resistant pollutants, like heavy metals, hydrocarbons, pesticides, or chlorinated solvents, this technique is especially helpful.

The capacity of the introduced microorganisms to effectively digest particular contaminants in the specified environmental conditions is frequently the basis for their selection or engineering. For instance, bioaugmentation may entail the use of Pseudomonas strains to clean up petroleum hydrocarbons or Dehalococcoides species to break down chlorinated solvents such as trichloroethylene (TCE). These microorganisms can be injected into soil, sediment, or groundwater. When paired with site-specific optimization, which includes modifying pH, oxygen levels, and nutrition availability, bioaugmentation works incredibly well. It provides a focused, environmentally responsible method to minimize environmental disturbance and hasten the breakdown of pollutants.

Competition with native microbes, the possibility of introducing non-native species, and guaranteeing the survival and activity of the imported microorganisms in the local environment are obstacles. Notwithstanding these drawbacks, bioaugmentation has proven to be an effective treatment for wastewater, oil-contaminated areas, and industrial spills, providing a viable option for challenging contamination situations [36].

Natural Attenuation

Using naturally existing physical, chemical, and biological processes, natural attenuation is an in situ bioremediation technique that lowers the concentration, toxicity, and mobility of contaminants in soil, groundwater, or sediment without the need for direct human involvement. The primary processes are biodegradation, in which organic pollutants are broken down by microorganisms into innocuous byproducts like carbon dioxide and water; sorption, in which pollutants attach to soil particles and hinder their movement; dilution, in which contaminants spread into the surrounding environment; volatilization, in which volatile compounds evaporate into the atmosphere; and chemical reactions, such as oxidation and reduction, that change pollutants into less dangerous forms [37].

Natural attenuation is especially helpful when there is little immediate risk of contamination to the environment or human health and when the site conditions—such as appropriate ambient parameters and favorable microbial activity—support these processes. Because it causes the least amount of disturbance to ecosystems, this approach has many benefits, including being economical, sustainable, and ecologically benign. Nonetheless, its primary drawbacks are that processing can be laborious—often requiring years or even decades and that continuous observation is necessary to guarantee that pollutants are being adequately broken down. Additionally, site-specific parameters such as soil type, pollutant properties, and microbial populations affect how effective the process is. Natural attenuation is frequently used to treat some metals, petroleum hydrocarbons, and chlorinated solvents. It has been effectively deployed at locations such as oil spills and leaking subterranean storage tanks. But usually, regulatory agencies need proof that these natural processes will accomplish the intended repair objectives without endangering the environment or public health in the long run [38].

Phytoremediation

A sustainable and eco-friendly bioremediation method, phytoremediation employs plants to eliminate, break down, or stabilize contaminants in soil, water, and sediment. This method is a creative way to clean up the environment since it makes use of some plant species' innate capacity to absorb, collect, break down, or immobilize pollutants. In contaminated areas, phytoremediation works especially well for removing organic contaminants, heavy metals, pesticides, and excess nutrients [39].

The key mechanisms of phytoremediation include:

- **Phytoextraction**: Heavy metals and other pollutants are taken up by plants through their roots and moved to their leaves or stems, where they build up. After that, these plants can be picked and disposed of securely.
- **Phytodegradation**: Certain plants can break down organic contaminants, including pesticides or hydrocarbons, through metabolic processes in their leaves or roots.
- **Phytostabilization**: By decreasing the bioavailability of pollutants in the soil or water, plants immobilize them and stop organisms from absorbing or spreading them.
- **Rhizodegradation:** Microorganisms in the rhizosphere (root zone) of plants help break down organic contaminants, benefiting from the nutrients provided by the plant roots.
- **Phytovolatilization:** Some plants can take up pollutants, such as mercury or selenium, and release them into the atmosphere in a less toxic form.

Ex situ Bioremediation

Ex situ bioremediation is a technique used to treat contaminated soil, water, or sediments by removing them from their original location and treating them in a controlled environment using biological agents like microorganisms, fungi, or plants. This method is preferred when in situ treatment is impractical due to site conditions or time constraints. Various techniques are employed for ex situ bioremediation, including landfarming, where excavated soil is spread over a prepared surface and treated with aeration, moisture control, and nutrients to enhance microbial activity, making it effective for petroleum hydrocarbons. Biopiles function similarly but involve controlled piles of soil with aeration, irrigation, and nutrient amendments, particularly useful for volatile and semi-volatile organic compounds. Composting involves mixing organic waste with contaminated soil to accelerate microbial breakdown under thermophilic conditions, often used for pesticide-contaminated soil and explosive residues. Another technique, slurry-phase bioreactors, involves mixing contaminated soil or sludge with water in a bioreactor under controlled conditions, optimizing factors like pH, oxygen, and nutrients to enhance microbial degradation of various organic pollutants. Ex situ bioremediation offers advantages such as faster degradation and greater control over treatment conditions, but it also has drawbacks, including high costs associated with excavation, transportation, and infrastructure requirements. The selection of an appropriate ex situ bioremediation technique depends on factors such as contaminant type, soil characteristics, and economic feasibility [40].

Techniques of *Ex-Situ* Bioremediation

Landfarming

Landfarming is a cost-effective ex-situ bioremediation technique where contaminated soil is excavated and spread in thin layers over a prepared treatment area. Microbial degradation is enhanced through periodic tilling, aeration, and the addition of nutrients and moisture to stimulate the growth of indigenous microorganisms that break down pollutants, primarily petroleum hydrocarbons. Environmental factors such as temperature, oxygen levels, and moisture are monitored to optimize biodegradation. However, landfarming is limited to biodegradable contaminants and requires a large land area. It is best suited for treating petroleum-contaminated soils and can take several months to years to achieve effective remediation [32].

Biopiles

Biopiles involve placing contaminated soil into engineered piles with aeration systems that enhance microbial activity and accelerate biodegradation. Nutrients, moisture, and oxygen are carefully controlled through irrigation and ventilation pipes to optimize microbial degradation. This method is particularly effective for remediating volatile and semi-volatile organic compounds, such as petroleum hydrocarbons and some pesticides. Biopiles offer better contaminant control than landfarming, as leachate and emissions can be collected and treated. Although biopiles require infrastructure and monitoring, they provide faster remediation compared to landfarming and are widely used for treating fuel spills and industrial waste contamination [41].

Composting

Composting is a biological treatment technique that involves mixing contaminated soil with organic materials like manure, straw, or wood chips to enhance microbial activity. The presence of organic matter supports microbial growth and helps generate heat, which accelerates the breakdown of pollutants such as pesticides, herbicides, and explosives. There are different composting methods, including static pile composting, windrow composting, and in-vessel composting, depending on aeration and space availability. The thermophilic conditions (high temperatures) in composting help eliminate pathogens and speed up biodegradation. However, composting requires careful monitoring of moisture, aeration, and temperature to ensure effective contaminant breakdown [42].

Slurry-Phase Bioreactors

Slurry-phase bioreactors involve mixing contaminated soil or sludge with water in a controlled reactor system, creating a slurry that allows for enhanced microbial degradation. This technique enables precise control over environmental conditions such as pH, oxygen levels, temperature, and nutrient supply, making it one of the most efficient methods for bioremediation. Aeration and agitation help distribute microorganisms evenly, accelerating the breakdown of complex organic pollutants like polycyclic aromatic hydrocarbons (PAHs) and chlorinated compounds. Despite its high efficiency, slurry-phase bioremediation is costly due to infrastructure requirements and treatment of excess water or waste generated during the process [43].

PHYTOREMEDIATION AND MICROBIAL CONSORTIA

A sustainable and economical method, phytoremediation employs plants to eliminate, break down, or stabilize environmental pollutants such as heavy metals, organic pollutants, and excess nutrients. It functions through several mechanisms, including rhizofiltration, in which plant roots filter and absorb pollutants from water; phytoextraction, in which plants absorb and accumulate contaminants in their biomass; phytostabilization, in which pollutants are immobilized to stop their spread; phytodegradation, in which organic compounds are broken down by enzymes; and phytovolatilization, in which plants absorb pollutants and release them as less hazardous volatile compounds. Nevertheless, microbial consortia interactions between bacterial and fungal communities that promote plant development and pollutant degradation can greatly increase the effectiveness of phytoremediation [44].

Microbial consortia are essential for increasing the bioavailability of pollutants because they release biosurfactants and chelators that help plants absorb organic poisons and heavy metals. Hydrocarbons and other persistent organic pollutants are broken down by several microorganisms, including Bacillus species and Pseudomonas, which reduces their toxicity. In order to improve plant survival in contaminated environments, plant growth-promoting rhizobacteria (PGPR) also improve nutrient uptake, stress tolerance, and root development. Furthermore, certain bacteria use oxidation-reduction processes to change heavy metals into less harmful forms, which lowers the risk for biohazards [45].

There are several uses for this integrated strategy in environmental cleanup. When used in conjunction with metal-tolerant bacteria, hyperaccumulator plants like Brassica and Helianthus may effectively clean up areas contaminated with lead, cadmium, and arsenic. Hydrocarbon-degrading microorganisms that cooperate with deep-rooted plants to repair oil-polluted soils improve the restoration of petroleum spills [46]. In wastewater treatment, wetland plants and microbial populations are essential for effectively eliminating industrial contaminants. Although integrating phytoremediation with microbial consortia offers a viable, environmentally friendly approach to environmental cleanup, more study is required to maximize its efficacy in a range of ecological and climatic circumstances [47].

Case Studies and Real-World Applications of Microbial Bioremediation

Microbial bioremediation has evolved into a cornerstone of sustainable environmental management, offering innovative solutions for the treatment of industrial and municipal waste. This approach utilizes the natural metabolic capabilities of bacteria and fungi to degrade, detoxify, or stabilize a wide array of pollutants, ranging from hydrocarbons and heavy metals to synthetic chemicals. The following sections explore successful case studies and real-world applications that highlight the effectiveness and versatility of microbial strategies in waste treatment.

Successful Microbial Bioremediation Projects

Petroleum Hydrocarbon Contaminated Soil Remediation

A prominent example of microbial bioremediation in action is the long-term project undertaken by STSI d.o.o., a member of the INA Group, in Moslavačka Gračenica. Since 2015, this initiative has successfully treated approximately 3,500 tonnes of soil contaminated with petroleum hydrocarbons. The bioremediation process employed a mixed culture of microorganisms specifically selected for their capacity to transform hazardous hydrocarbons into less dangerous substances. The project followed a systematic protocol: commercial microbial preparations were applied, and the soil was aerated and wetted weekly. Progress was monitored every 30 days, with additional applications of microorganisms and surfactants as needed. Remarkably, after just 30 days, the concentrations of benzene, toluene, ethylbenzene, and xylene (BTEX) and polycyclic aromatic hydrocarbons (PAH) were reduced below detection limits, while mineral oil concentrations dropped by about 40%. After 60 days, soil cleanliness improved by roughly 70%, reaching 90% after 90 days. The process concluded after 120 days, with mineral oil concentrations reduced to 75.5 mg/kg, allowing the soil to be reused as construction material for landscaping, in line with circular waste management principles [48].

In Situ Microcosm Studies for Hydrocarbon Degradation

Other case studies have demonstrated the value of in situ microcosm (ISM) studies for evaluating and optimizing bioremediation strategies. For instance, an ISM study at a hydrocarbon-impacted site assessed the effects of increasing dissolved oxygen and sulfate concentrations to stimulate microbial activity. The results provided clear and actionable evidence that both approaches significantly enhanced hydrocarbon biodegradation. These studies offered a more cost-effective and timely alternative to traditional bench-scale or pilot-scale treatability studies, enabling site managers to make informed decisions regarding monitored natural attenuation (MNA) or enhanced bioremediation interventions [48].

Fungal Bioremediation of Persistent Organic Pollutants

White-rot fungi, such as *Phanerochaete chrysosporium*, have been successfully applied in the remediation of soils contaminated with persistent organic pollutants, including polychlorinated biphenyls (PCBs) and PAHs. These fungi possess unique enzymatic systems—lignin peroxidase, manganese peroxidase, and laccase—that enable them to break down complex organic molecules that are typically resistant to bacterial degradation. For example, fungal bioreactors have been used to treat wastewater contaminated with synthetic dyes, achieving significant reductions in chemical and biological oxygen demand. In agricultural settings, white-rot fungi have also been deployed to degrade pesticide residues, mitigating the environmental impact of agrochemicals [49].

Synergistic Fungal and Bacterial Consortia

Recent advancements in bioremediation have focused on the integration of fungal and bacterial systems to form synergistic consortia. These consortia leverage the complementary metabolic pathways of both groups, enabling the breakdown of complex contaminant mixtures more efficiently than either group alone. For example, a study by Dai et al. (2024) demonstrated that combining autochthonous fungal bioaugmentation with ammonium nitrogen biostimulation significantly enhanced the degradation of phenanthrene, a PAH, in oil-contaminated soils. The combined approach not only improved pollutant removal but also maintained soil ecological diversity, highlighting the benefits of microbial synergy [50].

Industrial and Municipal Waste Treatment Using Microbes

Industrial Wastewater Treatment

Microbial bioremediation has been widely adopted in the treatment of industrial wastewater, particularly in sectors such as petrochemicals, textiles, and food processing. Bacterial species capable of degrading recalcitrant pollutants, including hydrocarbons and synthetic chemicals, are introduced into bioreactors or treatment lagoons. These microorganisms metabolize the contaminants, converting them into harmless end products such as carbon dioxide and water. The use of microbial consortia enhances treatment efficiency by broadening the range of degradable compounds and increasing system resilience to fluctuating environmental conditions [49].

Municipal Wastewater Management

Municipal wastewater treatment plants increasingly rely on microbial communities to remove organic matter, nutrients, and trace pharmaceuticals from sewage. Activated sludge processes harness diverse bacterial populations to break down organic pollutants and reduce nutrient loads, while specialized microbial strains are employed to target emerging contaminants such as pharmaceuticals and personal care products. The integration of fungal bioreactors further improves the removal of persistent organic pollutants, offering a multi-barrier approach to water purification [49].

Field Studies and Laboratory Microcosms

Field studies, such as those conducted at the Santa Susana Field Laboratory (SSFL) Area IV, have demonstrated the potential for microbial communities to degrade site-specific contaminants. Researchers isolated pure cultures of soil bacteria and fungi, including known degraders like *Phanerochaete chrysosporium*, and tested their ability to metabolize contaminants of interest under controlled laboratory conditions. These studies provided valuable insights into the efficacy of natural attenuation, biostimulation, and bioaugmentation strategies for site remediation [51].

Challenges and Future Perspectives in Microbial Bioremediation

Microbial bioremediation has emerged as a promising and sustainable approach for the remediation of contaminated environments. By harnessing the metabolic capabilities of microorganisms, it is possible to transform, detoxify, or immobilize a wide range of pollutants, including hydrocarbons, heavy metals, pesticides, and dyes. However, despite its potential, the field faces several significant challenges and limitations that must be addressed to enhance its effectiveness and applicability. Advances in genetic engineering and biotechnology are paving the way for future trends that may overcome these barriers and expand the scope of bioremediation technologies.

LIMITATIONS OF MICROBIAL BIOREMEDIATION

Limited Biodegradability of Certain Pollutants

Certain pollutants are resistant to microbial breakdown, including highly chlorinated chemicals (PCBs, dioxins) and heavy metals (lead, mercury, cadmium). Microbes can decompose organic pollutants, while inorganic pollutants, such as heavy metals, are persistent in the environment. Although microbes can change these metals into less harmful forms, further techniques like chemical precipitation or phytoremediation are frequently needed for full removal [52].

Dependency on Environmental Conditions

A number of variables, including temperature, pH, oxygen concentrations, and nutrition availability, affect microbial activity. Extreme settings that are extremely acidic or alkaline, excessive salinity, or extremely high or low temperatures can all hinder microbial metabolism. For instance, the efficacy of bioremediation is decreased in colder climes due to a considerable slowdown in microbial breakdown Given that the environment affects how aerobic and anaerobic microorganisms behave, oxygen availability is also very important [53].

Slow Process Compared to Other Methods

In order to achieve a considerable reduction in pollutants, microbial bioremediation is frequently a gradual process that takes weeks, months, or even years. On the other hand, pollutants can be quickly eliminated by chemical processes like oxidation or incineration. Bioremediation is less appropriate for emergency spill responses or quick site cleanups due to the slow rate of degradation of some contaminants, particularly persistent organic chemicals [53].

Toxicity of Pollutants to Microbes

The development and metabolic processes of microbial populations can be inhibited by high concentrations of pollutants. Certain contaminants, like industrial solvents and heavy metals, disrupt the action of microbial enzymes, causing cell damage and decreasing the effectiveness of bioremediation. Microbial communities may need bioaugmentation with more robust strains or extra nutrient supplementation in highly contaminated environments in order to survive and perform well [54].

Microbial Survival and Competition

Due to competition with native microbial communities, introduced microbes—including genetically engineered strains may find it difficult to survive in contaminated environments. It might be challenging for introduced species to establish and flourish since native microorganisms are frequently well-suited to site-specific circumstances. Furthermore, microbial survival may be restricted by environmental stressors such as nutrient scarcity or elevated pollutant levels, which would lower the overall efficacy of bioremediation [55].

Genetic Engineering for Enhanced Microbial Degradation

To overcome many of these limitations, advances in genetic engineering are being leveraged to create microbial strains with enhanced degradative capabilities. Through recombinant DNA technology, it is possible to introduce or optimize specific metabolic pathways in bacteria and fungi, enabling them to degrade a broader spectrum of pollutants or to function more efficiently under adverse environmental conditions [56].

Genetically engineered microorganisms (GEMs) can be tailored to express enzymes that break down otherwise recalcitrant compounds, such as polychlorinated biphenyls (PCBs), certain pesticides, and industrial solvents. For instance, genes encoding for oxygenases, dehalogenases, or other specialized enzymes can be inserted into microbial genomes, expanding their substrate range and improving their resilience to environmental stressors [36].

However, the deployment of GEMs in the field is not without challenges. Engineered strains often exhibit reduced fitness in natural environments due to the metabolic burden of maintaining foreign genetic material, and they may be outcompeted by native microbial populations. There are also regulatory and ethical considerations regarding the release of GMOs, including the potential for gene transfer to indigenous microbes and unintended ecological consequences [36].

Despite these hurdles, laboratory and pilot-scale studies have demonstrated that genetically engineered microbes can significantly enhance the degradation of specific pollutants. Ongoing research is focused on improving the stability, survivability, and safety of GEMs, as well as developing containment strategies to minimize environmental risks [56].

Future Trends in Bioremediation Technology

The future of microbial bioremediation is likely to be shaped by several emerging trends and technological innovations. One major direction is the integration of omics technologies—such as genomics, proteomics, and metabolomics to better understand microbial communities and their functional dynamics in contaminated environments. These approaches enable the identification of key degradative genes and pathways, facilitating the design of more effective bioremediation strategies [56].

Another promising trend is the development of microbial consortia, where multiple species with complementary metabolic capabilities are combined to tackle complex mixtures of pollutants. Such consortia can enhance degradation efficiency, resilience, and adaptability to fluctuating environmental conditions [56].

Advancements in bioreactor design and process engineering are also expanding the applicability of bioremediation. For example, the use of immobilized microbial cells, biofilms, and engineered wetlands can improve pollutant removal rates and allow for the treatment of larger volumes of contaminated water or soil.

Synthetic biology holds significant potential for the future of bioremediation. By designing synthetic microbial circuits and regulatory networks, scientists can create microbes with programmable functions, enabling precise control over degradation pathways and response to environmental cues [56].

Finally, there is growing interest in coupling bioremediation with other remediation technologies, such as phytoremediation, chemical oxidation, or nanotechnology-based approaches, to achieve synergistic effects and address a wider range of contaminants [56].

CONCLUSION

The report underscores the growing environmental challenges posed by pharmaceutical waste, which includes residues from manufacturing, healthcare facilities, and improper disposal of unused or expired medications. These pollutants are persistent, bioaccumulative, and potentially toxic, threatening aquatic ecosystems, soil health, and human safety. Conventional waste treatment methods such as incineration, landfilling, or chemical degradation often fail to eliminate these compounds, leading to their accumulation and adverse ecological impacts, including disruption of aquatic life and the promotion of antibiotic-resistant microorganisms. Bioremediation emerges as a promising, sustainable solution for mitigating these environmental hazards. It leverages the natural metabolic capabilities of microorganisms—primarily bacteria and fungi—to degrade complex pharmaceutical chemicals into less harmful or inert substances like carbon dioxide, water, and biomass. The process can be optimized through strategies such as biostimulation, which enhances native microbial activity, and bioaugmentation, involving the introduction of specific pollutant-degrading strains. Additionally, phytoremediation, which employs plants in concert with associated microbial communities, offers an environmentally friendly and cost-effective approach to extract and break down pollutants from contaminated soils and water bodies. Despite its potential, the application of bioremediation faces several challenges. These include the slow degradation rates owing to the complex chemical nature of pharmaceuticals, environmental factors such as pH, temperature, and oxygen levels that influence microbial activity, and the delayed breakdown caused by microbial community limitations. Furthermore, the diversity of pharmaceutical compounds necessitates tailored and integrated remediation strategies, complicating large-scale applications. Advances in biotechnology, including genetic engineering, could help overcome these hurdles by enhancing microbial abilities and accelerating degradation processes.

REFERENCES

[1] Sharma P, Bano A, Singh SP, Dubey NK, Chandra R, Iqbal HMN. Recent advancements in microbial-assisted remediation strategies for toxic contaminants. Cleaner Chemical Engineering 2022; 2: 100020.
[http://dx.doi.org/10.1016/j.clce.2022.100020]

[2] Ojha S, Mishra S, Vishwakarma P K. Pharmaceuticals and personal care products as contaminants of emerging concern: sources, nature, and possible health effects In: Vigneshwaran S, Preethi V, Eds. Advanced oxidation process-based integrated and hybrid technologies for degradation of

pharmaceuticals and personal care products. Amsterdam: Elsevier 2025; pp. 1-14.

[3] Ojha S, Tripathi S M, Vishwakarma P K, Mishra S. Pharmaceuticals in the water: emerging concerns and innovative remediation solutions Curr Green Chem 2024; 11(1): 50-62.

[4] Maglione G, Zinno P, Tropea A, *et al.* Microbes' role in environmental pollution and remediation: a bioeconomy focus approach. AIMS Microbiology 2024; 10(3): 723-55.

[5] Bala S, Garg D, Thirumalesh B V, *et al.* Recent strategies for bioremediation of emerging pollutants: a review for a green and sustainable environment. Toxics 2022; 10(8): 484.

[6] Shen Y, Stedtfeld RD, Guo X, *et al.* Pharmaceutical exposure changed antibiotic resistance genes and bacterial communities in soil-surface- and overhead-irrigated greenhouse lettuce. Environ Int 2019; 131: 105031.
[http://dx.doi.org/10.1016/j.envint.2019.105031] [PMID: 31336252]

[7] Murray AK, Zhang L, Yin X, *et al.* Novel insights into selection for antibiotic resistance in complex microbial communities. MBio 2018; 9(4): e00969-18.
[http://dx.doi.org/10.1128/mBio.00969-18] [PMID: 30042197]

[8] Chen Z, Zhang W, Yang L, *et al.* Antibiotic resistance genes and bacterial communities in cornfield and pasture soils receiving swine and dairy manures. Environ Pollut 2019; 248: 947-57.
[http://dx.doi.org/10.1016/j.envpol.2019.02.093] [PMID: 30861417]

[9] Kumar A, Tyagi PK, Tyagi S, Ghorbanpour M. Integrating green nanotechnology with sustainable development goals: a pathway to sustainable innovation. Discov Sustain 2024; 5: 48.

[10] Shah B A, Malhotra H, Papade S E, *et al.* Microbial degradation of contaminants of emerging concern: metabolic, genetic and omics insights for enhanced bioremediation. Frontiers in Bioengineering and Biotechnology 2024; 12: 1356070.

[11] Ayilara MS, Babalola OO. Bioremediation of environmental wastes: the role of microorganisms. Front Agron 2023; 5: 1183691.

[12] Kuppan N, Padman M, Mahadeva M, Srinivasan S, Devarajan R. A comprehensive review of sustainable bioremediation techniques: Eco friendly solutions for waste and pollution management. Waste Management Bulletin 2024; 2(3): 154-71.
[http://dx.doi.org/10.1016/j.wmb.2024.07.005]

[13] Eslami E, Joodat S H S. Bioremediation of oil and heavy metal contaminated soil in construction sites: a case study of using bioventing-biosparging and phytoextraction techniques. Ithaca (NY): Cornell University 2018.

[14] Filote C, Roşca M, Hlihor R M, *et al.* Sustainable application of biosorption and bioaccumulation of persistent pollutants in wastewater treatment: current practice. Processes 2021; 9(10): 1696.

[15] Gelagutashvili E, Ginturi E, Pataraia D, Gurielidze M. Biosorption of Cr(VI) and Cr(III) by Arthrobacter species. Appl Biochem Microbiol 2016; 52(4): 389-93.

[16] Tanasupawat S, Takehana T, Yoshida S, Hiraga K, Oda K. *Ideonella sakaiensis* sp. nov., isolated from a microbial consortium that degrades poly(ethylene terephthalate). Int J Syst Evol Microbiol 2016; 66(8): 2813-8.
[http://dx.doi.org/10.1099/ijsem.0.001058] [PMID: 27045688]

[17] Peng YH, Shih Y, Lai YC, Liu YZ, Liu YT, Lin NC. Degradation of polyurethane by bacterium isolated from soil and assessment of polyurethanolytic activity of a *Pseudomonas putida* strain. Environ Sci Pollut Res Int 2014; 21(16): 9529-37.
[http://dx.doi.org/10.1007/s11356-014-2647-8] [PMID: 24633845]

[18] Yao Z, Seong HJ, Jang YS. Degradation of low density polyethylene by Bacillus species. Appl Biol Chem 2022; 65(1): 84.
[http://dx.doi.org/10.1186/s13765-022-00753-3]

[19] Mor R, Sivan A. Biofilm formation and partial biodegradation of polystyrene by the actinomycete

Rhodococcus ruber. Biodegradation 2008; 19(6): 851-8. [http://dx.doi.org/10.1007/s10532-008-9188-0] [PMID: 18401686]

[20] Mehmood CT, Qazi IA, Hashmi I, Bhargava S, Deepa S. Biodegradation of low density polyethylene (LDPE) modified with dye sensitized titania and starch blend using *Stenotrophomonas pavanii*. Int Biodeterior Biodegradation 2016; 113: 276-86. [http://dx.doi.org/10.1016/j.ibiod.2016.01.025]

[21] Nikolopoulou I, Piperagkas O, Moschos S, Karayanni H. Bacteria Release from Microplastics into New Aquatic Environments. Diversity (Basel) 2023; 15(1): 115. [http://dx.doi.org/10.3390/d15010115]

[22] Yang J, Yang Y, Wu WM, Zhao J, Jiang L. Evidence of polyethylene biodegradation by bacterial strains from the guts of plastic-eating waxworms. Environ Sci Technol 2014; 48(23): 13776-84. [http://dx.doi.org/10.1021/es504038a] [PMID: 25384056]

[23] Sivasankari S. *In vitro* degradation of plastics (plastic cup) using *Micrococcus luteus* and *Masoniella sp.* Sch Acad J Biosci 2016; 4(3B): 265-71.

[24] Venisha C V, Zalak R R, Saraf M S. Biodegradation of polythene by novel bacteria Sphingomonas sp. VC1. Int Res J Eng Technol 2020; 7(8): 4737-40.

[25] Kitadokoro K, Kakara M, Matsui S, *et al.* Structural insights into the unique polylactate-degrading mechanism of *Thermobifida alba* cutinase. FEBS J 2019; 286(11): 2087-98. [http://dx.doi.org/10.1111/febs.14781] [PMID: 30761732]

[26] Bala S, Gupta S, Sharma S, *et al.* Recent strategies for bioremediation of emerging pollutants: a review for a green and sustainable environment. Front Microbiol. 2022; 13: 874439.

[27] Viel T, Manfra L, Zupo V, Libralato G, Cocca M, Costantini M. Biodegradation of plastics induced by marine organisms: future perspectives for bioremediation approaches. Polymers 2023; 15(16): 3340.

[28] Karigar CS, Rao SS. Role of microbial enzymes in the bioremediation of pollutants: A review. Vol. 2011. Enzyme Res 2011; 2011: 1-11. [http://dx.doi.org/10.4061/2011/805187]

[29] Udekwu C C, Francis U C, Ojetunde M M, Okakpu J C, Awah F M, Awe O B. A review of plastic pollution: conventional and recent bioremediation technologies. J Dev Food Energy Water Syst 2024; 5(1): 11-33.

[30] Olicón-Hernández DR, González-López J, Aranda E. Overview on the biochemical potential of filamentous fungi to degrade pharmaceutical compounds. Front Microbiol 2017; 8: 1792.

[31] Nancy KU, Kumari U. Biodegradation of Pharmaceutical Pollutants Using Fungal Enzyme. Int J Res Appl Sci Eng Technol 2024; 12(5): 827-33. [http://dx.doi.org/10.22214/ijraset.2024.61672]

[32] Jørgensen KS. *In situ* bioremediation. Adv App Microbio 2007; 61: 285-305.

[33] Sharma J. Advantages and Limitations of *in situ* Methods of Bioremediation. Recent Adv Biol Med 2019; 5: 9.

[34] Court E K, Chaudhuri R R, Kapoore R V, *et al.* Looking through the fog: microbiome characterization and lipolytic bacteria isolation from a fatberg site. Microbiology 2019; 167(12): 1123-35.

[35] Samborska-Goik K, Pogrzeba M. A Critical Review of the Modelling Tools for the Reactive Transport of Organic Contaminants. Appl Sci 2024; 14(9): 3675. [http://dx.doi.org/10.3390/app14093675]

[36] Gaur N, Narasimhulu K, Pindi PK, *et al.* Bioremediation of contaminated soil and groundwater by *in situ* biostimulation. Front Microbiol. 2023; 14: 1258148.

[37] Sharma P, Kumar S, Pandey A. Bioremediated techniques for remediation of metal pollutants using metagenomics approaches: A review. J Environ Chem Eng 2021; 9(4): 105684.

[http://dx.doi.org/10.1016/j.jece.2021.105684]

[38] Anjana M, Prajna R, Katti US, Kavitha RV. Bioremediation – the recent drift towards a sustainable environment. Environ Sci Adv. 2024; 3(8): 1097–1110. [http://dx.doi.org/10.1039/D3VA00358B]

[39] Li L, Wang H, Tang J, *et al.* Genome-resolved metagenomics provides insights into the ecological roles of the keystone taxa in heavy-metal-contaminated soils. Front Microbiol. 2023; 14: 1203164. [http://dx.doi.org/10.3389/fmicb.2023.1203164]

[40] Pandey J, Chauhan A, Jain R K. Integrative approaches for assessing the ecological sustainability of in situ bioremediation FEMS Microbiol Rev 2009 Mar 01; 33(2): 324-75.

[41] Stanojevic AB, Vrvić M, Száková J, Miletić S. Evaluation of the ex-situ bioremediation of the petroleum hydrocarbons contaminated soil. Bioremediation J 2023; 28: 553-63.

[42] Ayub F, Haider Naqvi SL, Zahra Naqvi SH, *et al.* Exploring Knowledge, Attitudes and Practices Regarding Single-Use Plastics in Lahore Workspaces. J Qua Assur Agri Sci 2023; 3(1): 16-27. [http://dx.doi.org/10.38211/jqaas.2023.3.23]

[43] Filote C, Roşca M, Hlihor RM, Cozma P, Simion IM, Apostol M, *et al.* Sustainable application of biosorption and bioaccumulation of persistent pollutants in wastewater treatment: Current practice 2021; 9(10): 1696.

[44] Viñas M, Sabaté J, Espuny MJ, Solanas AM. Bacterial community dynamics and polycyclic aromatic hydrocarbon degradation during bioremediation of heavily creosote-contaminated soil. Appl Environ Microbiol 2005; 71(11): 7008-18. [http://dx.doi.org/10.1128/AEM.71.11.7008-7018.2005] [PMID: 16269736]

[45] Cleophas FN, Zahari NZ, Murugayah P, Rahim SA, Mohd Yatim AN. Phytoremediation: A Novel Approach of Bast Fiber Plants (Hemp, Kenaf, Jute and Flax) for Heavy Metals Decontamination in Soil—Review 2023; 11(1): 5.

[46] Balcom IN, Crowley DE. Isolation and characterization of pyrene metabolizing microbial consortia from the plant rhizoplane. Int J Phytoremediation 2010; 12(6): 599-615. [http://dx.doi.org/10.1080/15226510903390437] [PMID: 21166284]

[47] Hussain F, Hussain I, Khan AHA, *et al.* Combined application of biochar, compost, and bacterial consortia with Italian ryegrass enhanced phytoremediation of petroleum hydrocarbon contaminated soil. Environ Exp Bot 2018; 153: 80-8. [http://dx.doi.org/10.1016/j.envexpbot.2018.05.012]

[48] Tang H, Dar ZA, Wang S, Chen S, Lin H, Wang J. Microbial mediated remediation of heavy metals toxicity: mechanisms, advancements and future prospects. Front Plant Sci. 2024; 15: 1420408.

[49] Thirumalaivasan N, Gnanasekaran L, Kumar S, *et al.* Utilization of fungal and bacterial bioremediation techniques for the treatment of toxic waste and biowaste. Frontiers in Materials 2024; 11: 1416445.

[50] Rezaei Z, Moghimi H. Fungal-bacterial consortia: A promising strategy for the removal of petroleum hydrocarbons. Ecotoxicol Environ Saf 2024 Jul 15; 280: 116543.

[51] Nielsen S G, Baker R S, Heron G, Lemming G. Making thermal remediation more sustainable: a detailed analysis [Internet]. Columbus (OH): Battelle Memorial Institute; 2015.

[52] Azubuike CC, Chikere CB, Okpokwasili GC. Bioremediation techniques–classification based on site of application: Principles, advantages, limitations and prospects. World J Microbiol Biotechnol 2016; 32(11): 180.

[53] Alori ET, Gabasawa AI, Elenwo CE, Agbeyegbe OO. Bioremediation techniques as affected by limiting factors in soil environment. Frontiers in Soil Science. 2022; 2: 937186.

[54] Bilal M, Iqbal HMN. Microbial bioremediation as a robust process to mitigate pollutants of environmental concern. Case Stud Chem Envir Eng 2020; 2: 100011 2020; 2: 100011.

[http://dx.doi.org/10.1016/j.cscee.2020.100011]

[55] Edwards SJ, Kjellerup BV. Applications of biofilms in bioremediation and biotransformation of persistent organic pollutants, pharmaceuticals/personal care products, and heavy metals. Appl Microbiol Biotechnol 2013; 97(23): 9909-21.
[http://dx.doi.org/10.1007/s00253-013-5216-z] [PMID: 24150788]

[56] Pant G, Garlapati D, Agrawal U, Prasuna RG, Mathimani T, Pugazhendhi A. Biological approaches practised using genetically engineered microbes for a sustainable environment: A review. J Hazard Mater 2021; 405: 124631.
[http://dx.doi.org/10.1016/j.jhazmat.2020.124631]

SUBJECT INDEX

A

B

C

Suman Gautam, Jai Narayan Mishra, Preeti Mishra, Preeti Verma & Sudhanshu Mishra (Eds.)

D

E

N

O

P

R

S

T

U

V

W

X

Z

www.ingramcontent.com/pod-product-compliance
Lightning Source LLC
LaVergne TN
LVHW070946210926
848482LV00002B/108
9798898815240